Pharmacy: Beyond the Basics

Pharmacy: Beyond the Basics

Edited by Winter Hayes

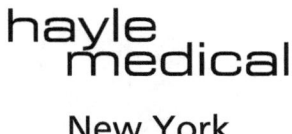

hayle medical

New York

Hayle Medical,
750 Third Avenue, 9th Floor,
New York, NY 10017, USA

Visit us on the World Wide Web at:
www.haylemedical.com

ISBN: 978-1-63241-794-7

Cataloging-in-Publication Data

Pharmacy : beyond the basics / edited by Winter Hayes.
   p. cm.
Includes bibliographical references and index.
ISBN 978-1-63241-794-7
1. Pharmacy. 2. Drugs. 3. Materia medica. 4. Pharmacology. I. Hayes, Winter.
RS153 .P43 2019
615--dc23

Table of Contents

Preface

The purpose of the book is to provide a glimpse into the dynamics and to present opinions and studies of some of the scientists engaged in the development of new ideas in the field from very different standpoints. This book will prove useful to students and researchers owing to its high content quality.

Pharmacy is an essential part of the healthcare system that deals with the manufacture of medicines, their supply, their use and potential effects and side-effects. The ultimate concern of pharmacy is the facilitation of appropriate medication to patients. The scope of pharmacy is wide, which includes various stages in the development and standardization of a drug, such as the synthesis of chemical compounds of therapeutic value, the analysis of medicinal agents, preparation of the dosage, etc. Pharmacy laws regulate the sale and labeling of narcotics, poisons and dangerous drugs. The delivery of pharmaceutical care delivered by pharmacists and other health care providers also come under the scope of pharmacy research. Medicinal policy and governance, medicine access and rational use, and quality assurance and safety are some of the main areas in focus in this field. Another emerging frontier of drug research is the exploration of the availability of various dosage forms of drugs to the body. The topics included in this book on pharmacy are of utmost significance and bound to provide incredible insights to readers. It studies, analyzes and upholds the pillars of pharmacy and its utmost significance in modern times. With state-of-the-art inputs by acclaimed experts of this field, this book targets students and professionals.

At the end, I would like to appreciate all the efforts made by the authors in completing their chapters professionally. I express my deepest gratitude to all of them for contributing to this book by sharing their valuable works. A special thanks to my family and friends for their constant support in this journey.

Editor

From Learning to Decision-Making: A Cross-Sectional Survey of a Clinical Pharmacist-Steered Journal Club

Sherine Ismail [1],*, Sara Al Khansa [1], Mohammed Aseeri [1], Hani Alhamdan [1] and K. H. Mujtaba Quadri [2]

[1] King Abdullah International Medical Research Center, King Saud bin Abdulaziz University for Health Sciences, Pharmaceutical Care Department, King Abdulaziz Medical City, Ministry of National Guard Health Affairs, Jeddah 21423, Saudi Arabia; khansasa@ngha.med.sa (S.A.K.); aseerima@ngha.med.sa (M.A.); hamdanhs@ngha.med.sa (H.A.)

[2] National University of Medical Sciences, The Mall, Rawalpindi 44000, Pakistan; deanresearch@numspak.edu.pk

* Correspondence: esmailss@ngha.med.sa or esmailse@gmail.com

Academic Editor: Yvonne Perrie

Abstract: Journal clubs have been traditionally incorporated into academic training programs to enhance competency in the interpretation of literature. We designed a structured journal club (JC) to improve skills in the interpretation of literature; however, we were not aware of how learners (interns, residents, clinical pharmacists, etc.) would perceive it. We aimed to assess the perception of learners at different levels of pharmacy training. A cross-sectional design was used. A self-administered online survey was emailed to JC attendees from 2010–2014 at King Abdulaziz Medical City, Jeddah, Saudi Arabia. The survey questions included: introduction sessions, topic selection, JC layout, interaction with the moderator, and decision-making skills by clinical pharmacists. The response rate was 58/89 (65%); 52/54 (96%) respondents believed that JC adds to their knowledge in interpreting literature. Topic selection met the core curriculum requirements for credentials exams for 16/36 (44.4%), while 16/22 (73%) presenters had good to excellent interaction with the moderator. JC facilitated decision-making for 10/12 (83%) of clinical pharmacists. The results suggest that clinical pharmacist-steered JC may serve as an effective tool to empower learners at different levels of pharmacy practice, with evidence-based principles for interpretation of literature and guide informed decision-making.

Keywords: journal club; learning; decision-making; clinical pharmacist; evidence-based practice

1. Introduction

Journal clubs have been traditionally incorporated into academic training programs to enhance competency in the interpretation of literature [1]. A systematic review highlighted the potential influence of a journal club to enhance critical thinking and promote knowledge in clinical research, bridging theory to practice and subsequently improving clinical practice [2]. Furthermore, several journal club models conducted over training periods have been reported to promote life-long learning and maintain certifications for residents and faculty [3]. Harris et al. (2011) conducted a systematic review of 18 studies to assess the effectiveness of JCs. Five studies (5/11) reported an improvement in reading behavior, (7/7) showed confidence in critical appraisal, (5/7) presented critical appraisal test scores, and (5/7) demonstrated an ability to implement study findings; however, pooling of the study results was difficult due to heterogeneous interventions and it was not obvious how JCs would guide evidence-based decisions [4]. Additionally, Matthews DC (2011) pointed that Harris et al. (2011)

identified two key points: first, the success of the JC is dependent on learner-centered approach; second, there is no standard layout for the journal club, despite identifying the essential elements such as skilled mentorship, structured format for literature review, and the use of active learning techniques [5].

The statement of the American Society of Health-System Pharmacist for formulary management identifies pharmacists as crucial members of multidisciplinary teams to nourish the Pharmacy and Therapeutics Committee (P & T) proceeding with critical evaluation of literature and to guide P & T evidence-based decisions for drug alternatives [6]. Therefore, it is prudent to promote critical thinking and sharpen critical appraisal skills for the interpretation of literature for pharmacy practitioners at different levels of training and expertise, through structured JCs to fulfill leadership obligations and organizational decisions [7].

The structure of an effective JC has been identified in literature with several features such as a trained leader to mentor the discussion and select scientific papers for review, mandatory attendance, regular scheduled meetings, disseminating JC materials, and the use of standard critical appraisal tools [8]. Mcleod RS et al. (2010) published a randomized control trial comparing moderated JCs versus Internet-based JCs for surgical residents and reported higher scores in critical appraisal skills with moderated JCs [9].

We designed a structured JC steered by a clinical pharmacist certified in clinical research to improve skills in interpretation of literature in the pharmaceutical care department at King Abdulaziz Medical City, Ministry of National Guard Health Affairs, Jeddah, Saudi Arabia. However, we were not aware of the perception of learners attending the JC (interns, residents, clinical pharmacists, etc.) on their practice, skills and decision-making process. Therefore, our aim was to assess the perception of learners at different levels of pharmacy training regarding the structure and utility of the JC steered by a clinical pharmacist. Additionally, we evaluated the perception of pharmacists regarding its role in guiding formulary decisions and informing clinical practice.

2. Materials and Methods

2.1. Development and Validation of the Survey Tool

An online survey was designed through SurveyMonkey by the clinical pharmacist in May 2014 and validated for language, wording, and content through a pilot study on 4 volunteering health care professionals (co-authors). Several changes have been adapted in the survey after validation. Inclusion Criteria: all participants who attended the monthly JC (pharmacy residents, interns, clinical pharmacists, pharmacists, and administrators) from 2010 to 2014 at King Abdulaziz Medical City, Jeddah, Saudi Arabia.

2.2. Administration of Survey

All participants were e-mailed the survey link in May 2014 explaining the objectives and were invited to respond to the survey. E-mail reminders were sent for non-responders on a regular basis.

2.3. Structure of the Survey

The survey comprised of several quantitative domains to assess the perception of learners/pharmacists towards the structured journal club including the introduction sessions presented at the beginning of each academic year, the selection of topics, the clinical pharmacist as a moderator, the layout of the journal club, the presenter's interaction with the moderator, and the perception of the practicing pharmacists towards the journal club. Each domain consisted of several questions. The first author was the same JC moderator who consistently organized the JC from 2010 to 2014. Additionally, structures of the JC and appraisal forms have been consistent during the same period. The survey allowed participants to omit and skip different patterns for questions to direct respondents to answer questions relevant to their level of practice (pharmacy interns versus clinical pharmacists, for example)

2.4. *Structure of the Journal Club*

We designed a structured journal club (Figure 1) since 2010 in the pharmaceutical care department accredited by the American Society of Health System Pharmacists (ASHP) for PGY1 residency. The aim of the journal club was to empower learners at different levels (interns, new practitioners, and residents) with basic principles of interpretation of literature via monthly sessions.

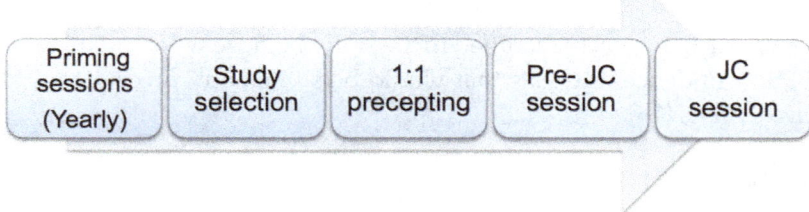

Figure 1. Structure of the journal club (JC).

1. The structure of the JC starts with each academic year by introducing evidence-based medicine principles through priming sessions prepared and presented by clinical pharmacists. These are composed of three interactive sessions to address: (1) the main JC objectives, structure, and layout; (2) the basic concepts of study designs and measures of associations; and (3) tools to assess internal validity, interpretation of study results and generalizability. Moreover, a monthly schedule for a JC meeting is planned and distributed to clinical pharmacists and learners at the beginning of each academic year. Each academic year, we have a new batch of interns and residents who typically attend priming sessions. Interns attend 1–7 sessions of scheduled monthly JC based on their rotations at our site. However, our PGY1 residency program is for 2 years; therefore, most residents attend on average 18–20 sessions during their residency, and it varies for clinical pharmacists according to their schedule.

2. The selection of the study question whether it is a "practice-based clinical question" or a "new drug request for formulary addition" used to be decided by the clinical moderator; however, the JC presenting pharmacy intern or resident were required to conduct a literature review and identify potential studies that best address the question raised by the JC. Subsequently, the selection of the JC study occurs after discussion with the JC moderator. Finally, the clinical pharmacist JC moderator sends an e-mail notification of the selected study to pharmacy interns, residents and all pharmacy staff at least 1–2 weeks prior to the scheduled JC.

3. A one-to-one precepting followed to aid the presenter to best interpret the study findings using specific appraisal tools adapted from critical appraisal skills programs (CASPs), a Center of Evidence-Based Medicine appraisal, and other literature resources for assessment of multiple treatment comparisons [10–12]. In addition, several other checklists for trials reporting were discussed with the learners, depending on the study design presented in JC, such as a Consolidated Standards of Reporting Trials (CONSORT) statement for reporting randomized controlled trials, a Strengthening the Reporting of Observational studies in Epidemiology (STROBE) statement and a Preferred Reporting Items for Systematic Reviews and Meta-Analyses (PRISMA) statement for the reporting of meta-analysis [13–15].

4. Before starting the journal club, a 30–60 min separate interactive group "pre-JC session" is delivered to the interns and residents to discuss general epidemiological concepts of the paper or to highlight various aspects of the study design. This is usually followed by the journal club session (1 h), which is attended by pharmacy interns and residents, practicing pharmacists at different levels, and administrators.

5. The JC session starts with a small presentation of 15–20 min prepared by the learner (intern or resident) and includes the background, the study question in a PICOT format

(patients/population, intervention, control, and time of the study), the main aspects of the study, and the critical appraisal of the topic. This was followed by an interactive group discussion moderated by the clinical pharmacist for critical appraisal of the study using the specific tools mentioned above. Sometimes the JC is presented again in a separate session to a multi-disciplinary team.

2.5. Sample Size Calculation

A sample of 86 participants were recruited to the study because we calculated that 86 respondents would provide 95% confidence intervals that would be sufficiently precise, to ±11%, even with a worst-case response of 50% [16].

2.6. Statistical Analysis

Responses are imported from SurveyMonkey [17] to Microsoft® Excel® for Mac 2011 version 14.7.0. Baseline demographics are presented as proportions; survey responses are also presented as proportions with 95% confidence intervals. Microsoft Excel® for Mac 2011 version 14.7.0 and STATA 2014 (StataCorp LLC, College Station, TX, USA) were used for statistical analysis.

2.7. Ethics

The study has an Institutional Review Board consent waiver (IRBC/598/15) by King Abdullah International Medical Research Center.

3. Results

The response rate was 58/89 (65%) of the invited participants, and only 3/58 (5%) refused to participate. Baseline characteristics of participants are presented in Figure 2.

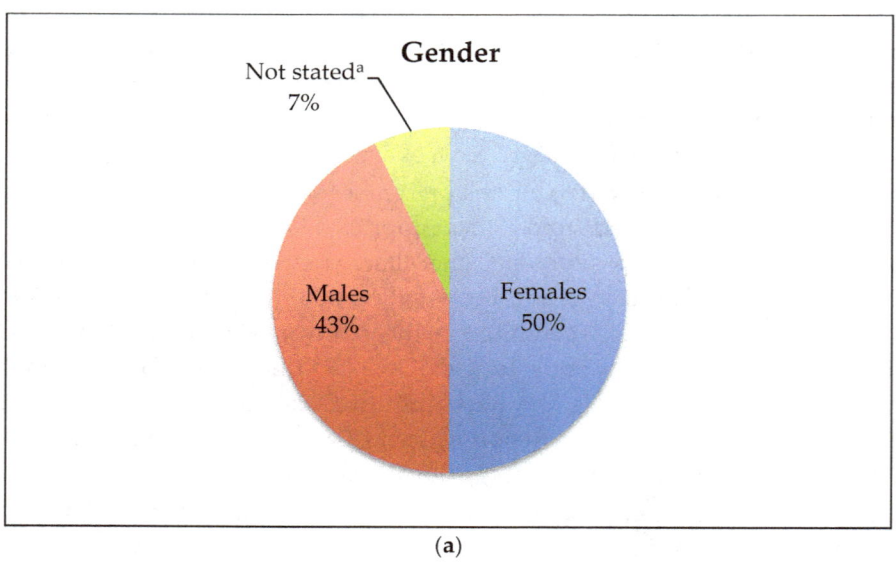

(a)

Figure 2. *Cont.*

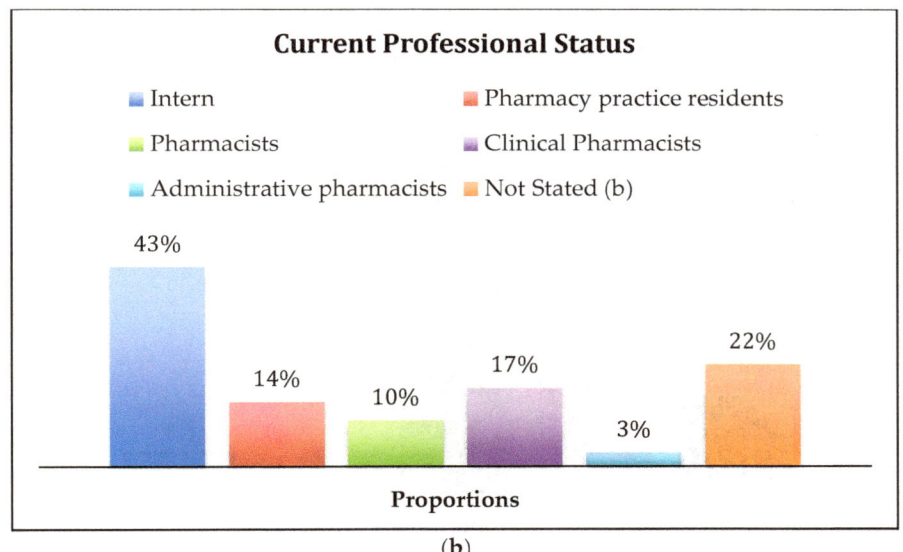

(b)

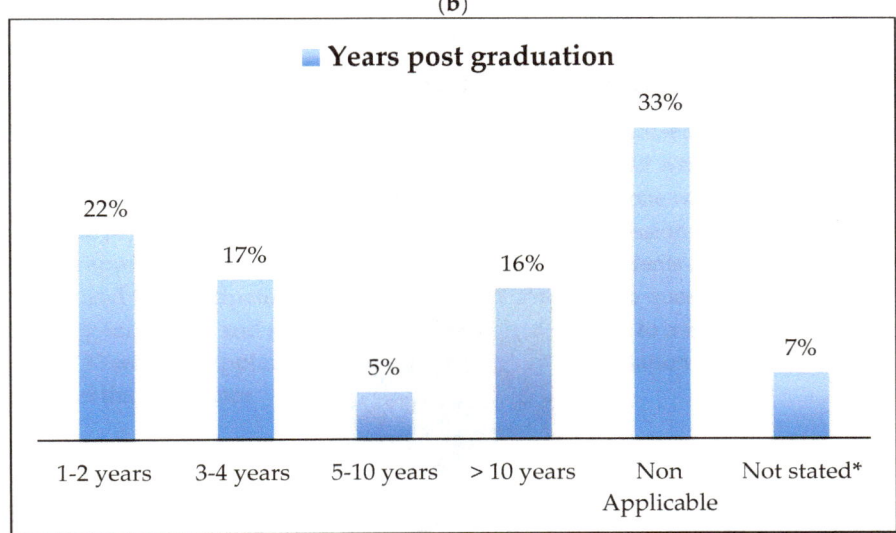

(c)

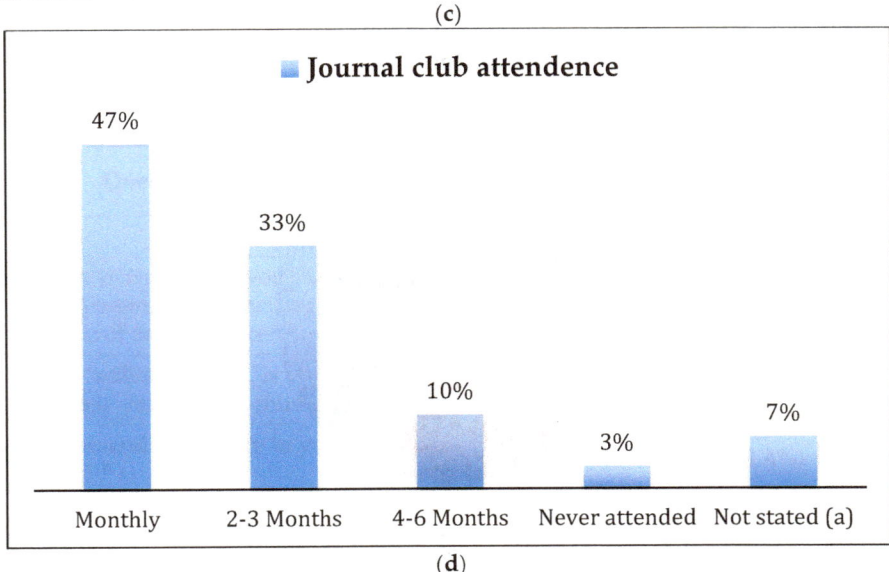

(d)

Figure 2. *Cont.*

Table 1. *Cont.*

Questions	Responses	Proportions *n/N* (%)	95% Confidence Interval
5. Do you think the clinical pharmacist steered JC idea is useful for you? [b]	Yes	52/58 (89.6%)	0.82–0.97
Introduction Sessions			
1. How do you describe the introduction sessions for JC? [e]	Poor [c]	0/31 (0%)	-
	Neutral	2/31 (6.5%)	−0.02–0.15
	Good [d]	29/31 (93.5%)	0.85–1.02
2. To what extent do you think the introduction session helped you to understand some basic concepts in critical appraisal skills? [e]	Poor [c]	0/31 (0%)	-
	Neutral	6/31 (19.4%)	0.055–0.33
	Good [d]	25/31 (80.6%)	0.67–0.95
Topic Selection			
1. How far do you think the selection of the topics meet your core curriculum requirements for your internship/residency/board exams? [f]	Rarely	7/36 (19.4%)	0.06–0.32
	Neutral	13/36 (36.1%)	0.20–0.52
	Always	16/36 (44.4%)	0.28–0.61
2. Do you think the topics discussed in the JC are current and help you to be updated with the literature?	Yes	35/36 (97.2%)	0.92–1.03
Assessment of 1:1 Percepting			
1. How do you evaluate your learning experience in preparation for JC? [g]	Poor [c]	0/22 (0%)	-
	Neutral	4/22 (18.2%)	0.021–0.34
	Good [d]	18/22 (81.8%)	0.66–0.98
2. How do you describe your interaction with the JC Moderator during the preparation phase? [g]	Poor [c]	1/22 (4.5%)	−0.04–0.13
	Neutral	5/22 (22.7%)	0.05–0.40
	Good [d]	16/22 (72.7%)	0.54–0.91
3. How do you find the quality of the materials provided to you by the moderator to facilitate your understanding of the paper presented in the JC? [g]	Poor [c]	4/22 (18.2%)	0.02–0.34
	Neutral	3/22 (13.6%)	−0.01–0.28
	Good [d]	15/22 (68.2)	0.49–0.88
Formulary Decisions and Clinical Practice			
1. Do you think JC activities facilitate formulary decisions? [h]	Yes	10/12 (83.3%)	0.62–1.04
2. Do you think JC activities are useful in changing your clinical practice? [h]	Yes [i]	9/12 (75%)	0.51–0.99
	Neutral	2/12 (16.7%)	−0.04–0.38
	No [j]	1/12 (8.3%)	−0.07–0.24

[a] Not stated: Three refused to participate and one was not applicable. [b] Not stated: Three refused to participate and two were not applicable. [c] Poor is a collapsed category for very poor and poor. [d] Good is a collapsed category of very good to excellent. [e] Twenty-seven not stated including 3 refused to participate and 24 were not applicable (not interns or residents). [f] Twenty-two not stated including 3 refused to participate and categories were collapsed to always for (mostly and almost always) and rarely for (sometimes and rarely). [g] Thirty-six not stated the questions including 3 refused to participate and 32 were not applicable (did not present). [h] Forty-six not stated including 3 refused to participate and 43 were not applicable. [i] Yes is a collapsed category for always and most of the times and [j] No is a collapsed category for not always and not at all.

4. Discussion

Our findings regarding our structured JC activity is consistent with various reports supporting the impact of JC on the perception of improving critical skills in interpretation of literature, and guiding decisions [2,3,5,18]. Additionally, its moderation by clinical pharmacist through imparting of specialized research training is unique in building competency in evidence informed decision-making. Priming sessions and 1:1 perceptorship were unique features in our JC with zero response for poor categories, which reflects the crucial role of clinical pharmacists in designing educational tools and mentoring.

Although 9/12 (75%) of clinical pharmacists believe that JC had been useful in changing clinical practice versus 3/12 (25%) disagreed. This might be explained by the small number of clinical pharmacists (12) in our survey and that many were not able to attend JC on a regular basis.

There are several limitations to our survey for assessment of the structured JC: (1) We used the webpage service and emailed the survey, which may have limited the response rate to only 65% due to outdated email lists for participants in the past five years and undeliverable emails; (2) The survey was designed and validated to assess learner's and pharmacist's perception based on our structured JC, which might lead to subjective responses rather then pre- and post-test scores for an objective assessment of learner's performance; (3) Our journal club did not host a biostatistician in most of our meetings, as is usually recommended for running effective journal clubs [8,19]; (4) The generalizability of our results for guiding formulary decisions and changing clinical practice shall be verified on a larger sample of practicing clinical pharmacists.

However, our structured journal club has several strengths: (1) Our JC is mentored by a skilled clinical pharmacist, which is consistent with previous literature in improving critical appraisal skills and is tailored to individual learners by providing 1:1 learner-centered precepting [5,9]; (2) The Pre-JC Interactive session is unique to our structured JC to stimulate critical reasoning skills and introduces new epidemiological concepts to interns and residents; (3) Additionally, the discussion is fostered with the expertise of clinical pharmacists having diverse backgrounds and expertise, which creates a unique opportunity to learn and enrich the environment for empowering learners with critical thinking and decision-making for changing practice-based settings. Over the past five years, we have noticed a great improvement in the critical appraisal skills of learners attending the JC suggesting that our structured JC is a successful tool to guide pharmacy practitioners in various critical formulary and practice-changing decisions.

5. Conclusions

Our results suggest that clinical pharmacist steered journal club may serve as an effective tool to empower learners at different levels of pharmacy practice with evidence-based principles for interpretation of literature and guide informed decision-making.

Future studies with qualitative data, pre- and post-test scores, and an assessment of learning metrics shall provide robust evidence on the utility of a clinical pharmacist-steered JC in reshaping clinical practice and guiding formulary decisions.

Acknowledgments: John Orav, Harvard T. H. Chan School of Public Health, Harvard Medical School for his valuable input and review of the manuscript. Pharmaceutical Care Department, King Abdulaziz Medical City, Jeddah, Saudi Arabia, for continuous support for journal club activity. Pharmacy preceptors, residents, and interns attending the pharmaceutical care department, King Abdulaziz Medical City, Jeddah, Saudi Arabia, from 2010 to 2014 for their valuable input to the journal club and participation in the survey. This study has been presented as a poster presentation and a pearl session at the National Pharmacy Preceptor Conference in Washington, DC, United States, in August 2014 as well as a poster at the King Abdullah International Research Center 5th Annual Forum, Jeddah, Saudi Arabia, in September 2014.

Author Contributions: All authors have read and approved the final version for publication.

References

1. Arif, S.A.; Gim, S.; Nogid, A.; Shah, B. Journal clubs during advanced pharmacy practice experiences to teach literature-evaluation skills. *Am. J. Pharm. Educ.* **2012**, *76*, 88. [CrossRef] [PubMed]

2. Honey, C.P.; Baker, J.A. Exploring the impact of journal clubs: A systematic review. *Nurse Educ. Today* **2011**, *31*, 825–831. [CrossRef] [PubMed]

3. Pato, M.T.; Cobb, R.T.; Lusskin, S.I.; Schardt, C. Journal club for faculty or residents: A model for lifelong learning and maintenance of certification. *Int. Rev. Psychiatry* **2013**, *25*, 276–283. [CrossRef] [PubMed]

4. Harris, J.; Kearley, K.; Heneghan, C.; Meats, E.; Roberts, N.; Perera, R.; Kearley-Shiers, K. Are journal clubs effective in supporting evidence-based decision making? A systematic review. Beme guide No. 16. *Med. Teach.* **2011**, *33*, 9–23. [CrossRef] [PubMed]

5. Matthews, D.C. Journal clubs most effective if tailored to learner needs. *Evid.-Based Dent.* **2011**, *12*, 92–93. [CrossRef] [PubMed]

6. American Society of Health-System Pharmacists. ASHP statement on the formulary system. *Am. J. Hosp. Pharm.* **1986**, *43*, 2839–2841.

7. American Society of Health-System Pharmacists. ASHP statement on leadership as a professional obligation. *Am. J. Health Syst. Pharm.* **2011**, *68*, 2293–2295.

8. Deenadayalan, Y.; Grimmer-Somers, K.; Prior, M.; Kumar, S. How to run an effective journal club: A systematic review. *J. Eval. Clin. Pract.* **2008**, *14*, 898–911. [CrossRef] [PubMed]

9. McLeod, R.S.; MacRae, H.M.; McKenzie, M.E.; Victor, J.C.; Brasel, K.J. A moderated journal club is more effective than an internet journal club in teaching critical appraisal skills: Results of a multicenter randomized controlled trial. *J. Am. Coll. Surg.* **2010**, *211*, 769–776. [CrossRef] [PubMed]

10. Critical Appraisal Skills Programme (CASP). Available online: http://www.casp-uk.net/casp-tools-checklists/c18f8 (accessed on 27 May 2015).

11. Center for Evidence Based Medicine by Oxford, UK. Available online: http://www.cebm.net/critical-appraisal/ (accessed on 27 May 2015).

12. Mills, E.J.; Ioannidis, J.P.; Thorlund, K.; Schunemann, H.J.; Puhan, M.A.; Guyatt, G.H. How to use an article reporting a multiple treatment comparison meta-analysis. *J. Am. Med. Assoc.* **2012**, *308*, 1246–1253. [CrossRef] [PubMed]

13. Moher, D.; Hopewell, S.; Schulz, K.F.; Montori, V.; Gøtzsche, P.C.; Devereaux, P.J.; Elbourne, D.; Egger, M.; Altman, D.G. Consort 2010 explanation and elaboration: Updated guidelines for reporting parallel group randomised trials. *Br. Med. J.* **2010**, *340*, c869. [CrossRef] [PubMed]

14. Von Elm, E.; Altman, D.G.; Egger, M.; Pocock, S.J.; Gøtzsche, P.C.; Vandenbroucke, J.P. The strengthening the reporting of observational studies in epidemiology (strobe) statement: Guidelines for reporting observational studies. *Lancet* **2007**, *370*, 1453–1457. [CrossRef]

15. Liberati, A.; Altman, D.G.; Tetzlaff, J.; Mulrow, C.; Gøtzsche, P.C.; Ioannidis, J.P.A.; Clarke, M.; Devereaux, P.J.; Kleijnen, J.; Moher, D. The prisma statement for reporting systematic reviews and meta-analyses of studies that evaluate healthcare interventions: Explanation and elaboration. *Br. Med. J.* **2009**, *339*, b2700. [CrossRef] [PubMed]

16. Raosoft. Sample Size Calculator. Available online: http://www.raosoft.com/samplesize.html (accessed on 15 May 2014).

17. SurveyMonkey Inc. [US]. Available online: https://www.surveymonkey.com (accessed on 27 May 2014).

18. Fowler, L.; Gottschlich, M.M.; Kagan, R.J. Burn center journal club promotes clinical research, continuing education, and evidence-based practice. *J. Burn Care Res.* **2013**, *34*, e92–e98. [CrossRef] [PubMed]

19. Wombwell, E.; Murray, C.; Davis, S.J.; Palmer, K.; Nayar, M.; Konkol, J. Leadership journal club. *Am. J. Health Syst. Pharm.* **2011**, *68*, 2026–2027. [CrossRef] [PubMed]

The Relevancy of Paracetamol and Breastfeeding Post Infant Vaccination

Nurain Suleiman [1,2,*], Siti Hadijah Shamsudin [2], Razman Mohd Rus [3], Samsul Draman [3] and Mai Nurul Ashikin Taib [4]

[1]   Pharmaceutical Services Division, Johor State Health Department, 81200 Johor Bahru, Johor, Malaysia
[2]   Kulliyyah of Pharmacy, International Islamic University Malaysia, 25710 Kuantan, Pahang, Malaysia; shadijah@iium.edu.my
[3]   Kulliyyah of Medicine, International Islamic University Malaysia, 25710 Kuantan, Pahang, Malaysia; razman@iium.edu.my (R.M.R.); nurin@iium.edu.my (S.D.)
[4]   Ara Damansara Medical Centre, 40150 Shah Alam, Selangor, Malaysia; dr.mai.nurulashikin@ramsaysimedarbyhealth.com
*   Correspondence: nurain.suleiman@moh.gov.my

Abstract: Background: Paracetamol may be used as an antipyretic agent for the treatment of fever, as well as an analgesic in the treatment of mild to moderate pain post-vaccination in infants. The use of paracetamol during fever may be or may not be recommended since it may alter the natural human body immune response, although it may reduce fever and fussiness. **Objectives:** The aims of this study are to describe the effectiveness of breastfeeding in reducing pain and paracetamol in reducing fever and pain post infant vaccination. **Methods:** Data sources and study selection was conducted by electronic searching of six databases. Manual reference checks of all articles on paracetamol and breastfeeding post infant vaccination published in the English language between 1978 and 2017. Two levels of screening were used on 9614 citations, which include screening of abstracts and titles followed by full text screening. The data synthesis were tabulated into study characteristics, quality, and effects. **Results:** Systematic review of breastfeeding included three studies from 9614 database searches found significant benefit from breastfeeding in pain scores and the duration of crying, as well as behavioural changes. None of the studies stated the detriment of breastfeeding before, during, and after immunization. Systematic review of paracetamol effectiveness included four studies from 1177 database searches found significant benefit from prophylaxis paracetamol in fever, one study found significant benefit from prophylaxis paracetamol in fussiness, and one study's results were found to be not significant. Two studies on evaluating the safety of prophylactic paracetamol in 2009 found that antibody responses to several antigens were significantly reduced, and the other study in 1988 found that antibody titres to DTP bacteria of placebo and PCM did not differ significantly. **Conclusions:** The relevancy of giving paracetamol post all types of vaccination may be questionable. Breastfeeding before, during, and after immunization are recommended for pain reduction and are proven effective. Further research is required in deciding if paracetamol is to be of rational use following infant immunization.

Keywords: paracetamol; breastfeeding; post; childhood; prophylactic; immunization; vaccination

1. Introduction

Paracetamol may be used as an antipyretic agent for the treatment of fever, as well as an analgesic in the treatment of mild to moderate pain on post vaccination in child [1]. Current recommendations of different guidelines [2–4] note the option to give paracetamol prophylaxis for childhood vaccinations, but neither promote nor discourage routine use of prophylaxis. The theoretical explanation on paracetamol is that it will inhibit the synthesis of prostaglandin in the hypothalamus, then inhibits the hypothalamic heat-regulating centre, and finally produces antipyeresis. It will also peripherally block pain impulse generation, thus producing analgesic effects [1]. These are the reasons why the use of paracetamol during fever may or may not be recommended since it may alter the natural human body immune response, although it may reduce pain.

The Medical News by The Lancet on 19 October 2009 stated that 'paracetamol (also known as acetaminophen) to reduce fever after vaccination is likely to be counterproductive'. There is a study to prove that that the antibody geometric mean concentration (GMC) is significantly lower in the paracetamol group than in the control group [5,6]. In fact, some evidence showed that prophylactic administration of an antipyretic drug around the time of vaccination may lower antibody responses to some vaccines [7,8]. Additionally, the vaccine, itself, may not be effective if paracetamol is given at an early stage to prevent fever following immunization. It may cause fewer antibodies to be produced, thus, it is possible that the vaccine may not work well [7]. Thus, this may suggest not to use paracetamol post vaccination in infants since it may contradict the Worlds Health Organization's Expanded Programme on Immunization's main aim.

The reduction of fever and pain following infant immunization is a high priority for the international community. Older recommendations for fever and pain treatment need to be revised since treating fever at an early stage and pain following infant immunization by paracetamol may be questionable since it may cause the vaccine injected to be less effective. Evidence-based health policies and programmes aiming to reduce fever and pain following infant immunization need reliable and valid information. Effective interventions to improve overall infant health need targeted health and social policies that are informed by reliable and valid epidemiological data. This study, using a systematic review, aimed to estimate the effectiveness of paracetamol for fever and natural intervention (e.g., breastfeeding) for pain following infant vaccination. Interventions used in the studies of antipyretic property of paracetamol were placed in two intervention categories. There are administration of prophylactic paracetamol and administration of paracetamol during fever. Meanwhile, interventions used in the studies of the analgesic property of breastfeeding were placed in two categories: breastfeeding and held in mothers' arms but not fed. The aim of this study is to determine the effectiveness of breastfeeding as an analgesic property, as well as the safety of paracetamol's antipyeretic properties post infants vaccination, and to provide evidence-based recommendations for clinical practice.

2. Method

2.1. Search Strategies

Medical, environmental, and scientific databases were search to identify primary studies of the effects of breastfeeding before, during, and after immunization, as well as the effects of antipyretic agent following infant immunization in order to capture as many relevant citations as possible. The electronic searches were supplemented by hand searching of six databases which were accessed through EzProxy for the Off Campus Access Online Database for the International Islamic University Malaysia (IIUM) Students and Staffs. The databases include the Ovid LWW Total Access Collection and Medline, CINAHL (Cumulative Index to Nursing and Allied Health Literature) Plus with Fulltext, Science Direct, Proquest Dissertations and Theses, Proquest Education Journal, and Proquest Health and Medical Complete. Additionally, manual reference checks were conducted of all articles on paracetamol and breastfeeding post childhood vaccination published in the English language between 1978 and 2017. Two levels of screening were used on 9614 citations. The keywords that were used included in Table A1.

The titles and abstracts of the articles were scanned by two reviewers (N.S. and S.H.S.). Articles selected by the reviewers were retrieved in full and assessed for eligibility by the two reviewers.

The reviewers did not contact the authors to identify additional studies, but the reviewers referred to reference lists from the identified trials. The reviewers were not blinded to the authors or settings of the scanned articles.

2.2. Study Selection: Inclusion Criteria

Only reports with information on infants (for this study defined as up to 1 year of age) were included. All randomized trials and cohort (non-randomized) studies that included a placebo or unexposed group were included for the determination of effectiveness. Trials of different designs, however, were handled separately. The effectiveness of breastfeeding as an analgesia and physical intervention of fever as antipyretic were reviewed for the immunization and/vaccination procedure only. All prospective studies that reported data on variables of noxious stimuli with behavioural, physiological, hormonal, and metabolic changes were included since infants respond to these variables. For the determination of safety, all prospective studies were included. Papers that have funding sources were also included in this study.

2.3. Study Selection: Exclusion Criteria

Reviews, meta-analyses, editorials, commentary, or conference abstracts were excluded in this study. Meta-analysis was excluded in this study because it was not feasible due to extensive variation in study features and methodological quality [9].

2.4. Data Collection and Analysis

There were two reviewers in this study. The study from World Health Organization also included two reviewers for systematic review [10]. The first reviewer screened all titles and abstracts of papers identified by the literature search. The second reviewer handled duplicate screening on a random selection of found titles or abstracts. The disagreements were discussed between both reviewers. All studies that had been identified as potentially relevant were retrieved and read in full to determine the eligibility for inclusion.

Data extractions were conducted by using a pre-defined data extraction template. Data that were extracted included design characteristics, study population and country, sample size, sample selection, age of participants, the exposure and outcome measures and results.

2.5. Primary Outcome

The primary outcome was pain and/fever following infant immunization. Examples of validated observational measures for pain were the Douleur Aigue du Nouveau-ne (DAN) Scale, Facial Pain Rating Scale, and Neonatal/Infant Pain Scale (NIPS), Children's Hospital of Eastern Ontario Pain Scale (CHEOPS), and cry duration. Examples of observational measures for fever were babies' fussiness and temperature reading 38 °C or greater.

2.6. Validity Assessment

The included trials were not masked to the reviewers (N.S. and S.H.S.). The methodological quality of each study was assessed by two independent reviewers using the Crowe Critical Appraisal Tool (CCAT) [11] to investigate internal validity (the extent to which the information is probably free of bias) with the following attributes. The CCAT was developed based on a wide number of previous critical appraisal tools, general research methods theory and reporting guidelines [11]. The tool was validated and has undergone testing for reliability and validity [11]. The CCAT appraised papers included in the review in eight categories. This tool uses scoring system in which each category is scored from zero in which no evidence to five in which highest evidence. Total scores of each study are presented as a percentage. The average scores of reviewers were reported.

2.7. Data Abstraction

Data from each eligible study were extracted individually on custom-made data collection forms (designed specifically for each intervention) by two (2) reviewers (N.S. or S.H.S.), and the results were compared. The reviewers resolved any disagreements through discussion.

2.8. Study Characteristics

Characteristics of included studies as well as the country of being conducted were displayed in Table A2 (for effectiveness of breastfeeding) and Table A3 (for effectiveness of prophylactic paracetamol and its safety). This study included research published in 1987 onwards.

2.9. Data Synthesis

Data syntheses were tabulated into study characteristics, quality, and effects. The original review of summarizing the evidence from studies of variable design will provide details how the differences between study results were investigated and how they were summarized [12].

Authors of trials were not contacted for further details or provision of original data if the published report contained insufficient information. The study findings, as reported by the authors, were included in this review.

The data in this research cannot be pooled due to insufficient data regarding odds ratios or relative risk, as well as confidence intervals in each study.

2.10. Secondary Outcomes

Local and adverse reactions following infant immunization was reviewed in the study of prophylactic paracetamol post infant vaccination.

3. Results

3.1. Effectiveness of Breastfeeding as an Analgesic Property for Pain Following Childhood Vaccination

3.1.1. Study Descriptions

Figure A1 presents a flow diagram of the search strategy. After duplicates were removed the search retrieved 9504 articles, of which 9481 are excluded (9400 on review of the abstracts/title and a further 81 after full-text paper assessment). Of the 23 reviewed full-text articles 19 were excluded because the outcome and exposure were not measured. Among these, one (1) was excluded because the age was not within the inclusion criteria. Finally, data from three (3) journal articles were included in the systematic review.

3.1.2. Study Characteristics

Overall, there were three (3) studies that met the inclusion criteria and eligibility for study of the effectiveness of breastfeeding's analgesic property for pain following immunization in infants. These studies were conducted mainly in the east coast country region, which include one (1) in Iran, one (1) in Jordan, and one (1) in Turkey. Studies began in 2007 and the latest study was in 2013.

These studies addressed two (2) of the intervention categories identified in the protocol: (i) breastfeeding; or (ii) held in mothers' arms but not fed. All studies included babies not more than one (1) year of age.

The researcher included randomized control trials and quasi-controlled trials that compared breastfeeding and combined interventions of interest with a placebo or control group for pain management during immunization in children aged from 0 months to 1 year of age. Among these, there were two (2) studies that were randomized controlled trials and only one (1) study that was a quasi-controlled trial. The primary outcome measure for pain was made by a health care worker or observer using observational methods; for example, the Douleur Aigue du Nouveau-ne (DAN) Scale,

Facial Pain Rating Scale and Neonatal/Infant Pain Scale (NIPS), Children's Hospital of Eastern Ontario Pain Scale (CHEOPS) and cry duration. However, all of these studies did not mention the duration of breastfeeding.

Among these three (3) studies, one (1) did not contain information about receiving approval by institutional review boards or ethics committees. On the other hand, two (2) of the three (3) studies mentioned that they obtained approval from institutional ethics review boards or committees. All of these studies mentioned that they obtained informed consent from the mothers.

3.2. Methodological Quality of the Included Studies

The percentage of agreement on all key items for assessment of the methodological quality of the three (3) studies was from 75% to 83%; disagreements were resolved by consensus. Three (3) trials which include 316 infants aged zero (0) to 12 months examined the analgesic effects of breastfeeding.

3.3. Effects of Breastfeeding Post Infants Vaccination

In all three (3) studies, infants who were breastfeed before, during, and after procedure were compared with infants who were not breastfed. The level of pain was measured using cry duration [13,14], Neonatal Infant Pain Scale (NIPS) [14], Douleur Aigue du Nouveau-ne (DAN) Scale, Facial Pain Rating Scale (FPS) [14], Children's Hospital of Eastern Ontarion Pain Scale (CHEOPS), as well as behavioural changes [13].

The reviews of all studies found significant benefit from breastfed in pain score and duration of crying, as well as behavioural changes. The pain score of one (1) study revealed a significant lower pain score in which $p < 0.001$ in the study by Razek et al., 2009 for the experimental group (breastfeeding group) than the control group (not breastfed). One study by Razek et al. in 2009 noted that the FPS for the intervention group represented "hurts little more" pain (38%) than the control group, which represented "hurts even more" (8.3%) Score 3 that indicate pain. Two (2) studies evaluated crying time and it was revealed that crying time was shorter in the intervention group rather than the control group [13,14]. Other than that, among two (2) studies that evaluated behavioural changes in heart rate and oxygen saturation, both were found to not differ significantly in mean heart rate elevation between control groups and experimental groups.

Breastfeeding was studied as an alternative to the painful procedure during immunization recently, with positive outcomes. Studies have demonstrated that breastfeeding [13–15], maternal holding [13], and skin to skin contact [13,14] statistically significantly reduced pain [15] and crying duration [13,14] in children following immunization.

These studies showed that breastfeeding is effective as pain relief following immunization in infants.

3.4. Effectiveness of Prophylactic Paracteamol's Antipyretic and Analgesic Properties and Its Safety for Fever Following Childhood Immunization

3.4.1. Study Descriptions

Figure A2 presents a flow diagram of the search strategy. After duplicates were removed the search retrieved 1176 articles, of which 1165 were excluded (1100 on review of abstracts/title and a further 65 after full-text assessment). Of the 11 reviewed full-text articles two (2) were excluded because the outcome and exposure were not measured. Among these, five (5) were excluded because the ages were not within the inclusion criteria. Finally, data from four (4) journal articles were included in the systematic review.

3.4.2. Study Characteristics

Overall, four (4) studies were assessed as being of sufficient quality to be included in the review. These studies were conducted mainly in Europe and east coast country regions, which include one (1) in the Czech Republic, one (1) in United States of America (USA), one (1) in Germany, and one (1) in Finland. Studies began in 1988 and the latest study was in 2013.

As mentioned before, these studies addressed two (2) intervention categories: (i) administration of prophylactic paracetamol; and (ii) non-prophylactic paracetamol for fever following childhood immunization.

All of these studies evaluated either the child was having fever or not [4,6,16,17], only one (1) study evaluated local systemic reactions [16], two (2) studies evaluated adverse reactions [16,17], and only one (1) study evaluated baby condition [4], as well as only two (2) studies evaluating the antibodies of children [6,17]. All studies included the age of babies from about six (6) weeks to around one (1) year of age [4,6,16,17]. All of these studies are also included in the systematic review.

The researcher (N.S.) included all randomised controlled trials that compared prophylactic paracetamol use and/no prophylactic paracetamol use post infant vaccination. The primary outcome measure for fever was made by parents completing the diary and/questionnaires given by the researcher of the study.

Among these four (4) studies, three (3) of them mentioned that they obtained approval from institutional ethics review boards or committees [4,6,16]. All of these studies mentioned that they obtained informed consent from parents and/legal guardian, except the study by Uhari et al. (1988) did not mention they obtained consent from guardians, however, they had obtained ethical approval from the Medical Faculty of Oulu University.

3.5. Methodological Quality of the Included Studies

The percentage of agreement on all key items for assessment of the methodological quality of the four (4) studies ranged from 65% to 88%; disagreements were resolved by consensus. Four (4) trials which include 1156 infants aged zero (0) to 12 months of age examined the antipyretic effect of paracetamol.

3.6. Effect of Prophylactic PCM for Fever and Pain Following Childhood Immunization

All studies compared children receiving prophylactic or non-prophylactic PCM post vaccination. Fever was measured using a body temperature $\geq38\,°C$ or $>39.5\,°C$ of axillary or rectal temperature. Meanwhile, baby condition was measured by the appearance of fussiness.

The reviews of two (2) studies found significant benefit from paracetamol prophylaxis in fever [6,16] and only one (1) study found significant benefit from paracetamol prophylaxis in fussiness [4]. On the other hand, there was one (1) study that found a non-significant benefit from prophylaxis paracetamol in fever [17].

3.7. Safety of Prophylactic paracetamol Post Infant Vaccination

Other than that, there were two (2) studies that evaluated the safety of prophylactic paracetamol [6,17]. These studies revealed different outcomes, in which the study by Prymula et al. in 2009 found that antibody responses to several antigens were reduced significantly, and the other study by Uhari et al. in 1988 found that antibody titres to DTP bacteria of placebo and PCM did not differ significantly. The study by Prymula et al. in 2009 also noted that prophylactic paracetamol at the time of vaccination should not be routinely recommended, although febrile reactions were significantly reduced since antibody responses to several antigens were significantly reduced.

Additionally, there was one (1) study by Jackson et al. in 2011 that was stopped because of the result of study by Prymula et al. in 2009. The study by Jackson et al. in 2011 also noted that the potential benefit of paracetamol prophylaxis in reducing the risk of fever and associated adverse events following contemporary infant immunizations appear to be outweighed by the potential harmful effects of paracetamol prophylaxis on vaccine immune responses.

4. Discussion

Paracetamol was used as an antipyeretic agent and analgesic post vaccination in infants. However, its use seems questionable since, in theory, the use of paracetamol at early stages of fever may alter the vaccine function and cause the vaccine to be less effective [6]. Theoretically, the use of paracetamol may interfere natural body immune response by inhibiting prostaglandins (PGs), which are involved in the natural human body defence mechanisms. Most of the vaccines injected in children originate from attenuated organisms, which may cause infection. The organism might replicate over days or weeks, then result in immunity.

This study found that breastfeeding before, during, and after immunization reduced pain, as assessed using cry duration, DAN scale, FPS, NIPS, CHEOPS, and/or behavioural changes (heart rate and oxygen saturation). The proposed mechanisms of breastfeeding providing analgesia include (i) breastfeeding; and (ii) maternal holding and skin to skin contact [13].

The findings of the systemic review were consistent with the effectiveness of breastfeeding as an analgesic property in reducing pain of injection immunization in neonates [18]. Breastfeeding is a natural, cost-neutral, time-efficient, and convenient intervention that could be easily adopted from the perspectives of health care providers and parents [18]. Other than the nutritional and psychological value of breastfeeding, the analgesic properties may encourage more mothers to breastfeed [18].

The prophylactic antipyretic of paracetamol significantly reduced the febrile reactions of $\geq 38\,°C$ after vaccinations. There were statistically significant differences in antibody responses between two groups which were lower in the prophylactic paracetamol group. One (1) recent study showed that there were significant reductions in the local and systemic symptoms in the prophylaxis group, but no significant difference between groups [16].

Only two (2) trials studied the antibody response [6,17], thus, the data cannot be pooled. Studies used different doses/schedules of antipyretic administration, and the age of participants or timing of administration were also markedly differed among studies.

There were no studies that were identified in the literature search that evaluated the effectiveness of oral analgesics in which paracetamol for immunization pain [18]. Paediatricians may recommend oral analgesics to parents as a pain-relieving intervention for vaccine injection pain [18]. However, no evidence was found to recommend the use of either agent as a method of pain relief for vaccine injections. There were no studies that identified the paracetamol effects on vaccine injection pain, however, this agent was widely used. Thus, a study that addresses this issue may be warranted.

5. Limitation

Methodological challenges and limitations of this review include the small number of studies for breastfeeding interventions, small sample size, limited age range of participants, limited number of vaccines evaluated, and variability in pain assessments. The included trials used various methods of assessing pain in infants, which made it difficult to combine and contrast the results.

6. Recommendation for Future Research

Further research is required in deciding paracetamol to be of rational use following infant immunization.

Based on the researcher's review, areas for future research were identified. The role of expressed breast milk has not been studied, and further research is needed. Finally, studies addressing whether the gap between research findings and clinical practice can be narrowed by communication and dissemination strategies aimed at practitioners, professional groups, and families will be important in establishing the common goal of pain-free, tolerable, and effective immunization for infants.

Future trials should focus on the timing (before, with, or after) and route (oral or rectal) of administration of paracetamol, as well as on the subgroup of infants (term or preterm) for any correlation with the immune response. Future trials should focus on trials examining the prophylactic effect of paracetamol post vaccination antibody response since there was lack of studies regarding this issue. The mechanism underlying the reduction in immune/antibody response should also be explored. Trials should also be conducted in developing countries where over-the-counter use of antipyretics (including prophylactic) are common. Other confounding factors that might affect the antibody response, such as infant sleep post-immunization, should also be studied.

7. Conclusions

The relevancy of giving, or the usage of, paracetamol post all types of vaccination is still questionable due to the safety issues this intervention might arise.

From this systematic review, breastfeeding before, during, and after immunization were recommended for pain reduction and is proven effective.

The reviews showed that prophylactic antipyretic paracetamol administration leads to reduce of fever and fussiness. However, there was a reduction in antibody responses to some vaccine antigens. Future study and surveillance programs should also aim at assessing the effectiveness of programs where prophylactic paracetamol is given. The timing of administration of paracetamol should be discussed with the parents after explaining the benefits and risks.

Acknowledgments: The author would like to thank the Director General of Health for his permission to publish this paper. The author also would like to thank International Islamic University Malaysia, Kuantan Campus for giving support in conducting this project.

Author Contributions: S.H.S. and N.S. analysed the data; N.S. wrote the paper; and S.H.S. reviewed the paper.

Appendix A

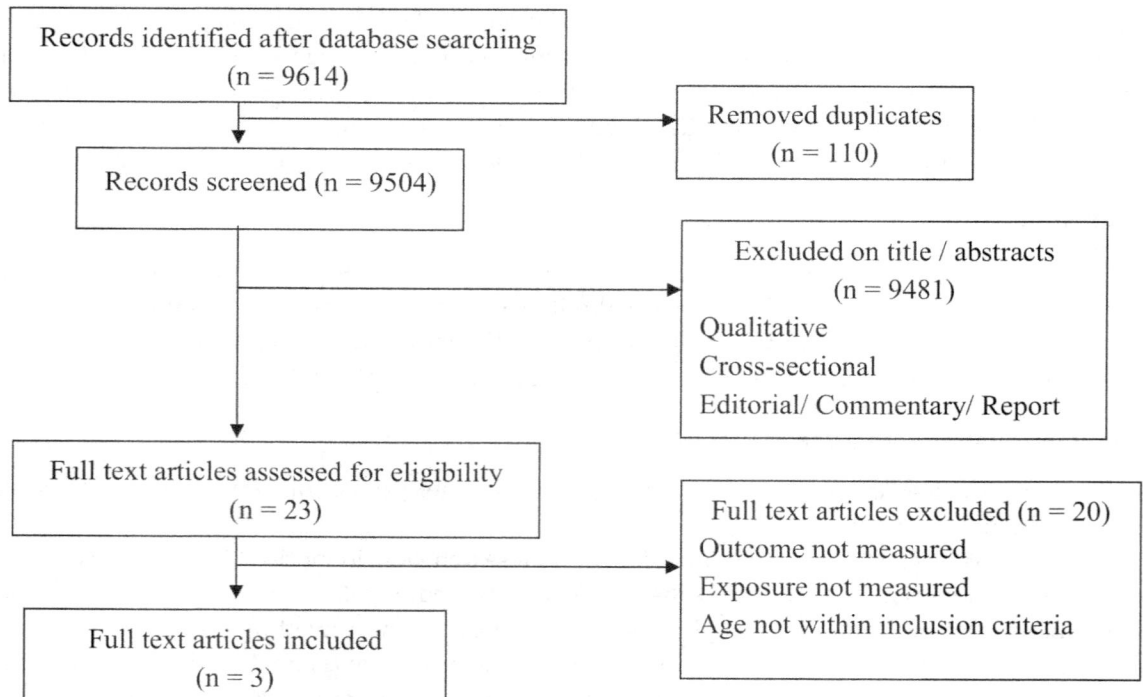

Figure A1. Flow diagramme of research strategy for effectiveness of breastfeeding as pain intervention.

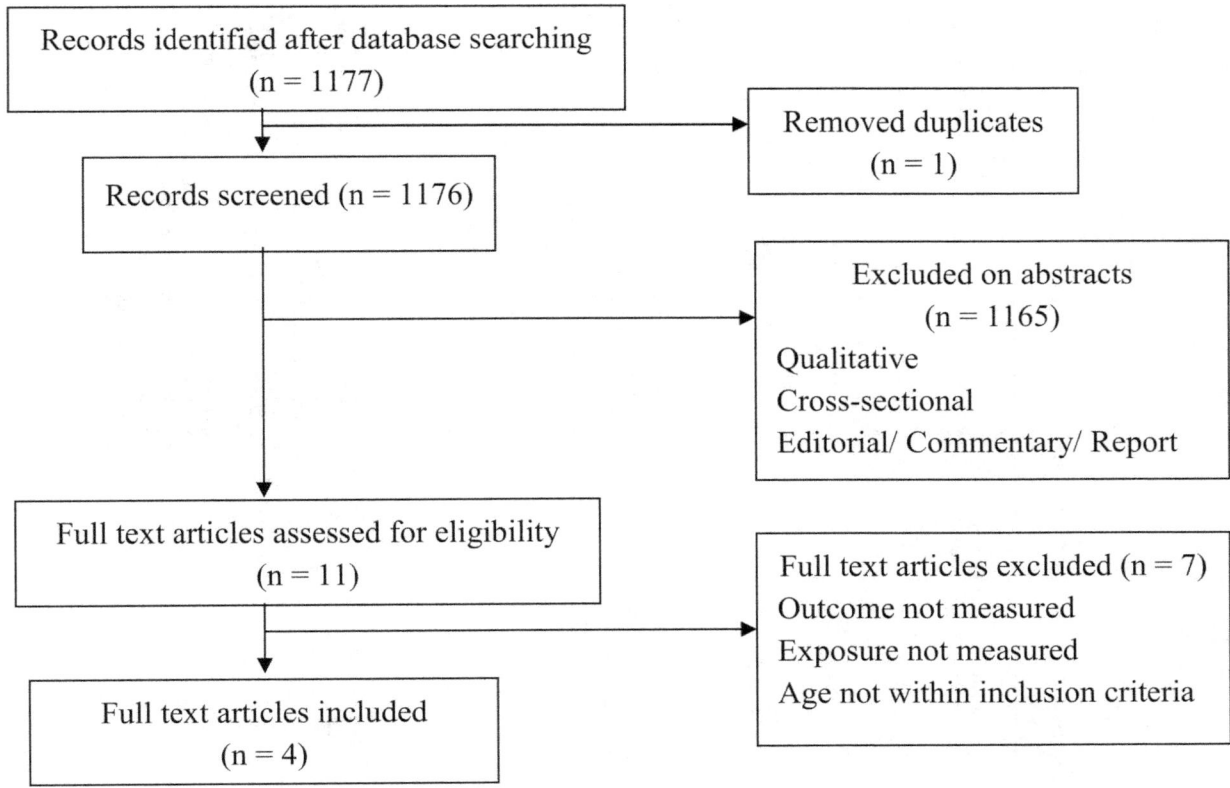

Figure A2. Flow diagram of research strategy for the effectiveness of prophylactic paracetamol for fever reduction post childhood vaccination.

Table A1. Keywords for systematic review.

Database Searches	Items Measure	Keywords
Ovid LWW Total Access Collection and Medline, CINAHL Plus with Fulltext, Science Direct, Proquest Dissertations and Theses, Proquest Education Journal and Proquest Health and Medical Complete (data collected from published paper from 1987 until 2017)	(1) Pain (2) Breastfeeding	'breastfeeding; pain or analgesia; following or post; immunization or vaccination; infant or newborn'
	(3) Fever and pain (4) paracetamol	'feverish or febrile or fever; breastfeeding; temperature decrease; antipyretic; analgesic; following or post; immunization or vaccination; infant or newborn; antibody'

Table A2. Summary of relevant research on effectiveness of breastfeeding used as an intervention to decrease pain in infants.

No.	Author; Country; Year of Publication	Research Design	Study Population; Care Recipient % Boys; Care Recipient Age Mean (SD)	Sample Size: Baseline; Follow-Up	Exposure Measure	Outcome Measure	Quality Score (%)	Statistical Results	Conclusion
1	Modarres, Jazayeri, Rahnama, Montazeri, Iran, 2013 [Funding Source: Instituitional Review Board of the Tehran University of Medical Sciences]	True experiment: Placebo controlled trial	Full term neonates breastfed 2 minutes before, during and after Hepatitis B immunization or held in mothers' arms but not fed; 83% boys; 39.4 (1.2) in control group and 39.1 (1.3) in experimental group weeks	130; 130; 130	Pain score measured using DAN scale (Facial expressions, limb movements and vocal expression)	Pain score	75	(1) Significant difference in mean of facial expressions of neonates between the control 2.58 (SD = 0.72) and experimental groups 1.39 (SD = 0.65). ($p < 0.001$). (2) Significant differences between two groups in mean of limb movements 1.92 (SD = 0.69) and experimental groups 0.83 (SD = 0.51). ($p < 0.001$) (3) Significant differences in mean of vocal expression between control 2.28 (SD = 0.57) and experimental groups 1.31 (SD = 0.68). ($p < 0.001$). (4) Significant difference in mean of Total DAN scores between control 6.78 (SD = 1.69) and experimental groups 3.52 (SD = 1.37). ($p < 0.001$)	Breastfeeding reduces pain and is effective way for pain relief during Hepatitis B injection
2.	Razek, El-Dein, Jordan, 2009 [Funding Source: None]	Quasi experiment: Counter balanced (cross-over)	Infants either breastfed or not; 64.2% boys; 1–12 months of age	120; 120; 120	(1) Pain score measured using Facial Pain Rating Scale before, during and after procedure (2) Duration of crying (3) Heart rates	(1) Pain rating scale (2) Crying time (3) Heart rate	75	(1) Significant difference in Facial Pain Rating Scale between control and experimental group ($p < 0.05$) (2) Significant difference in mean of Duration of Crying between control 148.66 s (SD 13.96) and experimental groups 125.33 s (SD 12.18). ($p < 0.005$) (3) Not differ significantly in mean of heart rate elevation between control group (before procedure 125.22 bpm SD 29.15, after procedure 162.25 bpm SD 40.22) and experimental group (before procedure 128.59 bpm SD 15.45, after procedure 149.210 bpm SD 20.510). p before procedure = 1.330, p after procedure=none	Breastfeeding and skin to skin contact significantly reduced the pain in infants receiving immunization. Pain Score also showed lesser in breastfeeding group.

Table A2. *Cont.*

No.	Author; Country; Year of Publication	Research Design	Study Population; Care Recipient % Boys; Care Recipient Age Mean (SD)	Sample Size: Baseline; Follow-Up	Exposure Measure	Outcome Measure	Quality Score (%)	Statistical Results	Conclusion
3.	Efe, Ozer, Turkey, 2007 [Funding Source: Akdeniz University Scientific Research Project Unit]	True experiment: Placebo controlled trial	Healthy infants receiving 2nd, 3rd or 4th immunization of IM DTP either breastfed before, during and after injection or given not breastfed; 56.1% boys; 3.08 ± 1.32 months control, 2.79 ± 1.13 months breastfed	66; 66; 66	(1) Length of crying (2) Heart rate (3) Oxygen saturation levels	(1) Crying time (2) Behavioural changes	83	(1) Significant difference in mean of Crying duration between control 76.24 s (SD 49.61) and experimental 35.85 s (SD 40.11). $p = 0.001$ (2) Not differ significantly in mean of heart rate elevation between control group (during procedure 129.58 bpm SD 38.32, after procedure146.36 bpm SD 31.06) and experimental group (during procedure 138.85 bpm SD 35.89, after procedure153.36 bpm SD 29.60). p during procedure = 0.31, p after procedure = 0.352 (3) Not differ significantly in mean of oxygen saturation between control group (during procedure 95.85% SD 4.18, after procedure 95.33% SD 4.17) and experimental group (during procedure 96.64% SD 2.93, after procedure 95.97% SD 3.08), p during procedure = 0.379, p after procedure = 0.483	Breastfeeding, maternal holding, and skin to skin contact significantly reduced crying time in infants receiving immunization injection for DTP

Table A3. Summary of relevant research on effectiveness of prophylactic antipyretic used as an intervention to decrease fever in infants and its safety issue.

No.	Author; Country; Year of Publication	Research Design	Study Population; Care Recipient % Boys; Care Recipient Age Mean (SD)	Sample Size: Baseline; Follow-Up	Exposure Measure	Outcome Measure	Quality Score	Statistical Results	Conclusion
1.	Rose, Juergens, Schmoele-Thoma, Gruber, Baker; Germany; 2013 [Funding Source: Pfizer Inc.]	True experiment: Placebo controlled trial	Healthy infants who received three-dose infant series of PCV-7 and DTPa-HBV-IPV/Hib plus a toddler dose either received prophylactic paracetamol at vaccination and at 6–9 h interval thereafter or a control group that received no paracetamol; 51.5% boys; 2.4–11.7 months	301; 286; 245	(1) Incidence of fever (2) Baby Conditions (3) Crying	(1) Fever (2) Drowsiness (3) Decreased appetite (4) Decreased activity (5) Persistent inconsolable crying	83	(1) Significant difference in temperature ≥38 °C to ≤39 °C of control 35.8% and experimental 9.3% groups: → after dose 1 ($p < 0.001$) (2) Significant difference in temperature ≥38 °C to ≤39 °C of control 43.7% and experimental 19.7% groups: → after dose 2 ($p = 0.000$) (3) Significant difference in temperature ≥38 °C to ≤39 °C of control 45.6% and experimental 19.3% groups: → after dose 3 ($p = 0.000$) (4) No significant difference in temperature ≥38 °C to ≤39 °C of control 60% and experimental 51.5% groups: → after toddler dose ($p = 0.221$) (5) No significant difference in temperature ≥39 °C to ≤40 °C of control 4% and experimental 0% groups: → after dose 1 ($p = 0.061$) (6) No significant difference in temperature ≥39 °C to ≤40 °C of control 1.8% and experimental 0% groups: → after dose 2 ($p = 0.238$) (7) No significant difference in temperature ≥39 °C to ≤40 °C of control 1.9% and experimental 1.0% groups: → after dose 3 ($p > 0.99$) (8) No significant difference in temperature ≥39 °C to ≤40 °C of control 13.1% and experimental 4.6% groups: → after toddler dose ($p = 0.072$) (9) No significant difference in temperature >40 °C of control 1.1% and experimental 0% groups: → after toddler dose ($p > 0.99$) (10) Significant difference in drowsiness of control 64.7% and experimental 50.4% groups: → after dose 1 ($p = 0.019$) (11) No significant difference in drowsiness of control 58.3% and experimental 46.5% groups: → after dose 2 ($p = 0.078$) (12) No significant difference in drowsiness of control 45.6% and experimental 36.4% groups: → after dose 3 ($p = 0.182$) (13) No significant difference in drowsiness of control 50.4% and experimental 43.5% groups: → after toddler dose ($p = 0.350$)	(1) PCM reduced incidence of fever ≥38 °C, reduction significant in infants but not in toddler (2) Fever >39 °C was rare during infant series, thus, too few cases for assessment (3) PCM reduced incidence of drowsiness, reduction significant in infants after dose 1 but not in dose 2 and 3 also in toddler (4) PCM reduced incidence of decreased appetite, reduction significant in infants after dose 2, but not after dose 1 and 3 also in toddlers (5) PCM reduced incidence of decreased activity, reduction significant in infants after dose 2, 3, and in toddlers, but not after dose 1 (6) PCM reduced incidence of persistent inconsolable crying, reduction significant in infants after dose 1, but not in dose 2 and 3 also in toddlers

Table A3. *Cont.*

No.	Author; Country; Year of Publication	Research Design	Study Population; Care Recipient % Boys; Care Recipient Age Mean (SD)	Sample Size: Baseline; Follow-Up	Exposure Measure	Outcome Measure	Quality Score	Statistical Results
1.	Rose, Juergens, Schmoele-Thoma, Gruber, Baker; Germany; 2013 [Funding Source: Pfizer Inc.]	True experiment: Placebo controlled trial	Healthy infants who received three-dose infant series of PCV-7 and DTPa-HBV-IPV/Hib plus a toddler dose either received prophylactic paracetamol at vaccination and at 6–9 h interval thereafter or a control group that received no paracetamol; 51.5% boys; 2.4–11.7 months	301; 286; 245	(1) Incidence of fever (2) Baby Conditions (3) Crying	(1) Fever (2) Drowsiness (3) Decreased appetite (4) Decreased activity (5) Persistent inconsolable crying	83	(14) No significant difference in decreased appetite of control 40% and experimental 30.3% groups: → after dose 1 ($p = 0.118$) (15) Significant difference in decreased appetite of control 42.7% and experimental 26.6% groups: → after dose 2 ($p = 0.011$) (16) No significant difference in decreased appetite of control 33.6% and experimental 23.0% groups: → after dose 3 ($p = 0.101$) (17) No significant difference in decreased appetite of control 45.2% and experimental 38.2% groups: → after toddler dose ($p = 0.336$) (18) No significant difference in decreased activity of control 46.3% and experimental 41.6% groups: → after dose 1 ($p = 0.457$) (19) Significant difference in decreased activity of control 48% and experimental 31% groups: → after dose 2 ($p = 0.007$) (20) Significant difference in decreased activity of control 40% and experimental 23.3% groups: → after dose 3 ($p = 0.007$) (21) Significant difference in decreased activity of control 48.3% and experimental 23.3% groups: → after toddler dose ($p = 0.005$) (22) Significant difference in persistent inconsolable crying of control 20% and experimental 9.5% groups: → after dose 1 ($p = 0.031$) (23) No significant difference in persistent inconsolable crying of control 15.8% and experimental 9.3% groups: → after dose 2 ($p = 0.171$) (24) No significant difference in persistent inconsolable crying of control 15.3% and experimental 14% groups: → after dose 3 ($p = 0.849$) (25) No significant difference in persistent inconsolable crying of control 17.1% and experimental 7.8% groups: → after toddler dose ($p = 0.056$)

Table A3. *Cont.*

No.	Author; Country; Year of Publication	Research Design	Study Population; Care Recipient % Boys; Care Recipient Age Mean (SD)	Sample Size: Baseline; Follow-Up	Exposure Measure	Outcome Measure	Quality Score	Statistical Results	Conclusion
2.	Jackson, Peterson, Dunn, Hambidge, Dunstan, Starkovich, Yu, Benoit, Dominguez-Islas, Carste, Benson, Nelson; Czech Republic; 2011 [Funding Source: Centre for Disease Control and Preventive (CDC) through America's Health Insurance Plans]	True experiment: Placebo controlled trial	Children received up to five PCM doses (10–15 mg/kg) or placebo following routine vaccinations; 51% boys; 31 weeks to 69 weeks	374; 352; 234	(1) Rectal temperature (2) Baby condition	(1) Fever (2) Fussiness (more than much more than usual and much more than usual)	83	(1) No significant difference in rectal temperature ≥38 °C between the control 22% and experimental groups 14% (p = 0.053) (2) No significant difference in rectal temperature ≥39 °C between the control 2% and experimental groups 0% (p = 0.08) (3) Significant difference in fussiness (more than much more than usual) between the control 62% and experimental groups 58% (p = 0.045) (4) Significant difference in fussiness (much more than usual) between the control 24% and experimental groups 10% (p = 0.001)	Acetaminophen may reduce risk of post-vaccination fussiness but not reduce fever
3.	Prymula, Siegrist, Chlibek, Zemlickova, Vackova, Smetana, Lommel, Kaliskova, Borys, Schuerman; Czech Republic; 2009 [Funding Source: GSK Biologicals]	True experiment: Placebo controlled trial	Children received 3 prophylactic PCM doses every 6 to 8 hours in first 24 h, or no prophylactic PCM after each vaccination with PHiD-CV co-administered with DTPa-HBV-IPV/Hib and oral human rotavirus vaccines; 51% boys; mean aged at time of 1st dose was 12.3 weeks (SD 2.13).	459; 459; 414	(1) Rectal temperature >39.5 °C after primary and after booster (2) Percentage of child with temperature ≥38 °C after at least one dose of prophylactic PCM after primary and after booster (3) Antibody GMC after primary and after boosting	(1) Fever (2) Antibody GMC	88	(1) Rectal temperature >39.5 °C was uncommon in both groups: → after primary: 1/226 participants (<1%) in prophylactic PCM group vs. 3/233 (1%) in no prophylactic group: → after booster: 3/178 (2%) vs. 2/172 (1%) (2) Percentage of child with temperature ≥38 °C after at least 1 dose of prophylactic PCM was significantly lower → after primary: 154/233 (66%) and → after booster: 64/178 (36%) in prophylactic PCM group than in no prophylactic PCM group: → after primary: 154/233 (66%) → after booster: 100/172 (58%) (3) Antibody GMC were significantly lower in prophylactic PCM group after primary vaccination for all ten pneumococcal vaccine serotypes, protein D, antipolyribosyl-ribitol phosphate, antidipthteria, antitetanus, and antipertactin.	Prophylactic administration of antipyretic drugs at time of vaccination should not routinely recommended, although febrile reactions significantly decreased since antibody responses to several antigens were reduced significantly

Table A3. *Cont.*

No.	Author; Country; Year of Publication	Research Design	Study Population; Care Recipient % Boys; Care Recipient Age Mean (SD)	Sample Size: Baseline; Follow-Up	Exposure Measure	Outcome Measure	Quality Score	Statistical Results	Conclusion
					(1) Temperature in the evening and the next morning (2) Percentages of temperature with no fever and fever in the evening and the next morning (3) Levels of IgG antibodies (for Diphtheria toxoid, Tetanus toxoid, Pertussis bacteria) (4) Frequency of fever during 24 h after DTP vaccination			(1) No significant difference in mean of temperature in the evening between the control 37.6 °C (SD 0.49) and experimental groups 37.6 °C (0.65). 95% confidence limits of the difference −0.1–0.1 (2) No significant difference in mean of temperature in the next morning between the control 37.6 °C (SD 0.53) and experimental groups 37.6 °C (0.53). 95% confidence limits of the difference −0.1–0.1 (3) No significant difference in mean percentages of temperature with no fever in the evening between the control 36.5% and experimental groups 37% (4) No significant difference in mean percentages of temperature with fever in the evening between the control 6.75% and experimental groups 6.75% (5) No significant difference in mean percentages of temperature with no fever in the next morning between the control 40% and experimental groups 35% (6) No significant difference in mean percentages of temperature with fever in the next morning between the control 5% and experimental groups 7.25% (7) No significant difference in mean levels of IgG antibodies (for Diphtheria toxoid) between the control 10.5 (SD = 6.3) and experimental groups 10.7 (SD = 6.6), 95% Confidence limits of differences −3.6–3.2 (8) No significant difference in mean levels of IgG antibodies (for Tetanus toxoid) between the control 16.6 (SD = 7.9) and experimental groups 14.2 (SD = 8.4), 95% Confidence limits of differences −1.9–6.7 (9) No significant difference in mean levels of IgG antibodies (for Pertussis bacteria) between the control 31.1 (SD = 20.0) and experimental groups 34.2 (SD = 25.3), 95% Confidence limits of differences −15.0–8.76 (10) No significant difference in frequency of fever during 24 h period after DTP vaccination between the control 48.5% and experimental groups 44.4%, 95% Confidence limits of differences −8.0–16.	
4.	Uhari, Hietala, Viljanen; Finland; 1988 [Funding Source: None]	True experiment: Placebo controlled trial	Healthy infants vaccinated with DTP or DTP-inactivated polio vaccine receive placebo or 75 mg PCM 4 h after vaccination; not mentioned; 5 months	295; 263; 263		(1) Fever (2) Antibody titres	65		Acetaminophen in a single dose schedule is ineffective in decreasing post-vaccination fever and antibody response also showed no significant difference in control and experimental groups

NS = Not significant; DTP = Diphtheria, Tetanus, and Pertussis; GMC = Geometric Mean Concentration.

References

1.   American Pharmacists Association. Acetominophen. In *Drug Information Handbook*; Lexi-comp: Hudson, OH, USA, 2006.

2.   Bahagian Pembangunan Kesihatan Keluarga. *Panduan Program Imunisasi Kebangsaan Kanak-Kanak Untuk Anggota Kejururawatan*; Kementerian Kesihatan: Kuala Lumpur, Malaysia, 2008.

3.   College of Paediatrics. *Malaysian Immunization Manual*; Academy of Medicine Malaysia: Kuala Lumpur, Malaysia, 2001.

4.   Jackson, L.A.; Peterson, D.; Dunn, J.; Hambidge, S.J.; Dunstan, M.; Starkovich, P.; Yu, O.; Benoit, J.; Dominguez-Islas, C.P.; Carste, B.; et al. A Randomized Placebo-Controlled Trial of Acetominophen for Prevention of Post-Vaccination Fever in infants. *PLoS ONE* **2011**, 6. [CrossRef] [PubMed]

5.   Paddock, C. Routine Use of Paracetamol (Acetaminophen) After Vaccination Not Recommended for Infants, Study. *Medical News Today*, 19 October 2009.

6.   Roman, P.; Siegrist, C.A.; Chlibek, R.; Zemlickova, H.; Vackova, M.; Smetana, J.; Lommel, P.; Kaliskova, E.; Borys, D.; Schuerman, L. Effect of prophylactic Paracetamol administration at time of vaccination on febrile reactions and antibody responses in children: Two open-label, randomised controlled trials. *Lancet* **2009**, *374*, 1339–1350.

7.   Cooper, C.; Atkinson, E.J.; O'fallon, W.M.; Melton, C.J., III. *Incidence of Clinically Diagnosed Vertebral Fractures: A Population-Based Study in Rochester, Minnesota, 1985–1989*; Department of Health Sciences Research, Mayo Clinic and Foundation: Rochester, MN, USA, 1992.

8.   Hirtz, D.G.; Nelson, K.B.; Ellenberg, J.H. Seizures following childhood immunization. *J. Pediatr.* **1982**, *102*, 14–18. [CrossRef]

9.   Centre for Clinical Practice at NICE. *Feverish Illness in Children Assessment and Initial Management in Children Younger Than 5 Years*; National Institute for Health and Care Excellence: Manchester, UK, 2013.

10. Katrin, S.K.; Michael, M.; Michael, B.; Marcy, C.J.; Ron, D.; John, H.; David, N.; Edward, R.; the Brighton Collaboration Fever Working Group. *Fever after Immunization: Current Comcepts and Improved Future Scientific Understanding*; Infectious Diseases Society of America: Arlington, VA, USA, 2004.

11. Das, R.R.; Panighari, I.; Naik, S.S. The effect of prophylactic antipyretic administration on post-vaccination adverse reactions and antibody response in children: A systematic review. *PLoS ONE* **2014**, *9*. [CrossRef] [PubMed]

12. Janice, E.; Sullivan, M.D.; Henry, C.; Farrar, M.D.; the Section on Clinical Pharmacology and Therapeutics, and Committee on Drugs. *Clinical Report: Fever and Antipyretic Use in Children*; American Academy of Peadiatrics: Itasca, IL, USA, 2011.

13. Coomarasamy, A.; Taylor, R.; Khan, K.S. A systematic review of postgraduate teaching in evidence-based medicine and critical appraisal. *Med. Teach.* **2003**, *25*, 77–81. [CrossRef] [PubMed]

14. Pisacane, A.; Continision, P.; Palma, O.; Cataldo, S.; Michele, F.D.; Vairo, U. Breastfeeding and risk for fever after immunization. *Peadiatrics* **2010**, *125*, e1448–e1452. [CrossRef] [PubMed]

15. Mathew, P.J.; Mathew, J.L. Assessment and management of pain in infants. *Postgrad. Med. J.* **2003**, *79*, 438–443. [CrossRef] [PubMed]

16. Rose, M.A.; Juergens, C.; Schmoele-Thoma, B.; Gruber, W.C.; Baker, S.; Zielen, S. An open-label randomised clinical trial of prophylactic paracetamol coadministered with 7-valent penumococcal conjugate vaccine and hexavalent diphteria toxoid, tetanus toxoid, 3-component acellular pertusis, hepatitis B, inactivated poliovirus, and Haemophilus influenzae type b vaccine. *BMC Peadiatr.* **2013**. [CrossRef]

17. Uhari, M.; Hietala, J.; Viljanen, M.K. Effect of prophylactic acetaminophen administration on reaction to DTP vaccination. *Acta Paedistr. Scand.* **1988**, *77*, 747–751. [CrossRef]

18. Rose, W.; Kirubakaran, C.; Scott, J.X. Intermittent clobazam therapy in febrile seizures. *Indian J. Peadiatr.* **2005**, *72*, 31–33. [CrossRef]

3

Exploring a Problem-Based Learning Approach in Pharmaceutics

Barbara McKenzie * **ⓘ** **and Alyson Brown**

School of Pharmacy and Life Sciences, Robert Gordon University, Aberdeen AB10 7GJ, Scotland, UK;
alyson.brown@rgu.ac.uk
* Correspondence: b.mckenzie1@rgu.ac.uk

Abstract: Objective. The basis of this study was to explore the impact of the initiation of a Problem-Base Learning (PBL) approach within a second-year pharmaceutics degree on a Master of Pharmacy programme, introduced as a way of improving deep learning and to foster independent learning. Design. A semi-structured interview was used to seek feedback from the students, and feedback from staff was secured though a focus group. A thematic approach was used for the analysis, once data saturation had been reached. Exam pass-rate statistics were also analysed. Assessment. Five parent themes were identified from the student interviews: Module structure, Promoting lifelong learning, Integration and future practice, Outcomes and Student experience. The third year exam pass rate improved by 12% in the year following the introduction of PBL in second year. Conclusions. Various recommendations were proposed to further improve the module, based on the findings of this study. These include improving feedback and support through tutorials, reducing the volume of directed study, as well as highlighting the relevance of pharmaceutics to the pharmacy degree. A long-term review would be needed to assess the full implications of PBL teaching within this course.

Keywords: problem-based learning; deep learning; pharmacy; pharmaceutics

1. Introduction

Medicine Design and Manufacture (MDM) is a second-year module at SCQF (Scottish Credit and Qualifications Framework) level 8 (in a 12-level scale) which runs over two semesters on the pharmacy Master's degree program. The module covers pharmaceutics, that is, the drug journey from raw ingredient to formulated drug-delivery system, such as a tablet or an ointment.

Prior to academic session 2013/2014, the MDM coursework was delivered as a series of set experiments, in which the students worked through a coursework based around a specific dosage formulation, such as an emulsion or a suppository. Each small group of students had a designated academic staff member to guide them through the process. The students were instructed how to perform relevant calculations, research the pre-formulation of the medicine and then complete the manufacturing stage, with the work structured around clear learning outcomes. The coursework assessment (two written short-answer coursework tests) was based around the four liquid and five tableting practical lab sessions, and contributed 20% of the overall module mark. The remaining 80% was allocated to the written exam, which was based around the lecture material.

For the 2013/2014 session, the coursework sessions were re-designed by the module team to follow a problem-based learning (PBL) approach using a set of mini-projects, which required students to explore a pharmaceutical formulation in a relevant problem. PBL is a teaching method used to develop skills such as team working, listening and self-directed learning [1]. The problem allows the use of research and reasoning in order to progress and complete the task in a contextualised way. The laboratory sessions were organised into groups of seven or eight students (130 students in total), who were each provided with a drug name, and a designated academic supervisor who was instructed to facilitate the work of the students. The coursework sessions ran as a series of six labs in semester one and dealt with liquid dosage forms, whilst semester two dealt with solid dosage forms, and ran as eight labs. Each lab was scheduled for three hours, with the designated staff member available throughout. These topics were complemented by parallel lecture sessions [2]. This format reflects other institutions, such as that described by Romero et al. [3]. Students undertaking the PBL sessions were provided with coursework sheets and questions on the pre-formulation and physicochemical aspects of their designated drugs. These served as a guide to the learning objectives that are essential to define the teaching and learning parameters for each module [4]. The coursework assessment for semester one was a formative report with feedback, and a summative report was submitted for semester two. The summative report contributed 50% towards the overall module grade, whilst the written exam after semester one provided the remaining 50% of the mark.

Initially, each group was assigned a drug at random, and students were expected to complete the coursework sheets on the physicochemical properties of this drug using appropriate literature sources. Successful completion of the coursework sheets was intended to provide the students with an information base to build on when deciding, with the guidance of the supervisor, on an appropriate formulation to be taken forward in the remaining laboratory sessions. After completing the appropriate COSHH (Control of Substances Hazardous to Health) and risk assessment (for physical risks) forms, each of the groups was able to create an appropriate drug-delivery system. Each supervisor mentored five groups over two sessions, and was able to work closely with each of the groups.

At this stage students were instructed to research their allocated drug. This was a change from the didactic approach students had experienced in their first year of study, and there was some initial uncertainty and reluctance. As this was the first year that the module had been taught this way, both staff and students were apprehensive. After an initial period of non-activity, the students appeared to behave in one of two ways; some realised that they had to organise themselves well and work together to gain the knowledge required to complete the project, whilst other students had a more negative reaction. The pressure of learning for themselves was a new experience for many of the students, and one which they did not appear to enjoy and reacted negatively to. Staff reassured students and helped build their confidence to make decisions and act on them. The students were encouraged to put effort into the formative report, in order to gain as much feedback as possible for the summative assessment. This formative report and the subsequent feedback received was essential in giving students the opportunity to improve and prepare for the summative report. Many of the students indicated that at first they did not see the point of the formative report, however the majority of students appreciated the value of the constructive feedback they received in helping them to complete the summative report.

The initial experience of PBL proved difficult and stressful for many of the students, who were not familiar with learning independently, and who were unsure of how to approach the formative report. Despite an end-of-year tutorial to give specific guidance on this aspect to students, many of the groups did not follow this guidance.

As the module delivery was novel, it was difficult to predict how the students would react to this new mode of teaching. There were also other issues to deal with, such as the School's relocation to another campus within the city. Students were required to manage their group workload appropriately to complete tasks. Problem-based learning requires motivation and cooperation from the whole group to complete the task [5–7]. Without this, the group can quickly break down into sub-groups, where a minority do the majority of the work, and the others do little to organise themselves and manage their time. Initially, several of the students made little contribution to the group effort and had to be given a reminder that their cooperation and engagement was an essential requirement of this form of learning. This highlighted that some of the students lacked group work and engagement skills, with many having had minimal experience of this approach prior to entering their second year. To help overcome this problem, engagement became part of the assessment structure for the second semester, and greatly improved the students' approach as a result. This was achieved by introducing an individual summary (30% weighting for the coursework assessment). The students were also exposed to scientific literature for the first time, which was daunting to begin with, however many students coped well and incorporated this information into their reports without prompting from staff. These are essential for progression through the degree program and into professional practice. Being able to work independently as well as part of a team are important skills for pharmacists, and also for lifelong learning [8–11].

When the students write their summative report for the coursework assessment, there is a requirement to link background theory to the lectures and directed study to the practical lab work, giving references and discussing the rationale behind their work [1]. This gives a context and a scientific basis for what they are trying to achieve. During semester two, all of the coursework related to tablet manufacture, so that all of the students were provided with the opportunity to go through the process. However, in semester one, each group chose a different type of liquid formulation and only manufactured one type of liquid. This meant that they could not build on the relevant lecture material in a practical way. This limits the deep learning which could occur, as the constructivism and connectivism mechanisms are restricted to theory only [12]. Many students need the practical aspect to fully understand and appreciate the information provided in lectures, and therefore these students could be disadvantaged. Mayes' learning framework describes this in more detail (Figure 1) [13].

The teaching of background theory prior to practical lab experience involving PBL permits the assimilation of knowledge through reasoning and reflection [14]. This is the basis of Mayes' learning framework [15], which deals with learning in a constructivist way. Constructivist learning is often problem-based, and allows students to build their own knowledge through supported tasks. This is compared to instructivism, which is a more traditional method of material delivery and requires rote learning. The structure of the new MDM module also allows cyclical learning to take place, from conceptualisation, through construction and finally to application, which is frequently dialogue in education (Figure 1) [15].

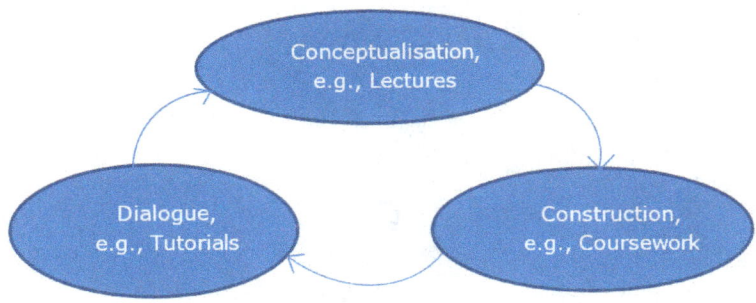

Figure 1. Mayes' learning cycle.

Conceptualisation is the interaction of new information with a student's existing knowledge. Construction is the process of building knowledge through practical tasks. Finally, application is the testing of this new knowledge in applied contexts. There is a general trend in pharmacy education in the US towards PBL, as outlined in the Accreditation Council for Pharmacy Education (ACPE) Standards, and in the 2004 revision of the Centre for the Advancement of Pharmaceutical Education (CAPE) Educational Outcomes [16]. There is a move away from the simple transmission of facts, towards critical thinking and problem solving [17].

Conceptualisation begins when the students are introduced to new information during the lectures. This new knowledge is then built upon during the construction phase, where the students work through practical examples of the theory, and apply the theory to a practical context. This is now limited to the liquid which they choose to manufacture, however there is directed study which may help with this stage of learning. These two stages are then consolidated in the identification phase, which links the theory and relates it directly to the practical [18]. The current structure of the Master of Pharmacy (MPharm) degree is an upward spiral, allowing basic knowledge to be built on and reinforced, further promoting 'deep learning' (Figure 2). The old method of working through set coursework covered all of the lecture material in a practical way; however, this was not an ideal way to teach the subject. Certainly the feedback from students was that they preferred the new method of PBL compared to the more traditional approach which had an element of 'spoon-feeding', however, while they welcomed the PBL approach, they were of the view that it had gone from one extreme to the other, and would have preferred more input from staff. This was not helped by a lack of drug formulation in year one of the course. They also do not like that each staff member gave them a different answer to their questions, based on personal preference or experience. This is unfortunately undermining the students' trust in the staff, and led to some major problems half way through the coursework. As this was the first year that MDM had been delivered in this way, there were always going to be teething problems, however, many of the students felt angry that they were 'guinea pigs' for this new method of module delivery.

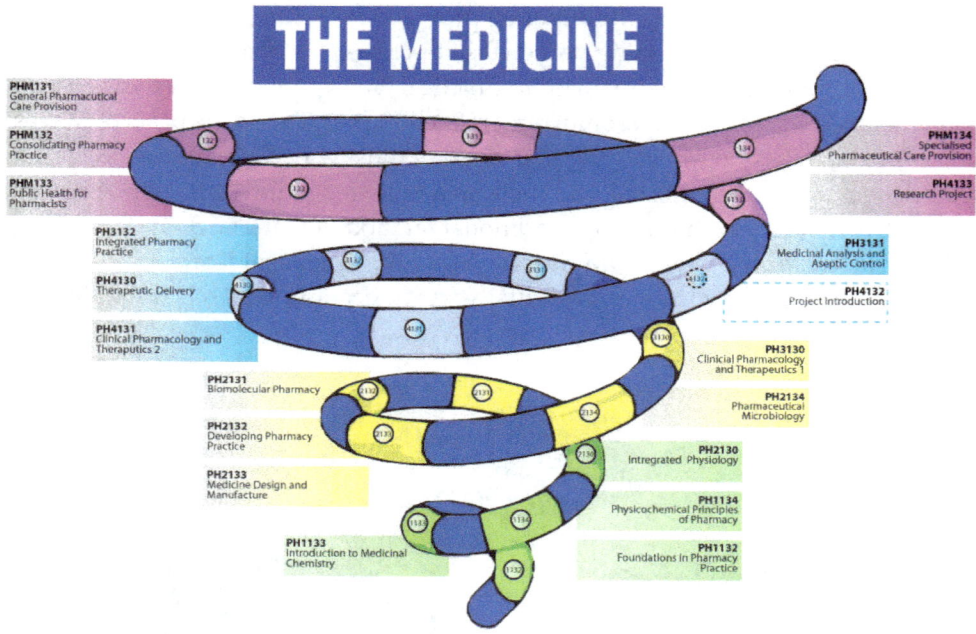

Figure 2. Schematic showing vertical learning through the MPharm degree course.

As a direct result of feedback received from the students, this year (2014/2015 session) the module was altered. Seminars and coursework covering some basic background and general techniques (didactic delivery of material) are carried out in semester one, before the summative work begins in semester two, which will be run as PBL. It is believed that this will improve the student experience, so that they are more prepared for the PBL, developing the relevant underpinning knowledge and improving the opportunity for deep learning with increased confidence. The basis of this study is to explore the impact of and reflect upon the 2014/2015 approach as compared to the 2013/2014 approach. It is the intention to seek feedback from the students at a later date on whether they consider their introduction to the PBL approach and associated independent learning helped them perform better in subsequent modules and in their third year of study. It is hoped that, by introducing PBL and a more independent learning style earlier in the degree, this form of teaching is made easier as they progress into other modules such as Therapeutic Delivery.

1.1. Design

This study explored student and staff views and attitudes on the introduction of PBL to the MDM module using a qualitative methodological approach. Semi-structured interviews were conducted with undergraduate pharmacy students followed by a focus group with staff involved in the delivery of the module. Ethical approval was obtained from the School of Pharmacy and Life Sciences Ethical Review Committee.

1.2. Recruitment

An invitation email was sent to all 2nd year ($n = 130$) and 3rd year ($n = 128$) undergraduate pharmacy students registered on the Master of Pharmacy program at the Robert Gordon University (RGU) in April 2015. An information leaflet (Appendix A) was attached to the email. A reminder email was sent to students after 2 weeks.

Pharmaceutics staff were invited by email to participate in a focus group. The information leaflet (Appendix A) was attached to the email, which was sent to all of the pharmaceutics staff ($n = 6$).

Informed consent was obtained from all participants prior to data being collected. Students were assured that their involvement would have no influence on their progression through the course.

1.3. Data Collection

Semi-structured interviews were conducted with students. Interviews lasted up to 20 min and were recorded on a digital voice recorder. An interview schedule was developed from existing literature and student feedback that had been gathered from existing module review processes, and reviewed by the research team before use. This was used as a guide for each interview and answers were explored further where appropriate.

A focus group was conducted with staff to validate themes that emerged from student interviews. The focus group topic guide was informed by the themes emerging from student interviews and the feedback gathered through the module review process.

1.4. Participants

Second-year students: Five second-year students volunteered to participate in the study (3.8%), and initially, five interviews were conducted. A further 2 interviews were then conducted to confirm data saturation.

Third-year students: Fifteen third-year students volunteered to participate in the study (11.7%), and initially, fifteen interviews were conducted. A further 2 interviews were then conducted to confirm data saturation.

1.5. Analysis

Each interview was transcribed verbatim following the conclusion of the interview, and analysis took place to identify emerging themes. Once data saturation was reached (i.e., no further themes were emerging), transcripts were independently analysed by another member of the research team to confirm no new themes were emerging and to validate the existing themes, and a further two interviews conducted to confirm saturation. The focus group transcript was analysed independently by two members of the research team and emerging themes validated [19–21].

1.6. Data Protection

All study materials were stored, processed and destroyed in accordance with Pharmacy and Life Sciences standard operating procedures. All data collected was stored securely and participants were assigned an anonymous code to ensure they could not be identified.

2. Evaluation and Assessment

Five parent themes were identified from the student interviews: Module structure (17 comments in total), Promoting lifelong learning (7 comments in total), Integration and future practice (16 comments in total), Outcomes (12 comments in total) and Student experience (18 comments in total) (Figure 3).

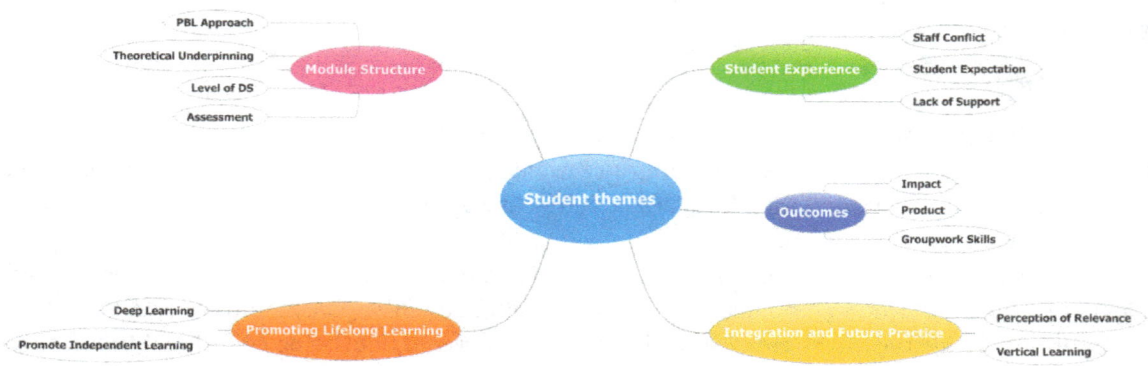

Figure 3. Mind map of the themes raised from the student interviews.

Module structure is concerned with the use of PBL as a teaching method, how the module is assessed, the level of directed study (DS) and theoretical underpinning. Promoting lifelong learning is the overarching theme for deep learning and promoting independent learning. Integration and future practice involves the topics of vertical learning and the student's perception of relevance. Outcomes are definable outputs such as group work skills, pharmaceutical product production and impact. Student experience involves student expectation, staff conflict and lack of support.

"Being able to apply your knowledge is the best way of learning."
Participant 3.2F.

"It prepares you for the future . . . It's what you need to do in reality."
Participant 10.3F.

"There needs to be some sort of integration in terms of stepping up."
Participant 3.3F.

"Our group made eye drops in first semester, but we didn't learn about them until second semester . . . when it wasn't really relevant anymore."
Participant 2.3F.

"One DS had 40 questions . . . with no feedback."
Participant 4.2F.

"That's what employers look for, problem solving . . . you just need to get on with it, use your initiative."
Participant 10.3F.

"Finding out the information yourself is sometimes more effective than someone just telling it all to you. You probably remember it better if you went and looked it up."
Participant 2.3F.

"A lot of what I was reading and studying wasn't relevant to be a pharmacist."
Participant 5.2M.

"Vertical learning is starting to make sense now. I know that I have material from last year that I can look at."
Participant 4.3F.

"It has improved my group work skills."
Participant 4.2F.

"The best bit was finishing the tablet. I used my knowledge over 5–6 weeks, and made a tablet that could be used."

Participant 3.2F.

"I felt like I knew a lot about suspensions at the end, but I didn't really know a lot about the other formulations. Limited focus."

Participant 8.3F.

"I felt I had no base knowledge."

Participant 1.3F.

"I think it's great, and it's really useful to have the scope to be able to do things outside of constraints . . . it's nice to be given the responsibility."

Participant 7.2M.

"Misunderstanding between staff and students . . . that's what caused the stress and frustration."

Participant 3.3F.

Three overarching themes were identified from the staff focus group: Impact of building move (6 comments in total), Staff experience (7 comments in total) and Module structure (7 comments in total) (Figure 4).

Impact of building move encompasses issues such as the larger student cohort, larger lab, travel and equipment issues. Staff experience covers staff and student expectation and time management. Module structure involves staff preparation, module amalgamation (in the case of Therapeutic Delivery, TD) and clarity of processes.

"It was intensive, it required a lot of staff support."

Participant 2SF.

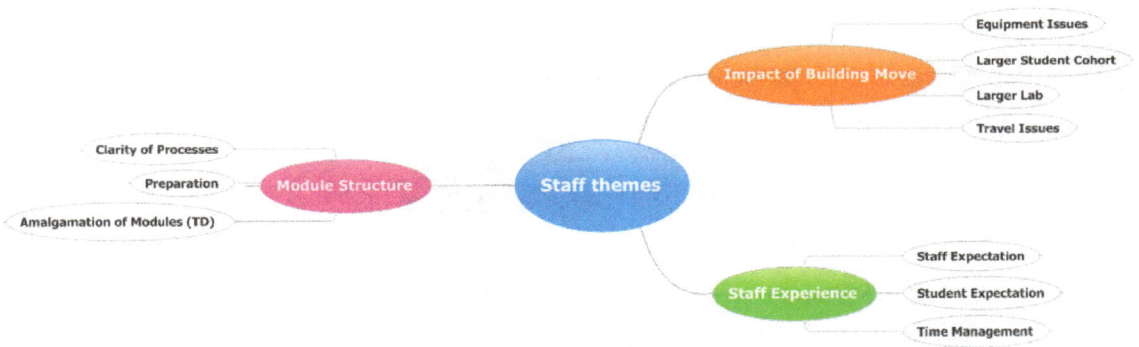

Figure 4. Mind map of the themes raised during the staff focus group.

"It was a perfect storm of a new, large lab, bigger cohort, a lot of walking, disorientation, not knowing where equipment is . . . I found that quite stressful."

Participant 3SM.

"There was a lot of confusion amongst the students, because they are dealing with different individuals, with different experiences."

Participant 3SM.

"Generally I don't think students understand the concept that they are not being assessed on the quality of the products produced."

Participant 2SF.

"It would be beneficial for us not to have 10 groups doing 10 different things. It's exhausting."

Participant 1SM.

"They've been exposed to the background, and because of it they are applying it and therefore they are more likely to remember it for next year."

Participant 2SF.

3. Exam Results

For the MDM module (2nd year), there was no significant difference between the results for 2015/2015 and 2013/2014. The assessment outcome was a pass rate of 82% in 2014/2015, compared to 79% in 2013/2014. The overall mean for 2013/2014 was 54% compared to 56% for 2014/2015 (Figure 5).

The therapeutic delivery module (TD, 3rd year) enjoyed a significantly higher pass rate for session 2014/2015 compared to 2013/2014 (79% compared to 67%) (Figure 6).

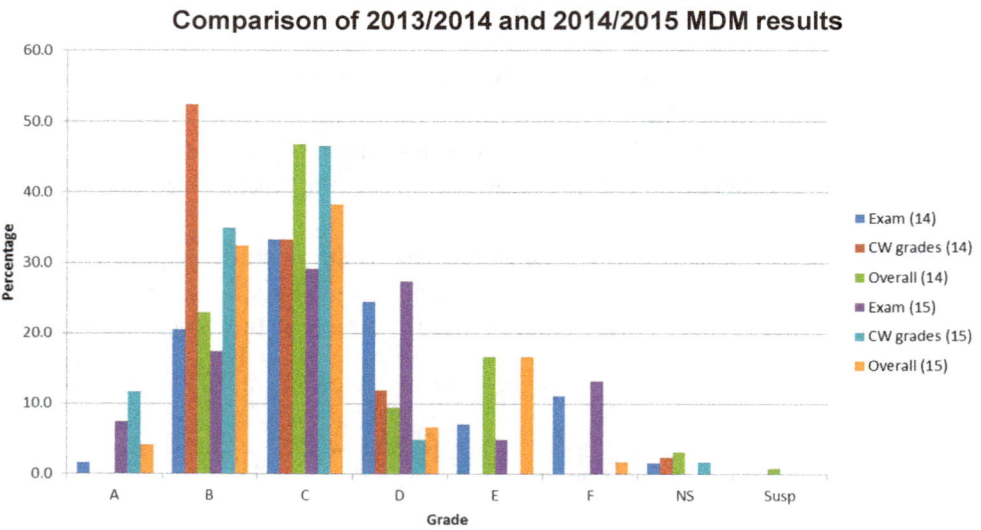

Figure 5. Comparison of Medicine Design and Manufacture (MDM) exam results between 2013/2014 and 2014/2015.

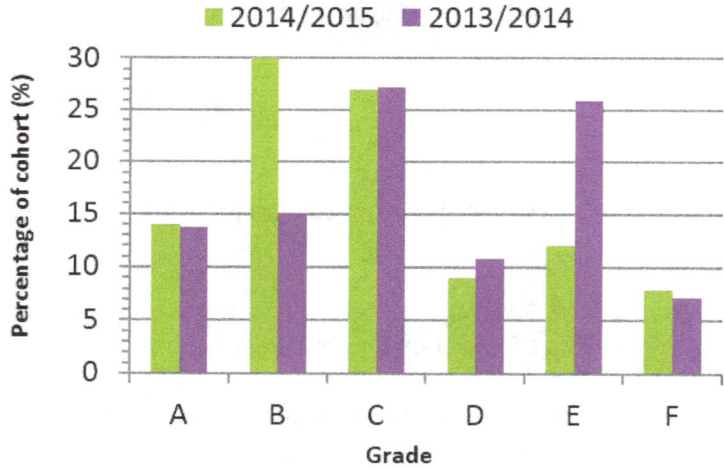

Figure 6. Comparison of Therapeutic Delivery (TD) exam results between 2013/2014 and 2014/2015.

4. Discussion

Key findings:

- Students enjoy the freedom of PBL, however, they need a lot of support to make this method successful.
- The level of DS needs to be reviewed.
- The relevance of the topics taught in MDM and TD needs to be emphasised to students.
- Communications between staff and students need to be improved, and outcomes clarified.

Overall, there were both positive and negative outcomes of the teaching year, and this is reflected in the positive and negative themes which emerged from interviews. The use of PBL in the new module structure was welcomed by the students. The 2013/2014 students enjoyed the freedom of the MDM module, and felt that having a structure where they were given the opportunity to put their skills and knowledge into practice benefitted their learning and their future practice; however, they also felt that they lacked support. This is not unusual for students undertaking problem-based or student-led learning for the first time. It is a different method of delivery and requires a lot of input from both staff and students. Giving the students this degree of responsibility so early in the course was a cause for concern during the planning stage, as some members of staff believed that the students were too inexperienced and used to being 'spoon-fed' to be able to deal with PBL effectively. However, after preparing the students during the first semester with set laboratory experiments, which covered all of the material they would be likely to encounter during semester two and was further backed up with tutorials and lectures, the students coped remarkably well. As a result of changes made to the module, the 2014/2015 students felt supported, although they felt that there could be more clarity in the expected outcomes. The level of DS came under scrutiny, as many students stated that they didn't complete any of the DS, and nevertheless achieved over 60% in the exam. Many of the students completed the DS, but were unsure of the correct answers from a lack of feedback. With regard to the module exam, many students expressed concern that, out of eight questions, two were almost identical and one came from one lecture. They felt that it wasn't representative of the module as a whole, nor of their future likelihood of dealing with the topics. The students also identified a lack of clarity regarding the module outcomes. Many students believed they were being assessed on the quality of the medicine that they made.

As part of the module reorganisation, the written exam was moved to the end of the first semester. This required that the students learn the material from semester one, before undertaking the practical project in semester two. It was believed that this would allow the 'deep learning' to fully occur. The third-year TD module enjoyed a significantly higher pass rate for 2014/2015 compared to 2013/2014 (79% compared to 67%) (Figure 6). There are many possible reasons for this. Firstly, the new amalgamated module had time to 'bed in', whereas last year was the first iteration of it. Staff were much more comfortable with the new lab layout, the larger student cohort and the projects they were running this year. This was also the first year of students who had been through the new PBL MDM module previously, so there is a possibility that the previous experience of a mini-project had prepared the students for the third-year module. These short-term improvements in pass rates have been seen previously in other studies [3].

For the MDM module, the assessment outcome was a pass rate of 82% for 2014/2015, compared to 79% for 2013/2014. The overall mean for 2013/2014 was 54% compared to 56% for 2014/2015 (Figure 5). There was no significant difference in short-term outcomes between the two academic years. When the MDM module was delivered as set coursework, before the 2013/2014 session, there were on average 20–30% of students who failed every year. For the 2013/2014 session, 18% of students failed. Further follow-up studies are required to determine if these affects are anomalies, and also if they have any impact on the third-year module TD.

Long-term outcomes are unknown at this point, and would require further study of postgraduates [22]. There is a possibility that PBL enhances students' critical thinking and problem-solving skills, as well as their ability to learn independently.

Many of the students felt that they had experienced 'deep learning' due to the module's structure. By making the students find out information for themselves, independent learning was also encouraged, which will be a vital career skill [10,11]. It is also a useful skill in many other areas of life. The results of this project are aligned with that of other studies that assess the outcome of PBL compared to a lecture-based module [22]. This study also reports that students feel significantly better-prepared for their future careers as a result of the PBL design, with regard to lifelong learning. There are many other published cases of successful PBL implementation [23].

Many of the students who were interviewed questioned the relevance of learning pharmaceutics in such detail, when they want to be career pharmacists. As the degree is at Master's level, it incorporates surrounding elements of other relevant disciplines, such as human physiology, cell biology, sterile production and quantum mechanics. This is to provide a wide knowledge base, and allows many varied career options for our graduates. Having an underpinning knowledge of pharmaceutics allows our students to be medicine experts, and fully prepares them for whatever they might come across during their careers. Unfortunately, the implications of a strong background in science to underpin their knowledge as a pharmacist were not clear to them. There is therefore a clear need to further contextualise the module. Knowledge of the journey involved in making a medicine, from base chemical through manufacture to the patient administration, is of critical importance to the career of a pharmacist. The underpinning science of the MPharm degree serves not only to provide background knowledge—indeed, all pharmacists, whether they are working in industry, community, regulation or clinical settings will require in-depth knowledge of the area—but also the ability to utilise this knowledge on a daily basis. It is that which sets pharmacists aside from doctors, nurses and all other healthcare professionals; a deep and thorough understanding of all aspects of the medicines with which they work.

The vertical learning framework on which the MPharm course is based became apparent to the students (Figure 2). By introducing ideas slowly, and reinforcing them over the four-year course, ideas are built on and reinforced, becoming 'deep' knowledge.

Group work skills are important in the students' future careers, as outlined in the General Pharmaceutical Council's (GPhC) outcomes [10]. Being able to work effectively as part of a team is also attractive to future employers. During the first year of the MPharm degree course, there are very few group work exercises. Many students reported positive improvement in their group work skills during the second year. They also expressed pride over manufacturing their own dosage forms. Unfortunately, for those students who had a negative overall experience, the option of pharmaceutics as a final-year project was made untenable.

Key findings:

- There is a requirement for staff equipment training.
- The students need to be reminded of the relevance and importance of knowledge in pharmaceutics to their future careers.
- There is a need for improvement in the clarity of objectives and outcomes.
- The module structure in terms of learning outcomes and level of DS needs to be examined.
- The group sizes should be reduced in order to enhance lab experience.

There were a number of unique issues which came together to affect the overall student experience in the 2013/2014 semesters. In the new lab, 70 students could be taught at once, permitting a twice-a-week teaching schedule. As a result of this, more staff were required than originally thought. Students also discovered that staff have different areas of expertise, particularly with regard to equipment. This may have impacted on the students' ability to work effectively in the lab sessions [23]. This feedback has identified a potential opportunity for staff training. In previous years it has been all too easy to ask for technical help from support staff during labs. In order to lessen that burden, staff training will be undertaken over the summer of 2015. There was also more pressure on staff, and some equipment was damaged during the move, impacting greatly on teaching. Despite highlighting the relevance of pharmaceutics as a module during the module introduction, students deemed the modules unnecessary and irrelevant. This produced a lack of engagement in some students, as well as disinterest and bad attitudes towards staff. Other science modules have reported the same problem, and therefore there is a need to emphasise the importance of a pharmaceutics background. Perhaps recently graduated students would be able to give an insight into how the science modules are useful in an everyday way for every pharmacist, whether they be working in community, hospital or industrial settings.

There was some confusion amongst students over outcomes of the module, particularly with regard to the coursework and what material was examinable. The amount of unsupported DS was a source of great frustration to the students, and was one of the most frequent topics raised by students during interviews. There needs to be improved communication generally between staff and students, and processes streamlined.

Due to the new lab size, many students and staff reported anxiety caused by too-large groups and too many people in the lab. Staff time had to be divided between the groups equally, which was challenging, and students felt there was not enough work for such large group sizes, which led to problems and resentment. This has been discussed at module review meetings, and will be reviewed for 2015/2016 semesters.

The implementation of PBL needs a lot of initial input from both staff and students, and so it was perhaps unsurprising that there were difficulties faced during the first year of the new module [24]. The first year of PBL implementation was a learning curve for both staff and students, and it is perhaps ill-advised to use it as a comparison. The second year of teaching the new module was much easier, and the students also had fewer criticisms, as the staff were also more comfortable with the new method of teaching. There is also the possibility that the previous year's students gave feedback to the new cohort, easing anxieties and lessening unknowns. Only over time will we be able to monitor accurately for short-term outcomes [25].

Long-term outcomes are unknown at this point, and would require further study of postgraduates [25]. There is a possibility that PBL enhances students' critical thinking and problem-solving skills, as well as their ability to learn independently.

As a result of the student interviews and staff focus group, the following recommendations are suggested to address the issues raised by staff and students.

1. The relevance of the pharmaceutics aspect of the course must be highlighted to the students, in terms of their future careers. MDM is not the only module which the students deem 'irrelevant', and therefore a course-wide initiative is being planned with other staff from a science background.
2. The individual nature of each staff member's experience and expertise can be utilised to create 'equipment champions', whereby each member of staff becomes a designated expert on certain pieces of equipment. This may help to eliminate frustration amongst students.
3. The volume of material included as directed study should be reviewed, and support such as feedback offered.
4. The exam set-up should be revised, and more multi-disciplinary questions included.
5. There should be an improvement in the clarity of objectives and outcomes made available to students.
6. Students should be introduced to all staff early in the module, and given an overview of their areas of expertise.
7. All staff involved in the MDM module are to be issued with coloured lab coats, to aid visibility during labs.
8. Student group sizes should be reduced, as many students are reporting having little to do.

To complete the cyclical process of review and reflection, further interviews and focus groups should be held to determine if any improvements have been made to overall module performance after the implementation of the above recommendations. Assessment results can also be compared from year to year, as a benchmark of learning.

5. Summary

Last year saw the introduction of a new remodelled PBL version of the MDM module. There were some issues raised by students at the time, and as a result of that feedback, improvements were made to the module. This is the second year that the module has been run, and the feedback was more positive. Staff are more comfortable with the module set-up, and there are less confounding issues. There are, however, still some issues which have come to light as a result of this project, and recommendations have been made to continue the process of continual module improvement. Despite a seemingly positive introduction to the MPharm degree, the results of this study are limited inasmuch as it only examines a short-term, cross-sectional outcome of the new MDM module, and it would require further, long-term reviews to determine the full impact of this method of module delivery.

Acknowledgments: Many thanks go to Ruth Edwards, for the loan of materials and reviewing the project plan. My mentor Colin Thompson has also been very supportive during this project.

Author Contributions: Barbara McKenzie researched and carried out this project, and wrote up the manuscript. Alyson Brown contributed to this research, and also to the write up of this manuscript.

References

1. Wood, D. ABC of learning and teaching in medicine: Problem based learning. *BMJ* **2003**, *326*, 328–330. Available online: http://www.bmj.com/content/326/7384/328 (accessed on 26 May 2014). [CrossRef] [PubMed]

2. Biggs, J.; Tang, C. *Teaching for Quality Learning at University*, 3rd ed.; Open University Press: Berkshire, UK, 2007; Chapter 4.

3. Romero, R.M.; Eriksen, S.P.; Haworth, L.S. Quantitative Assessment of Assisted Problem-based Learning in a Pharmaceutics Course. *Am. J. Pharm. Educ.* **2010**, *74*, 66. [CrossRef] [PubMed]

4. Adam, S. Learning Outcomes Current Developments in Europe: Update on the Issues and Applications of Learning Outcomes Associated with the Bologna Process. 2008. Available online: http://www.ond.vlaanderen.be/hogeronderwijs/bologna/BolognaSeminars/documents/Edinburgh/Edinburgh_Feb08_Adams.pdf (accessed on 26 May 2014).

5. Giving Effective Lectures: Transforming Information into Learning. Available online: http://www.westminster.ac.uk/__data/assets/pdf_file/0008/30230/EffectiveLectures_WEx.pdf (accessed on 26 May 2014).

6. O'Neill, G.; McMahon, T. Student-Centred Learning: What Does it Mean for Students and Lecturers? In *Emerging Issues in the Practice of University Learning and Teaching*; O'Neill, G., Moore, S., McMullin, B., Eds.; AISHE: Dublin, Ireland, 2005.

7. Kirk, K. A 'Holistic' Approach to Support for Learning. Learning and Teaching in Action 1(3): Student Support, 1–7. 2002. Available online: http://www.celt.mmu.ac.uk/ltia/issue3/kirk.pdf (accessed on 26 May 2014).

8. Submission to General Pharmaceutical Council: MPharm Reaccreditation January 2013. Available online: S:HSC/pharmacy/accreditation2013 (accessed on 12 September 2017).

9. General Pharmaceutical Council. Accreditation and Recognition of Pharmacy Technician Level 3 Knowledge-Based and Competence-Based Qualifications. Scottish Qualifications Authority, 2011. Available online: www.pharmacyregulation.org (accessed on 4 February 2012).

10. General Pharmaceutical Council. Future Pharmacists: Standards for Initial Education and Training of Pharmacists. 2011. Available online: www.pharmacyregulation.org (accessed on 4 February 2012).

11. Mayes, T.; Freitas, S.D. "Review of E-Learning Theories, Frameworks and Models." JISC E-Learning Models Desk Study 1. General Pharmaceutical Council (2013) Annual Report 2012/2013. 2004. Available online: http://www.pharmacyregulation.org/sites/default/files/Annual%20Report%2013.pdf (accessed on 29 February 2012).

12. Jonassen, D.; Mayes, T.; McAleese, R.A. *Manifesto for a Constructivist Approach to Technology in Higher Education*; Duffy, T., Jonassen, D., Lowyck, J., Eds.; Designing Constructivist Learning Environments; Springer: Heidelberg, Germany, 1999.

13. Entwistle, N.; Thomson, S.; Tait, H. *Guidelines for Promoting Effective Learning in Higher Education*; Centre for Research on Learning and Instruction, University of Edinburgh: Edinburgh, UK, 1992.

14. Saidu, A.; Ukwumonu, A.J.; Soba, B.M.; Akeem, S. Maximising the use of multimedia for effective teaching and learning in Nigerian tertiary institutions. *Int. J. Manag. Sci.* **2014**, *3*, 254–259.

15. Mayes, J.T.; Fowler, C.J. Learning technology and usability: A framework for understanding courseware. *Interact. Comput.* **1999**, *11*, 485–497. [CrossRef]

16. Accreditation Council for Pharmacy Education. Accreditation Standards and Guidelines for the Professional Program in Pharmacy Leading to the Doctor of Pharmacy Degree. Available online: https://www.acpe-accredit.org/pdf/s2007guidelines2.0_changesidentifiedinred.pdf (accessed on 29 June 2015).

17. American Association of Colleges of Pharmacy. Educational Outcomes. Available online: http://www.aacp.org/resources/education/cape/Pages/default.aspx (accessed on 29 June 2015).

18. Choi, S.-H.; Cairncross, S.; Kalganova, T. Use Interactive Multimedia to Improve Your Programming Course. 2011. Available online: http://www.hull.ac.uk/engprogress/Prog1Papers/NapierChoiS.pdf (accessed on 26 May 2014).

19. Ritchie, J.; Lewis, J.; McNaughton Nicholls, C.; Ormston, R. *Qualitative Research Practice: A Guide for Social Science Students and Researchers*, 2nd ed.; Sage: London, UK, 2014.

20. Creswell, J.W. *Research Design: Qualitative, Quantitative, and Mixed Methods Approaches*, 2nd ed.; Sage: Los Angeles, CA, USA, 2009.

21. Francis, J.J.; Johnston, M.; Robertson, C.; Glidewell, L.; Entwistle, V.; Eccles, M.P.; Grimshaw, J.M. What is an adequate sample size? Operationalising data saturation for theory-based interview studies. *Psychol. Health* **2010**, *25*, 1229–1245. [CrossRef] [PubMed]

22. Whelan, A.M.; Mansour, S.; Farmer, P.; Yung, D. Moving from a lecture-based to a problem-based learning curriculum-perceptions of preparedness for practice. *Pharm. Educ.* **2007**, *7*, 239–247. [CrossRef]

23. Cheng, J.W.; Alafris, A.; Kirschenbaum, H.L.; Kalis, M.M.; Brown, M.E. Problem-based learning versus traditional lecturing in pharmacy students' short-term examination performance. *Pharm. Educ.* **2003**, *3*, 117–125. [CrossRef]

24. Robson, C. *Real World Research*, 2nd ed.; Blackwell publishing: Cornwall, UK, 2004; Chapter 9.

25. Cohen, L.; Manion, L.; Morrison, K. *Research Methods in Education*, 6th ed.; Routledge: Oxon, UK, 2007; Chapter 16.

4

Medication Reviews by a Clinical Pharmacist at an Irish University Teaching Hospital

Alan Kearney [1,*], **Ciaran Halleran** [1], **Elaine Walsh** [2], **Derina Byrne** [1], **Jennifer Haugh** [1] **and Laura J. Sahm** [1,3]

[1]   Pharmacy Department, Mercy University Hospital, Cork T12 WE28, Ireland; challeran@muh.ie (C.H.); dbyrne@muh.ie (D.B.); jhaugh@muh.ie (J.H.); l.sahm@ucc.ie (L.J.S.)

[2]   Department of General Practice, School of Medicine, University College Cork, Cork T12 YN60, Ireland; elaine.walsh@ucc.ie

[3]   The Pharmaceutical Care Research Group, School of Pharmacy, University College Cork, Cork T12 YN60, Ireland

*   Correspondence: akearney@muh.ie

Abstract: Purpose: Pharmacist-led medication reviews in hospitals have shown improvement in patient outcomes. The aim of this study is to describe the prevalence and nature of pharmacist interventions (PIs) following a medication review in an Irish teaching hospital. **Methods:** PIs were recorded over a six-month period in 2015. PIs were assessed by a panel of healthcare professionals ($n = 5$) to estimate the potential of adverse drug events (ADEs). Descriptive statistics were used for the variables and the chi square test for independence was used to analyse for any association between the variables. **Results:** Of the 1216 patients (55.8% female; median age 68 years (interquartile range 24 years)) who received a medication review, 313 interventions were identified in 213 patients. 412 medicines were associated with PIs, of which drugs for obstructive airway disease ($n = 82$), analgesics ($n = 56$), and antibacterial products for systemic use ($n = 50$) were the most prevalent. A statistically significant association was found between PI and patient's age ≥ 65 years ($p = 0.000$), as well as female gender ($p = 0.037$). A total of 60.7% of the PIs had a medium or high likelihood of causing an ADE. **Conclusion:** Pharmacist-led medication review in a hospital setting prevented ADEs. Patients ≥ 65 years of age and female patients benefited the most from the interventions.

Keywords: hospital pharmacy; pharmacist intervention; medication review; adverse drug event; Ireland

1. Introduction

Whilst medication is used to prevent, treat, and manage disease and illness, medication management is the most common intervention in order to prevent adverse drug events (ADEs) [1]. The use of medication has inherent risks, and medication errors compound these risks and can lead to increased morbidity and mortality [1]. The traditional role of a pharmacist as a compounder and a dispenser of medicines resulted in the pharmacist being quite detached from other healthcare professionals (HCPs) [2]. The profession has since evolved and the pharmacist is now recognised as an essential member of a multidisciplinary healthcare team [2]. The joint guidelines from the International Pharmaceutical Federation and the World Health Organisation (WHO) on good pharmacy practice have identified that multidisciplinary collaboration among HCPs is paramount to improving patient safety and outcomes [3]. In addition to sourcing, compounding, and dispensing medicines, pharmacists also provide tailored advice to both HCPs and patients on the optimal and safe use of medicines [2]. A pharmacist-led medication review and the communication of subsequent interventions to HCPs is an example of non-traditional pharmacy services provided by pharmacists [2].

Medication review is defined as "a structured, critical examination of a patient's medicines with the objective of reaching an agreement with the patient about treatment, optimising the impact of medicines, minimising the number of medication related problems, and reducing waste" [4]. Medication review is a key element of medicines management to detect and reduce medical errors and to optimise medical treatment [4]. Due to their clinical knowledge and expertise, pharmacists are the ideal choice to undertake medication reviews [4,5]. A recent systematic review by Graabaek et al. identified that a pharmacist-led medication review in a hospital setting showed improvement in patient outcomes [6]. For our study, we adopted the following definition of a pharmacist intervention (PI): "any action taken by a pharmacist that aims to change patient management or therapy" [7,8].

Whilst medication reviews already occur within this hospital, there has been no official audit of what type of errors are occurring or their prevalence. This paper will describe the prevalence and nature of PIs following a pharmacist-led medication review in an Irish teaching hospital.

2. Methods

2.1. Setting

The study was undertaken in the Mercy University Hospital (MUH) which is a 350-bed general acute university teaching hospital in Cork in the south of Ireland. Data from this study cover a six-month time period from 1 May 2015 to 1 November 2015 inclusive. A hospital pharmacist reviewed patient's medications prospectively, once or twice per week. Inclusion criteria were inpatients whose drug kardex was available for review. Patients were excluded if aged ≤17 years and those on specialty wards e.g., oncology, as they receive chemotherapy using a specific prescription form.

2.2. Intervention

The pharmacist-led medication review at the MUH consisted of a patient drug kardex review and, if required, was supported by the patient notes and laboratory data, but did not involve the patient as a source of data. When a PI(s) was identified, it was brought to the attention of the patient's medical or surgical team for review.

2.3. Data Collection

Age, gender, type of care (medical/surgical), and length of hospital stay were collected for all patients. In addition, allergy status, co-morbidities, and the number of regular and "as required" (*pro re nata* (PRN)) medicines were recorded for patients with PI(s) only. A coding system was used to ensure confidentiality and data protection was guaranteed. The time taken for the pharmacist to conduct the medication review was also measured.

2.4. Classification of the PIs

PIs were classified by the hospital pharmacist according to type, based on the classification system employed by Gallagher et al. in a recent Irish study, but with minor modifications; the addition of two extra subheadings; duplication and poor prescribing practice, and the removal of rate of drug administration [8]. Poor prescribing practice reflects ambiguous prescribing which could be interpreted in more than one way, thus potentially affecting patient safety. Examples of these included illegible prescriptions.

The medicines associated with PIs identified were classified using the Anatomical Therapeutic Chemical (ATC) classification system [9].

2.5. Assessment of Potential Clinical Harm

PIs were reviewed and assigned a probability score, reflecting the likelihood of an ADE occurring in the absence of the PI, by five HCPs (three hospital pharmacists, an academic pharmacist and a general practitioner) using Table 1 as an example of how to assess potential clinical harm [8,10].

The median probability score for each intervention was used for analysis. An interrater reliability (IRR) analysis using the Kappa statistic was performed to determine absolute agreement between raters [11].

Table 1. Probability scores with examples for the assessment of potential clinical harm of the PIs provided to raters.

Probability of ADE Occurring	Probability Score	Example
No harm expected	0	Pharmacist suggests changing a person from esomeprazole to omeprazole exclusively for economic reasons
Very low	0.01	Patient regularly takes a bisphosphonate, but medication omitted from hospital kardex
Low	0.1	Patient takes an antibiotic twice daily, when recommended dose would be three times daily
Medium	0.4	Metformin dose not reduced despite patient demonstrating renal impairment
High	0.6	Patient prescribed amiodarone while taking digoxin without any reduction in digoxin dose

ADE: adverse drug event.

2.6. Data Analysis

Descriptive statistics were used to report the variables and the chi square test for independence was used to analyse for any association between the variables using the Statistical Package for the Social Sciences (SPSS) Version 20 (IBM Corp., New York, NY, USA).

The a priori level of statistical significance was set at $p < 0.05$. A test of normality of the continuous variables reported, patient age, length of hospital stay, number of co-morbidities, and number of regular and PRN medicines prescribed was performed. The chi-square test for independence was used to determine if there was a significant association between PI and patient's age ≥ 65 years or patient gender. The Kappa measure of agreement was used to assess the strength of interrater agreement of assignment of probability scores to the PIs.

2.7. Ethical Approval

Ethical approval was granted by the Clinical Research Ethics Committee of the Cork Teaching Hospitals, University College Cork (UCC) and the local MUH management committee.

3. Results

3.1. Patient Characteristics

A total of 1216 patients received a medication review; PIs were identified in 213 patients. The demographics of the patients with and without PIs are displayed in Table 2.

A significant result for the Kolmogorov-Smirnov statistic ($p < 0.05$) for the continuous variables reported, patient age, length of hospital stay, number of co-morbidities, and number of regular and PRN medicines prescribed indicates that the data does not follow a normal distribution. A total of 843 co-morbidities were identified in patients with PIs with a median of 4 per patient and an interquartile range (IQR) range of 2. The most common co-morbidities identified included hypertension ($n = 88$), chronic obstructive pulmonary disease (COPD) ($n = 74$), dyslipidaemia ($n = 56$), cardiovascular disease ($n = 54$), and atrial fibrillation or flutter ($n = 53$). Those with PIs were prescribed a median of 11 regular medicines (IQR 7 medicines) per patient and a median of 2 PRN medicines (IQR 2 medicines) per patient.

Table 2. Demographics of study patients.

Demographic	Description	Patients with PI(s)	Patients with no PI(s)
		n = 213	*n* = 1003
Gender (n)	Male	80 (37.6%)	458 (45.7%)
	Female	133 (62.4%)	545 (54.3%)
Specialty (n)	Medicine	191 (89.7%)	820 (78.2%)
	Surgery	22 (10.3%)	229 (21.8%)
Age (years)	Median	74	65
	IQR	15	25
	≥65 years	*n* = 164 (77.0%)	*n* = 521 (51.9%)
Length of hospital stay (days)	Median	10.4	4.7
	IQR	11.4	6.9

PI(s): pharmacist intervention(s); *n*: number of patients; IQR: interquartile range.

3.2. PI Prevalence

A total of 313 PIs were identified in 213 patients. This represents an average of 0.26 PIs per patient who received a medication review(s), and an average of 1.47 PIs per patient who received a PI(s). The time taken for the pharmacist to conduct medication reviews was calculated as 180 h, which approximates to 0.19 Full Time Equivalent (FTE).

3.3. Types of PIs

Duplication, poor prescribing practice, frequency, dose, and interaction represents >70% of the PIs identified. The types of PIs and their prevalence are displayed in Table 3.

Figure 1 displays a snapshot from a patient drug kardex reflecting poor prescribing practice.

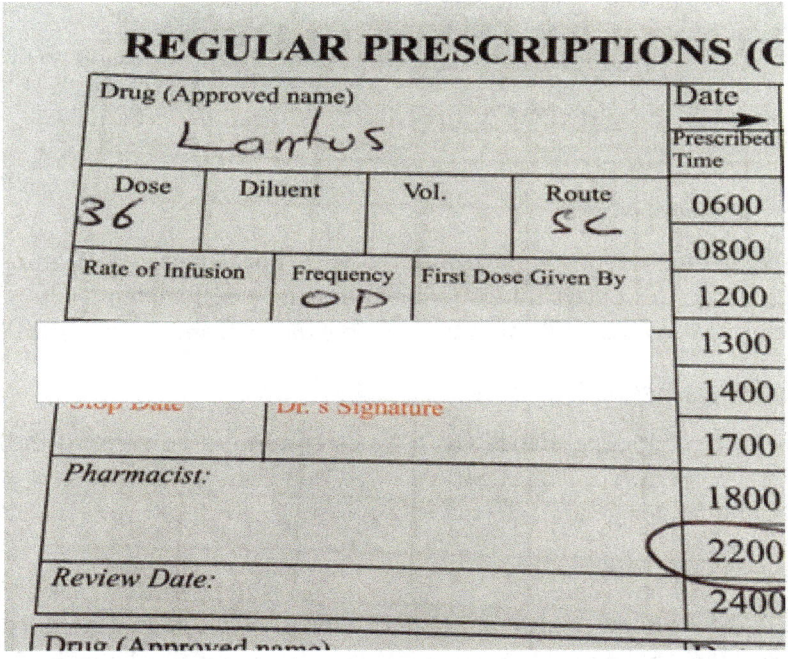

Figure 1. Example of unclear insulin dose.

Table 3. Types and prevalence of PIs ($n = 313$) in 213 patients.

Type of PI	No. of PIs (%)
Duplication	**87 (27.8%)**
Co-prescribe same drug class	45 (14.38%)
Co-prescribe same drug	42 (13.42%)
Poor Prescribing Practice	**41 (13.1%)**
Frequency of administration unclear	24 (7.67%)
Dose charted unclear	13 (4.15%)
Drug charted unclear	4 (1.28%)
Frequency [1]	**38 (12.14%)**
More than approved normal frequency	21 (6.71%)
Less than approved normal frequency	17 (5.43%)
Dose [1]	**33 (10.54%)**
More than approved normal dose	25 (7.99%)
Less than approved normal dose	8 (2.56%)
Interaction [1]	**32 (10.22%)**
Pharmacokinetic	30 (9.58%)
Pharmacodynamic	2 (0.64%)
Timing [1,2]	**27 (8.63%)**
Review Therapy	**23 (7.35%)**
Omission [3]	**12 (3.83%)**
Route	**4 (1.28%)**
Duration	**3 (0.96%)**
Other [4]	**13 (4.15%)**
Total	**313 (100%)**

PI: pharmacist intervention; PIs: pharmacist interventions. [1] As per Summary of Product Characteristics; [2] As per British National Formulary 71 [12]; [3] Relative to admission notes, this intervention was opportunistic; [4] For example, this includes medicines incorrectly transcribed.

3.4. Medicine Types Associated with PIs

A total of 412 medicine types were associated with PIs. The most common medicine types identified included drugs for obstructive airway disease ($n = 82$), analgesics ($n = 56$), antibacterial products for systemic use ($n = 50$), antithrombotic agents ($n = 31$), and drugs used in diabetes ($n = 19$).

3.5. Patient Characteristics Associated with PIs

A chi-square test for independence (with Yates continuity correction) indicated there was a significant association between: PI and patient's age ≥ 65 years, χ^2 (1, $n = 1216$) = 43.809, $p = 0.000$, phi = 0.192; and PI and female gender, χ^2 (1, $n = 1216$) = 4.355, $p = 0.037$, phi = -0.062.

3.6. Potential for Adverse Drug Events

A total of 60.7% of PIs had a medium or high likelihood of causing an ADE. The prevalence and examples of PIs based upon the likelihood of an ADE occurring is displayed in Table 4. The Kappa measure of agreement values ranged from 0.114 to 0.324.

Table 4. Prevalence and examples of PIs identified in this study based upon the likelihood of an ADE occurring.

Likelihood of an ADE Occurring	Number (%) of PIs [1]	Example
Zero (no harm expected)	1 (0.32%)	Omeprazole prescribed as a PRN medicine with no doctor's signature
Very low	11 (3.51%)	Thiamine prescribed 200 mg OD as a regular medicine and two administration times circled
Low	111 (35.46%)	Combivent®[2] and Tiotropium both prescribed as regular medicines
Medium	169 (53.99%)	Solpadol®[3] II QDS prescribed as a regular medicine and Paracetamol 1 g QDS prescribed as a PRN medicine
High	21 (6.71%)	Enoxaparin and Rivaroxaban both prescribed as regular medicines

ADE: adverse drug event; PRN: "as required"; OD: once daily; QDS: four times daily. [1] This is based on taking the median probability score of the five healthcare professionals who rated the PIs; [2] Combivent® is a combination product licensed in Ireland that contains ipratropium and salbutamol; [3] Solpadol® is a combination product licensed in Ireland that contains paracetamol and codeine.

4. Discussion

This study describes the prevalence and nature of PIs following a pharmacist-led medication review in an Irish teaching hospital. A prevalence of 0.26 PIs per patient, who received a medication review, was found, which is within the range of 0.13 to 10.6, of the studies reported in a recent systematic review by Graabaek et al. [6]. The rate reported in this study was at the lower end of the scale which may be explained by time constraints, as the kardexes studied received a pharmacist-led medication review at a maximum of twice weekly. A total of 180 h was spent delivering the clinical pharmacy service during the six-month study period, which equates to approximately one fifth of a full time equivalent (FTE) of a hospital pharmacist. In comparison, in a similar study by Spinewine et al. that had 0.8 of a FTE of a clinical pharmacist, a higher PI rate was identified, indicating the time the pharmacist spends undertaking the intervention as a variable that influences the PI rate [13]. The number of PIs per patient who received a PI(s) was 1.47, which was lower than the 1.98 reported in a similar Irish study by Gallagher et al., who also reported that medicine omissions, relative to admission notes, represented 43% of the PIs compared to 4% of the PIs in this study [8]. Medication reconciliation, identifying medicine omissions relative to admission notes, was only opportunistically performed for patients in this study. This highlights that the definition used to categorise the intervention will influence the PI rate reported, indicating that a broader definition will lead to a higher PI rate [6].

Advancing age leads to an increase in the prevalence of chronic diseases and consequently drug consumption [14]. Increasing drug consumption together with patient metabolic changes with age predisposes older people to medication-related problems e.g., reduced elimination due to renal impairment, and ADEs [14,15]. Studies using the Screening Tools of Older People's Prescriptions (STOPP) criteria have identified high levels of inappropriate prescribing in patients' ≥65 years in the secondary care setting in Ireland [16,17]. Over three quarters (77%) of patients with PIs were ≥65 years of age in comparison to 52% of patients with no PIs. A statistically significant association was established between PI and patient's age ≥65 years, which is in agreement with a recent systematic review by Graabaek et al., showing increasing age as an important variable [6].

Almost two thirds (62%) of patients with PIs were female, in comparison to 54% of patients with no PIs, leading to a statistically significant positive association. This is also supported by Krahenbuhl-Melcher et al., who identified female sex as a risk factor for ADEs or adverse drug reactions (ADRs) in hospitalised patients [18]. The reasons for the increased risk include gender differences in immunological and hormonal physiology that influence the pharmacodynamic and the pharmacokinetic response [19].

Duplication, poor prescribing practice, frequency, dose, and drug-drug interactions were the most common PI types identified. Medication for obstructive airway disease, analgesics, antibacterial products for systemic use, antithrombotic agents, and drugs used in diabetes were the most common medicine types associated with PIs. Despite the PI classification system for this study based on that employed by Gallagher et al., the prevalence of PI types and the medicine types associated with PIs differed between both studies [8]. These differences may be explained by the study population, design, and setting. In the study by Gallagher et al., medication reconciliation, identifying medicine omissions relative to admission notes, represented 43% of the PIs, and the study was undertaken across all wards of the hospital including the maternity unit [8].

Duplication, in this case the co-prescribing of a long-acting and a short-acting antimuscarinic bronchodilator as regular medicines, was the most common PI associated with drugs for obstructive airway disease in this study. The risk of a patient experiencing anticholinergic adverse effects is increased with combination therapy [20]. While the use of combination therapy may provide spirometry improvements in lung function, the clinical significance of these improvements has not been demonstrated [20]. Neither the British National Formulary 71st edition (BNF 71) nor the National Institute for Health and Care Excellence (NICE) clinical guideline for the management of COPD recommend concomitant use of long-acting and short-acting antimuscarinic bronchodilators [12,21].

Dose, in this case the prescribing of intravenous (IV) paracetamol at a dose of >60 mg/kg/day for patients <50 kg, and duplication, whereby paracetamol is prescribed as regular and PRN medicine with the cumulative dose exceeding the maximum daily approved normal dose, were the most common PIs associated with analgesics in this study. Paracetamol over dosage may result in hepatic injury, which could lead to hepatic failure requiring a liver transplant [22]. The risk of hepatic injury is increased in patients with hepatic impairment, in patients suffering from chronic alcoholism or chronic malnutrition, and in patients receiving enzyme-inducing drugs [12]. Annual reports available from the National Poisons Information Centre (NPIC), Ireland, identifies paracetamol as the most common drug involved in human poisoning (accidental and non-accidental) [23]. In Ireland, hospital pharmacists have responded to this danger by forming the Irish Medication Safety Network (IMSN) and have published a safety alert on the risks associated with IV paracetamol [24].

Drug-drug interactions, for example the inhibition of the cytochrome P450 metabolic enzymes by clarithromycin, was the most common PI associated with antibacterial products for systemic use in this study. Clarithromycin is a potent inhibitor of the cytochrome P450 3A4 metabolic enzyme [25]. In this study, the statins (3-hydroxy-3-methyl-glutaryl-coenzyme A reductase inhibitors) were the most common class that interacted with clarithromycin, with a subsequent risk of statin-induced myopathy [25]. This myopathy should be avoided where possible as it is an unpleasant and potentially debilitating experience and can lead to reduced patient compliance with possible discontinuation of therapy [26].

Anticoagulants are defined as a high alert medicine class in the acute care setting by the Institute of Safe Medication Practices (ISMP) in the United States of America (USA) [27]. Non-vitamin K oral anticoagulants (NOACs) are non-inferior and potentially superior to the vitamin K antagonist, warfarin, for stroke prevention in atrial fibrillation and for the prevention of venous thromboembolism [28]. NOACs are associated with lower rates of major bleeding, intracranial bleeding, clinically relevant but non-major bleeding, and total bleeding; however, with the exception of dabigatran, antidotes to reverse their effect are not available [29]. The prescribing of NOACs at subtherapeutic or supratherapeutic doses, as well as the timing and conversion between NOACs and parenteral anticoagulants and vice versa, were the most common PIs associated with antithrombotic agents in this study. NOACs require dose adjustment with changes in renal function and have a rapid onset of action therefore do not require overlap with parenteral anticoagulants [12,30]. Inappropriate use of the NOACs can lead to under anticoagulation or over anticoagulation, leading to increased risk of a thrombotic event or a haemorrhagic event, respectively. In Ireland, the IMSN has produced a safety alert on the risks associated with the NOACs [30].

Insulins are defined as a high alert medicine class in the acute care setting by the ISMP in the USA [27]. Insulin is a narrow therapeutic index medication and errors related to insulin are twice as likely to cause patient harm in comparison to errors involving other medications [31]. Poor prescribing practice, as evidenced by ambiguous dosing of insulin, was the most common PI associated with drugs used in diabetes in this study. The failure to specify any unit and the use of "U" as an abbreviation for "unit" were reasons identified. In the case of failure to specify any unit, the dose may be measured in terms of "unit", "mL", "mg", or even "vial" or "pen". The use of "U" as an abbreviation can lead to confusion as it can be mistaken for a trailing zero, leading to a ten-fold overdose. In Ireland, the IMSN has produced a best practice guideline on the safe use of insulin in Irish hospitals [32].

In the study by Gallagher et al., almost one fifth (19.73%) of the PIs were estimated to have a zero likelihood of causing an ADE, in comparison to a mere 0.32% of the PIs in this study [8]. Additionally, in the work by Gallagher et al., 28.7% of the PIs were estimated to have a medium or high likelihood of causing an ADE, in contrast to a much higher percentage of 60.7% in this study [8]. Differences in panel composition and the types of PIs identified may explain the results reported. As per Gallagher et al., the panel was composed of three academic pharmacists, and in this study the panel was composed of three hospital pharmacists, an academic pharmacist, and a general practitioner [8]. The high alert medicine class in the acute care setting published by the ISMP in the USA included two of the five most prevalent medicines types associated with PIs in this study, in comparison to none of the five most prevalent medicine types associated with PIs in the work of Gallagher et al. [8,27]. The results of our study have been presented at the Drugs and Therapeutics Committee and to the Chief Pharmacist of the MUH, with a view to gaining additional pharmacists who would undertake these medication reviews as part of usual care. In addition, a seminar for all prescribers on the key findings and implications for safe prescribing will be delivered biannually in January and July to coincide with the intern doctors' educational programme. Medication reconciliation, identifying medication omissions relative to admission notes, was only opportunistically performed in this study. A formal medication reconciliation programme has proven to be successful for the patients of the geriatric ward and is planned to be rolled out to all wards in the hospital, once adequate resources are in place.

This study is not without its limitations, which include a single site, a small sample size, and the absence of a sample size calculation. The lack of a matched control group, to allow comparison, is a further limitation.

5. Conclusions

This study identified a prevalence of 0.26 PIs per patient who received a pharmacist-led medication review in an acute secondary care setting in Ireland. The results of this study confirmed previous work and supplemented the body of evidence that pharmacist-led medication reviews in a hospital setting reduce ADEs. Future studies may benefit from focusing on patients aged ≥65 years of age and female patients due the results observed in this study.

Acknowledgments: We would like to thank the staff of the MUH pharmacy department, Gavin Keogh of MUH information technology department, Joe Murphy of MUH medical library, and Carmel Walsh of MUH bed management department, who all contributed to the study.

Author Contributions: Alan Kearney, Ciaran Halleran and Laura J. Sahm devised the study design. Alan Kearney performed the intervention and classified both the PIs and the medicines associated with PIs. Alan Kearney, Elaine Walsh, Derina Byrne, Jennifer Haugh and Laura J. Sahm assessed the interventions to measure potential clinical harm. Alan Kearney performed the data analysis with assistance from Laura J. Sahm. Alan Kearney and Laura J. Sahm devised the concept of the manuscript, Alan Kearney was the primary author and drafts were revised by Laura J. Sahm. All authors read and approved the final manuscript.

References

1. National Medicines Information Centre. Medication Safety. 2004. Available online: http://www.stjames.ie/GPsHealthcareProfessionals/Newsletters/NMICBulletins/NMICBulletins2004/Medication%20Safety%20Vol.10%20No.6%202004.pdf (accessed on 29 December 2015).

2. Pearson, G.J. Evolution in the practice of pharmacy—Not a revolution! *CMA J.* **2007**, *176*, 1295–1296. [CrossRef] [PubMed]

3. World Health Organisation. Joint FIP/WHO Guidelines on Good Pharmacy Practice: Standards for Quality of Pharmacy Services. 2011. Available online: http://apps.who.int/medicinedocs/documents/s18676en/s18676en.pdf (accessed on 29 December 2015).

4. NHS Cumbria Medicines Management Team. Clinical Medication Review: A Practice Guide. 2013. Available online: http://www.cumbria.nhs.uk/ProfessionalZone/MedicinesManagement/Guidelines/MedicationReview-PracticeGuide2011.pdf (accessed on 29 December 2015).

5. Kaboli, P.J.; Hoth, A.B.; McClimon, B.J.; Schnipper, J.L. Clinical pharmacists and inpatient medical care: A systematic review. *Arch. Intern. Med.* **2006**, *166*, 955–964. [CrossRef] [PubMed]

6. Graabaek, T.; Kjeldsen, L.J. Medication reviews by clinical pharmacists at hospitals lead to improved patient outcomes: A systematic review. *Basic Clin. Pharmacol. Toxicol.* **2013**, *112*, 359–373. [CrossRef] [PubMed]

7. Alderman, C.P.; Farmer, C. A brief analysis of clinical pharmacy interventions undertaken in an Australian teaching hospital. *J. Qual. Clin. Pract.* **2001**, *21*, 99–103. [CrossRef] [PubMed]

8. Gallagher, J.; Byrne, S.; Woods, N.; Lynch, D.; McCarthy, S. Cost-outcome description of clinical pharmacist interventions in a university teaching hospital. *BMC Health Serv. Res.* **2014**, *14*, 177. [CrossRef] [PubMed]

9. WHO Collaborating Centre for Drug Statistics Methodology. ATC/DDD Index 2016. Available online: http://www.whocc.no/atc_ddd_index/ (accessed on 3 August 2016).

10. Nesbit, T.W.; Shermock, K.M.; Bobek, M.B.; Capozzi, D.L.; Flores, P.A.; Leonard, M.C.; Long, J.K.; Militello, M.A.; White, D.A.; Barone, L.D.; et al. Implementation and pharmacoeconomic analysis of a clinical staff pharmacist practice model. *Am. J. Health Syst. Pharm.* **2001**, *58*, 784–790. [PubMed]

11. Landis, J.R.; Koch, G.G. The measurement of observer agreement for categorical data. *Biometrics* **1977**, *33*, 159–174. [CrossRef] [PubMed]

12. British Medical Association & Royal Pharmaceutical Society. *BNF 71*; BMJ Group & Pharmaceutical Press: London, UK, 2016.

13. Spinewine, A.; Dhillon, S.; Mallet, L.; Tulkens, P.M.; Wilmotte, L.; Swine, C. Implementation of ward-based clinical pharmacy services in Belgium—Description of the impact on a geriatric unit. *Ann. Pharmacother.* **2006**, *40*, 720–728. [CrossRef] [PubMed]

14. Corsonello, A.; Pedone, C.; Incalzi, R.A. Age-related pharmacokinetic and pharmacodynamic changes and related risk of adverse drug reactions. *Curr. Med. Chem.* **2010**, *17*, 571–584. [CrossRef] [PubMed]

15. Beers, M.H. Aging as a Risk Factor for Medication-Related Problems. *Consult. Pharm.* **1999**, *14*, 1337–1341.

16. Hamilton, H.; Gallagher, P.; Ryan, C.; Byrne, S.; O'Mahony, D. Potentially inappropriate medications defined by STOPP criteria and the risk of adverse drug events in older hospitalized patients. *Arch. Intern. Med.* **2011**, *171*, 1013–1019. [CrossRef] [PubMed]

17. O'Sullivan, D.; O'Mahony, D.; O'Connor, M.N.; Gallagher, P.; Cullinan, S.; O'Sullivan, R.; Gallagher, J.; Eustace, J.; Byrne, S. The impact of a structured pharmacist intervention on the appropriateness of prescribing in older hospitalized patients. *Drugs Aging* **2014**, *31*, 471–481. [CrossRef] [PubMed]

18. Krahenbuhl-Melcher, A.; Schlienger, R.; Lampert, M.; Haschke, M.; Drewe, J.; Krähenbühl, S. Drug-related problems in hospitals: A review of the recent literature. *Drug Saf.* **2007**, *30*, 379–407. [CrossRef] [PubMed]

19. Soldin, O.P.; Chung, S.H.; Mattison, D.R. Sex differences in drug disposition. *J. Biomed. Biotechnol.* **2011**, *2011*, 187103. [CrossRef] [PubMed]

20. Cole, J.M.; Sheehan, A.H.; Jordan, J.K. Concomitant use of ipratropium and tiotropium in chronic obstructive pulmonary disease. *Ann. Pharmacother.* **2012**, *46*, 1717–1721. [CrossRef] [PubMed]

21. NICE. Chronic Obstructive Pulmonary Disease in over 16s: Diagnosis and Management (CG101). 2010. Available online: https://www.nice.org.uk/guidance/cg101/ (accessed on 24 July 2016).

22. Yoon, E.; Babar, A.; Choudhary, M.; Kutner, M.; Pyrsopoulos, N. Acetaminophen-Induced Hepatotoxicity: A Comprehensive Update. *J. Clin. Transl. Hepatol.* **2016**, *4*, 131–142. [PubMed]

23. National Poisons Information Centre. NPIC Annual Reports. 2010–2014. Available online: http://www. poisons.ie/ (accessed on 25 July 2016).

24. IMSN. Risks with Intravenous Paracetamol (Safety Alert). 2012. Available online: http://www.imsn.ie/alerts (accessed on 24 July 2016).

25. IPHA. Klacid Forte 500 mg FC Tablets SPC. 2016. Available online: http://www.medicines.ie/ (accessed on 14 November 2016).

26. Bhardwaj, S.; Selvarajah, S.; Schneider, E.B. Muscular effects of statins in the elderly female: A review. *Clin. Interv. Aging* **2013**, *8*, 47–59. [PubMed]

27. Institute for Safe Medication Practices (US). ISMP List of High Alert Medications in Acute Care Settings. 2016. Available online: http://www.ismp.org/Tools/institutionalhighAlert.asp (accessed on 27 July 2016).

28. Vilchez, J.A.; Gallego, P.; Lip, G.Y. Safety of new oral anticoagulant drugs: A perspective. *Ther. Adv. Drug Saf.* **2014**, *5*, 8–20. [CrossRef] [PubMed]

29. Hu, T.Y.; Vaidya, V.R.; Asirvatham, S.J. Reversing anticoagulant effects of novel oral anticoagulants: Role of ciraparantag, andexanet alfa, and idarucizumab. *Vasc. Health Risk Manag.* **2016**, *12*, 35–44. [PubMed]

30. IMSN. Novel Oral Anticoagulants (Safety Alert). 2015. Available online: http://www.imsn.ie/alerts (accessed on 25 July 2016).

31. Lamont, T.; Cousins, D.; Hillson, R.; Bischler, A.; Terblanche, M. Safer administration of insulin: Summary of a safety report from the National Patient Safety Agency. *BMJ* **2010**, *341*, c5269. [CrossRef] [PubMed]

32. Irish Medication Safety Network. Best Practice Guidelines for the Safe Use of Insulin in Irish Hospitals (Guideline). 2010. Available online: http://www.imsn.ie/guidelines (accessed on 27 July 2016).

5

Thinking in Pharmacy Practice: A Study of Community Pharmacists' Clinical Reasoning in Medication Supply Using the Think-Aloud Method

Hayley Croft [1,*], Conor Gilligan [2], Rohan Rasiah [3], Tracy Levett-Jones [4] and Jennifer Schneider [1]

[1] School of Biomedical Sciences and Pharmacy, Faculty of Health and Medicine, The University of Newcastle, Callaghan, NSW 2308, Australia; Jennifer.Schneider@newcastle.edu.au
[2] School of Medicine and Public Health, The University of Newcastle, Callaghan, NSW 2308, Australia; Conor.gilligan@newcastle.edu.au
[3] Western Australian Centre Rural Health, Geraldton, WA 6530, Australia; Rohan.rasiah@uwa.edu.au
[4] Faculty of Health, University of Technology Sydney, Ultimo, NSW 2007, Australia; Tracy.Levett-Jones@uts.edu.au
*   Correspondence: Hayley.croft@newcastle.edu.au

Abstract: Medication review and supply by pharmacists involves both cognitive and technical skills related to the safety and appropriateness of prescribed medicines. The cognitive ability of pharmacists to recall, synthesise and memorise information is a critical aspect of safe and optimal medicines use, yet few studies have investigated the clinical reasoning and decision-making processes pharmacists use when supplying prescribed medicines. The objective of this study was to examine the patterns and processes of pharmacists' clinical reasoning and to identify the information sources used, when making decisions about the safety and appropriateness of prescribed medicines. Ten community pharmacists participated in a simulation in which they were required to review a prescription and make decisions about the safety and appropriateness of supplying the prescribed medicines to the patient, whilst at the same time thinking aloud about the tasks required. Following the simulation each pharmacist was asked a series of questions to prompt retrospective thinking aloud using video-stimulated recall. The simulated consultation and retrospective interview were recorded and transcribed for thematic analysis. All of the pharmacists made a safe and appropriate supply of two prescribed medicines to the simulated patient. Qualitative analysis identified seven core thinking processes used during the supply process: considering prescription in context, retrieving information, identifying medication-related issues, processing information, collaborative planning, decision making and reflection; and align closely with other health professionals. The insights from this study have implications for enhancing awareness of decision making processes in pharmacy practice and informing teaching and assessment approaches in medication supply.

Keywords: pharmacists; reasoning; medication supply; cognitive skills

---

1. Introduction

Dispensing is a core part of the medication management cycle and the role played by pharmacists [1]. The health system provides a safety mechanism by ensuring that pharmacists are responsible for providing an independent review of prescriptions before treatment commences, a critical check that remains separate from the prescribing process. In addition to the technical skills of labelling and supply of a medicine, dispensing also involves complex cognitive processes. The interpretation and evaluation of the prescription, including assessing the safety and appropriateness of the dosage, checking for contraindications and drug interactions, are examples of cognitive processes that occur during the process [1]. The ability to ensure that medicine dispensing is safe, accurate and appropriate requires a combination of thinking and decision-making, recognised as clinical reasoning. These skills have a profound impact on patient safety, yet this remains an unexplored area in the pharmacy domain [2].

The scope of pharmacy practice has extended beyond the supply of medicines in recent times, to include a growing range of patient-centred professional health services, however the traditional dispensing of medicines still remains an important priority for the majority of pharmacists. The expansion in the number and diversity of prescription medicines, including the exponential growth in complicated biological agents and generic drug brands, requires community pharmacists to determine the appropriateness of a wider range of medicines than ever before. There is a growing trend in pharmacies installing robotic dispensing systems to improve efficiency in medicine dispensing and while this approach removes some of the technical processes, supply of medicine still requires cognitive input by pharmacists to ensure the appropriateness of medicines for each patient and to deliver enhanced patient-centred consultations [3]. High level cognitive skills are required to decide whether the medication should be handed to the patient cannot currently be undertaken by automated dispensing systems [4]. Furthermore, integral to new and expanding roles for pharmacists, which include new responsibilities such as extending or modifying prescriptions is the responsibility for making clinical decisions, both independently and collaboratively [5].

Clinical reasoning is a complex process that depends on the ability of humans to process, memorise, recall and synthesise huge amounts of data. These are all vulnerable areas that ultimately impact on healthcare professionals' competency and clinical performance [6]. For pharmacists, the process of reviewing a prescription or a medication chart and responding to patient symptoms are processes that are considered to be logical and systematic. However, clinical reasoning is complex and includes many overlapping and parallel processes [7,8]. The ability for a health professional to provide safe, high-quality care can be dependent on their ability to reason, think and judge. The World Health Organisation (WHO) stipulate that decision-making is a critical component of workplace safety in relation to minimising errors [9]. A majority of research in decision-making relates to doctor's diagnosis or treatment decisions [10], however there is increased published literature for factors affecting the pharmacists performance, including decision making and the incidence of dispensing errors [2,11–13]. The need for scientific evaluation of decision-making processes has become increasingly apparent in order to address the unexplained variability in performance, high rates of medication error and increased health expenditure. As a result, increased attention is being directed towards the development of valid and reliable methods to assess healthcare professionals' decision making and clinical reasoning skills [14].

Clinical reasoning is a core competency for all healthcare professions but it is not always clear how the reasoning processes used in each profession differ from each another. Current knowledge of pharmacists' clinical decision-making largely draws on studies undertaken in other health disciplines [8,15]. Several theories exist in the literature that relate to the reasoning processes that clinicians use throughout a consultation [15]. The information-processing/hypothetico-deductive approach to cognitive reasoning has a long history in medical education and practice [16]. This approach involves several stages including cue recognition (collate clinical patient information), hypothesis generation (tentative explanation based on initial information), cue interpretation (focus on information from a number of sources) and hypothesis evaluation (collate and evaluate evidence that supports or rejects the original hypothesis). By comparison, the intuitive-humanist model focuses on intuition and takes into account the impact of clinical experience on decision-making processes [15]. The evolution of these theories suggests that clinicians may use a combination of intuition and analysis in their consultations [15]. More recently, clinical reasoning models have been used to describe the complex process by which nurses collect cues, process information, understand the patients' problem, implement interventions, evaluate outcomes and reflect on the process [17].

The clinical consultation is the practical embodiment of the clinical reasoning process [15]. Various models of consulting have been identified in the literature, however they rarely focus on medication-related issues and are not ideal for evaluating medication-specific consultations. One exception to this is the Medication Related Consultation Framework (MRCF), a validated tool developed specifically for teaching and evaluating patient-centred, medication-related consultation skills by pharmacists [18]. However, whilst it provides a framework for the consultation process, the MRCF does not take into account the specific decision-making processes pharmacists use when reviewing a prescription and deciding if the prescribed medicine may be safely supplied to the patient, such as establishing if the medication order meets legal requirements; verifying the appropriateness of the drug, brand, form, strength, quantity; or decisions that relate to selection and assembly of a dispensed medicine.

Through key stakeholder consultation the pharmacy profession has already developed guidelines that inform the key steps that a pharmacist should follow when supplying a prescription [1]. There are similar guidelines in other jurisdictions [19] as well as internationally accepted standards for dispensing practice [20]. However, this framework does not detail the complex reasoning processes used by pharmacists to inform each of the steps. Compared to other professions, there is a lack of understanding and knowledge of the many processes used by pharmacists as they unravel the myriad of cues and leads associated with determining the appropriateness of a medicine order for a given patient [21].

The think-aloud method has been previously used to for providing insights into pharmacists' decision making patterns and has functioned effectively in this context [5,7]. In 2015, community pharmacists in the United Kingdom (UK) setting were asked to think-aloud their thoughts while establishing the cause of a simulated patient's symptoms. This study effectively highlighted that although most pharmacists arrived at the right diagnosis, the ability to clinically reason were limited. More recently, in a preliminary exploratory study in Canada, community pharmacists were asked to verbally reason through their decision-making process when presented with a paper-based case study dealing with challenging situations. This study too was able to highlight opportunities for educators to consider new ways of preparing pharmacists [5]. The aim of this study was to explore the reasoning processes community pharmacists undertake when presented with a prescription in a simulated patient scenario.

2. Materials and Methods

A qualitative, descriptive study was used to analyse cues associated with the decision-making processes pharmacists used while reviewing and supplying prescribed medicine in a simulated patient-pharmacist encounter. This methodology has previously been used to examine the clinical reasoning process used by other healthcare professionals [22–24].

Each pharmacist was asked to verbalise their thoughts spontaneously while performing tasks in patient management (concurrent think aloud using short term memory (STM)), which incorporates narration on medicines related aspects of patient care during the patient counselling component to facilitate clinical reasoning. This initial simulated patient-pharmacist encounter was video/audio-recorded. Each participant also then completed a post-task interview with the researcher to further investigate the rationale for specific actions or to elaborate on comments made during the simulation. During the follow up interview the video was played back to the pharmacist with an iPad to enable video-stimulated recall, in addition to a series of semi-structured interview questions, as prompts for thinking aloud (Appendix A) (retrospective think aloud using long-term memory (LTM)) [25–27]. The post-task interview was also audio-recorded to facilitate data analysis.

A scenario was developed (Box 1) between two pharmacy academics and a simulation expert, with objectives that closely align with the professional competency standards in Australia for medication supply. The scenario was further developed iteratively following input from two practicing community pharmacists, prior to being used in the think aloud study. The simulation scenario represents a typical patient-pharmacist encounter, with decision-making focused on a request for a prescription-only medication supply to a female type 2 diabetic patient. The simulation was conducted in a simulated community pharmacy at the University of Newcastle, Australia (UON). The scenario involves a range of concepts that have a direct or indirect impact on the safe management of diabetes including monitoring of blood glucose levels, assessment of renal function, responding to patient signs and symptoms, management of medication related issues and information required for patient counselling. The study was limited to one clinical scenario because the aim of the study is to explore the core cognitive processes used to make decisions about prescribed medicines, which should apply to any given scenario.

Box 1. Simulation scenario in prose.

A 60-year-old female patient presents to a community pharmacy to collect insulin glargine (10 units nocte, Qty 5) and amoxicillin + clavulanic acid (875/125mg BD, Qty 10) on a prescription written by her regular GP. These prescriptions have been handed to a pharmacy dispensary technician who has processed the prescriptions using FRED dispense and generated labels for each item in preparation for the pharmacist to complete the dispensing procedure. Pharmacist participants are to assume they are in their community pharmacy and their role is to manage this patient who would like to pick up her prescriptions. As the pharmacist manages the patient, they 'think aloud' about what they are doing by verbalising their thoughts and behaviours.

Ten Australian registered community pharmacists who are currently practicing in a community pharmacy were recruited using a mixture of non-probability sampling methods - convenience and snowball sampling. Each pharmacist individually participated in a simulation and evaluation for saturation of the data was conducted after each observation. [27]. The competencies embedded in the reasoning task are those that are expected of all entry level graduates and therefore no additional training was required for pharmacists in order to engage in the scenario, however, prior to data collection, participants were given instructions and a briefing about the think aloud technique [27].

The deductive approach used for the directed content analysis provided initial coding categories informed by a preliminary analysis of clinical decision-making literature. Two existing clinical reasoning frameworks for health professionals: the *clinical reasoning cycle* for nursing practice and the *biopsychosocial model of clinical reasoning* underpinning physiotherapist's assessment and management of a patient, were identified as existing frameworks that would provide an initial approach to organising the research data. Through observation the data showed that the pharmacist's decision-making processes correlated closely with the categories derived from the existing clinical reasoning cycle in nursing practice. The initial coding categories for clinical reasoning (consider patient situation; collect cues/information; process information; identify medication-related issues; set goals; take action; and evaluate outcomes) were applied to the data to conduct a preliminary analysis [8,17,18,27,28]. The data was then mapped to the specific component of the clinical reasoning cycle, which included a general description of the pharmacists cognitive process and evidence using specific dialogue examples from concurrent and retrospective think aloud data.

The codes were further developed iteratively and adapted to the pharmacy context by drawing on key themes from the biopsychosocial model of clinical reasoning used in physiotherapy and the Pharmacy Guild of Australia Medicine Dispensing Process [1]. The initial analysis of the decision-making process was based on the concurrent think aloud data for all participants. Once this was complete, the retrospective think aloud data was analysed to fill gaps and provide further explication. Ethical approval was granted from the Human Research Ethics Committee, University of Newcastle.

3. Results

Ten pharmacists participated in the think aloud study and Table 1 summarises the characteristics of the participant group. The results are presented in two sections. Firstly, how the pharmacists' thought processes correlated with existing medicine dispensing processes and secondly, key themes in clinical reasoning identified for pharmacists to make a decision.

Table 1. Demographic data for pharmacist participants.

Demographic		Number of Pharmacists
Gender	Male	3
	Female	7
Pharmacy experience	<2 years	1
	2–10 years	6
	11–20 years	1
	>20 years	2

3.1. Pharmacist Performance

All of the pharmacists demonstrated distinct patterns in verbalisation about the required tasks and each of them dispensed the medicines in accordance with the *Medicine Dispensing Process* model [1]. There were two distinct patterns in the order in which actions were performed. Seven pharmacists initially performed a check of the prescription and the dispensed product and then engaged the patient to further clarify patient specific details. Three pharmacists engaged the patient immediately after accepting the prescription to gather information, prior to performing a final check of the dispensed medicine. There were no differences in expected outcome for the patient irrespective of the process used by the pharmacist (see Table 2).

Table 2. Order of processes/actions taken by each pharmacist participant.

Step in Medicine Dispensing Process	Pharmacist Participant									
	1	2	3	4	5	6	7	8	9	10
1. Check prescription details	1	1	1	1	1	1	1	1	1	1
2. Script validity	3	2	3	6	5	7	2	2	2	2
3. Safety and appropriateness	4	4	5	7	4	6	5	4	4	5
4. Review dispensing history	2	3	4	3	3	4	3	3	3	3
5. Patient specific factors	5	6	2	2	2	5	4	5	5	4
6. Select product/check selected product	6	5	6	4	6	2	6	6	6	6
7. Dispensing check [a]	7	7	7	5	7	3	7	7	7	7
8. Supply prescription to patient/carer: re-check	8	8	8	8	8	8	8	8	8	8
9. Counsel patient on safe and appropriate use	9	9	9	9	9	9	9	9	9	9
Expected Outcome For Patient [b]	Yes	Yes	Yes	Yes	Yes	Yes	Yes	Yes	Yes	Yes

[a] Step 8 in the medicine dispensing process "label and assemble dispensed products" was completed by a dispensary assistant prior to pharmacists undertaking their checking procedure; [b] Defined as to whether the pharmaceutical needs of the patient have been met.

3.2. Key Themes in Clinical Reasoning in Describing How Pharmacists Arrived at Their Decision

Here, the results are presented using descriptors that relate to the clinical reasoning framework developed for nursing practice [17] and adapted for the reasoning task as it relates to a community pharmacist performing medication supply. The descriptors include: review of prescribed medicine order, retrieving information, processing information, identifying medication-related issues, collaborative planning, decision making and reflection.

3.2.1. Review of Prescribed Medicine Order

All pharmacists initially reviewed the prescription to understand and interpret the information and then place it in context by establishing a sense of what the patient situation was. Pharmacists at this point were initially concerned with the issues outlined in Table 3 which are common to the review process:

Table 3. Immediate review by pharmacist.

Issue Category	Common thought Processes	Example from Data
Nature of Medication	Does the drug have a narrow therapeutic window? Is this a new medication with limited experience, or one that I have not dispensed before? Will this medication require additional/specific counselling requirements such as device demonstration?	*'Amoxycillin is a common medication with a wide margin of safety'* *'The patient has not used insulin before and there is lots of information I will need to go through including demonstrating the injection'*
Patient	Is this for an adult or a child? Is this patient acutely unwell? Do I know the patient—am I likely to have a good dispensing history? Is the patient in a hurry?	*'The prescription appears to be for an adult—they are a local patient so may have been to this pharmacy before'*
Prescription	Is the prescription legal? Is there any information missing? Does the medication attract financial subsidy or is it expensive for the patient?	*'My first concern is if the prescription is legitimate and legal'* *'I usually glance at the prescription to see if there is anything that stands out as unusual or if there is missing information'* *'I always check if it is a medication that attracts a government subsidy because then there will be extra details that I need to check such as concession details'*

3.2.2. Retrieving Information

This is defined as the process of collecting cues from a source of information to use as a foundation for planning patient-orientated decisions relating to medicine management. Pharmacists collected information from a number of sources, including the patient, dispensing software and drug information resources, as well as drawing on their own discipline-specific knowledge, as outlined in Table 4. This thinking process involves noticing (*e.g., pharmacist 3, 'I noticed in your dispensing history that you are already using an injection'*); and reflecting (*e.g., pharmacist 6, 'it is quite a broad-spectrum antibiotic and I have seen it used for a number of different infectious conditions'*).

Table 4. Sources of information pharmacists retrieved and used in reasoning.

1. Dispensing history	✓	✓	✓	✓	✓	✓	✓	✓	✓	✓
2. Prescription–legalities	✓	✓	✓	✓	✓	✓	✓	✓	✓	✓
3. Patient–medication history	✓	✓	✓	✓	✓	✓	✓	✓	✓	✓
4. Patient–medical history	✓	✓	✓	✓	✓	✓	✓	✓	✓	✓
5. Patient–pathology/diagnostic data	✓	✓		✓	✓	✓	✓	✓		
6. Patient–preferences	✓	✓	✓	✓	✓	✓		✓	✓	✓
7. Patient–other e.g., financial entitlements, compliance	✓	✓	✓	✓			✓			
8. Propositional knowledge derived from theory	✓	✓	✓	✓	✓	✓	✓	✓	✓	✓
9. Non-propositionalknowledgederivedfromprofessional/personalexperience	✓	✓	✓	✓	✓	✓	✓	✓	✓	✓
10. Drug information sources–evidence-based guidelines	✓							✓	✓	
11. Drug information sources–product information	✓	✓								

3.2.3. Process Information

This is defined as the process of interpreting and clarifying information. This was mainly observed when the pharmacists compared more than one piece of information to another and drew comparisons in order to further organise information (*e.g., pharmacist 8 'the patient has an antibiotic prescribed and they are diabetic so I know if they are acutely unwell this can affect their blood glucose levels and the subsequent need for insulin'*). Table 6 outlines the cognitive processes that pharmacists used in interpreting information.

Seven of the pharmacists verbalised that when collecting cues and information provided on the prescription they were looking for information that stood out as unusual or different compared to what they were used to seeing in their practice role (*e.g., pharmacist 10 'so when I am looking at the prescription I am checking to see if all the medicine details are consistent with standard dosing guidelines and what you would normally see in practice'*).

3.2.4. Identification of Medication Related Issues

During the dispensing process pharmacists recognised key issues that were directly relevant to their role in meeting the pharmaceutical care needs of the patient. These issues have been broadly classified into two groups: (1) medication-related issues that relate to the presenting prescription which need to be addressed for the patient to achieve optimal benefits from their medicines with minimal risk of adverse events; and (2) co-existing issues which do not directly affect the decision about the supply of the prescribed medicine. There were four immediate issues and two co-existing issues that were common to all pharmacists in the simulation outlined in Table 5.

Table 5. Immediate issues and co-existing issues identified and action(s) taken by pharmacists.

IMMEDIATE ISSUES IDENTIFIED	ACTION(S) TAKEN BY PHARMACISTS
1. Recent unstable glycaemic control (pathology, patient) and the need for changed/additional pharmacological intervention	Determine the rationale for the prescribed medication (insulin) and check appropriateness before supply
2. Current infection (venous leg ulcer) and the need for pharmacological intervention	Determine the rationale for the prescribed medication (antibiotic) and check appropriateness before supply
3. Drug-related precaution—duplication of hypoglycaemic agents predisposes to increased risk of hypoglycaemia	Clarify with patient changes to existing medicines that include cessation of gliclazide and exenatide with continued metformin use
4. The patient is commencing on new medicines requiring explanation of any changes/recommendations/device demonstration	Provide medicines information for patient including administration, dose, insulin injection technique
Co-existing Issues Identified	**Action(s) Taken by Pharmacists**
1. Patient is complacent towards non-pharmacological management of diabetes	Provide lifestyle advice to aid management, offer some education as to the importance of good self-management of diabetes
2. Patient has not been referred to diabetes educator and has not seen a diabetes specialist for a couple of years	Recommend referral to diabetes educator

3.2.5. Collaborative Planning

All pharmacists engaged in mutual decision making with the patient during the process of considering various choices of actions and explaining the options available. Pharmacists actively sought the patient's opinions and relied on this information to inform their decision making. This process incorporated two main cognitive processes; eliciting the ideas and opinions of the patient and anticipating what to expect. Table 6 provides examples of the cognitive processes that pharmacists used in collaborative planning.

Table 6. The phases of clinical reasoning process [1] with descriptions for the pharmacy context and examples from the think aloud data.

Process	Description	Example of Pharmacists' Thinking
1. Consider prescription in context	**Review** legal and therapeutic aspects of prescribed medicine order **Describe** patient and context	*I can see that an adult female patient is collecting a prescription for a penicillin antibiotic and insulin. I'm just checking the script to see if it is legal and valid—if it's in date and the medication order is signed by the prescriber.*

Table 6. *Cont.*

Process	Description	Example of Pharmacists' Thinking
2. Retrieving information	**Gather** medication history from patient	*Do you have any allergies, particularly to penicillin?*
	Review dispensing history, laboratory/diagnostic information	*"I would establish if these are new medicines for this patient or if they have changed by looking up their dispensing history." "I am asking about BSL levels to ascertain the level of diabetes control and look at medication administration in the context of overall disease management."*
	Recall information from past/previous experience	*"I have seen diabetic patients with infections have fluctuating and higher than usual blood glucose levels."*
	Investigate new information e.g., directed searching in drug information databases	*I am just going to check the therapeutic guidelines to see if this is the right duration of antibiotic treatment for a diabetic leg ulcer.*
3. Processing information	**Recognise** the difference between normal and abnormal by comparing information	*What I'm looking for is if there is anything unusual or different about this prescription that stands out compared to what I am used to seeing.*
	Distinguish between information which is relevant from irrelevant;	*The antibiotic prescribed is penicillin, so I need to be looking for allergies but Matilda has no history of penicillin allergy. For this script we don't need be concerned about her morphine allergy.*
	Relate information to identify patterns of information	*I see that oral hypoglycaemic agents have not achieved optimal [diabetes] control and lifestyle interventions have not helped BSL levels and now there are some complications of high blood sugar starting to appear, including leg ulcer. So Matilda's diabetes control is deteriorating.*
	Match similar information and/or: identifying a **mismatch** between two pieces of information	*Matilda has been using the Byetta and that requires injections, so this information tells me how acceptable administering a new drug [insulin] in the same form would be. So that immediately makes me pull up as to why a doctor would be prescribing an antifungal for an ulcer. I can't think of any kind of therapeutic reason why that would be the case so that would require further investigation.*
	Prioritise information by ranking its importance	*Matilda has a number of chronic health conditions, so it is about prioritising what information you are able to give her in the short time you have available.*
4. Identifying medication-related issues	**Synthesise** information to formulate immediate issues that need to be addressed	*There is a duplication of hypoglycaemic agents that makes hypoglycaemia more likely in this patient.*
	Secondary issues that need to be addressed	*I can see the patient is complacent about their lifestyle aspects of diabetes management.*
5. Collaborative planning	**Elicit** ideas and opinions	*Tell me how you feel about starting insulin and going home tonight to administer for the first time.*
	Anticipate what to expect	*The antibiotic is broad spectrum and may cause diarrhoea or thrush. I could recommend a probiotic to minimise the chance of this occurring and am asking how Matilda would feel about this, because it will be an extra expense and extra medication to take.*
6. Decision making	**Verify** correct information	*I look at the drug information on the script and check that against the dispensed item. I am checking the name of the medication [amoxycillin + clavulanic acid] and its strength [875/125] against both the label on the product and the box itself. Then the directions [1 tablet every 12 h]. Then I check the quantity [10] so this is all correct.*
	Justify thoughts and actions	*Insulin and metformin is an acceptable combination for Type 2 diabetes and the prescription is entirely legitimate.*
	Select appropriate interventions to optimise patient outcomes	*I recommend Matilda go back to her GP and the GP will measure the outcomes of the new medications. A diabetes educator can assist with overall disease state management. She could also come back to the pharmacy, to get her blood glucose measured, have a HMR or diabetes MedsCheck, have their BP monitored.*

Table 6. *Cont.*

Process	Description	Example of Pharmacists' Thinking
7. Reflection	**Contemplate** what was done well and what could have been done differently	*I should have asked more about their reflux—it could have been related to diabetic gastroparesis.* *I would not usually have this long to spend with a patient in the pharmacy.*

[1] Adapted from [17,29–31].

3.2.6. Decision Making

All 10 pharmacists met the patient's pharmaceutical needs and correctly arrived at the final decision that the prescribed medicines were safe and appropriate to supply to the patient. All pharmacists decided to provide pharmacological management, by recommending that the patient be supplied with both prescribed medicines and they provided verbal counselling and written information. The pharmacists also decided the patient would require specific follow up on the medications that were being supplied, including review of diabetic leg ulcer in 5 days' time, more frequent ambulatory blood glucose monitoring and referral to diabetes educator. They also confirmed that gliclazide should be ceased to minimise the additive risks of hypoglycaemia when starting insulin. The main cognitive process used was rationalisation, defined as the process of justifying the thoughts and actions. Table 6 provides examples of the cognitive processes that pharmacists used in decision making.

3.2.7. Reflection

Each of the pharmacists showed metacognitive skills, an awareness of their own thinking, during both concurrent and retrospective think aloud processes. They reflected on their management of the patient, agreed that this was a common scenario that they were likely to face in their usual practice role and contemplated what this situation may have been like if encountered in real practice (e.g., pharmacist 2 *'if it were a real situation and I took the time I needed to ensure the patient was managed appropriately, I'd probably have about 10 more prescriptions from other consumers waiting for me to check, so in reality sometimes there is an inability to provide a complete consultation with patients, especially if you are the only pharmacist on duty'*). The pharmacists also noted that prioritising their time was one of the key influences on how they managed the medication supply (e.g., pharmacist 9 *'it is important to make judgement of your own time pressures and those of the patient about whether they are in a hurry to catch a bus or need to go to work or whether they are happy to keep talking because when they have a number of health conditions and chronic health conditions it is about prioritising what information you are able to give them in the short time you have available'*).

3.3. Other Observations

Pharmacists with more than 20 years' experience were on average faster at arriving at their decision that supply of the medications to the patient was appropriate. The average time for pharmacists with more than 20 years' experience was 6 min and the average time for pharmacists with less than 20 years' experience was 12 min. However, many other factors may have influenced their dispensing efficiency such as recency of practice, current work load, usual practice model etc. There were no differences noted between male and female pharmacists.

4. Discussion

Our findings identified seven different processes that were sequentially performed by pharmacists to ensure the pharmaceutical needs of the patient were met when presented with a written prescription. The results show that all pharmacists essentially apply the steps recommended in the Medicine Dispensing Process model and arrived at the decision that the prescribed medicines were safe and appropriate to supply to the patient. However, the focus of this study was to unravel the processes involved in a pharmacist arriving at this decision. Using a community pharmacy simulation, the pharmacists progressed from one form of thinking to another, moving back and forth among various thinking processes, in arriving at a decision on the safety, accuracy and appropriateness for dispensing a medication.

The seven reasoning processes are drawn from existing frameworks and modified to suit the medication supply context in a community pharmacy. The key themes aligned well with other models of clinical reasoning and demonstrated similarities between the way pharmacists and other health professionals think. The clinical reasoning process developed from a body of research undertaken by [17,29] was used as a basis for categorising the reasoning processes shown by pharmacists in the think aloud study, with a high degree of correlation. Like physiotherapists and nurses, a pharmacists' reasoning begins with the initial collection of cues and information, which forms the basis of the working interpretations as the reasoning process continues. For instance, when pharmacists initially reviewed the prescription, the initial interpretations include hypothesis about what condition the patient is likely requiring medication for; and then this information is considered against subsequent information that is obtained throughout the consultation that supports or refutes the initial impressions.

Further similarities with physiotherapists and nurses were the element of routine that pharmacists demonstrated in their decision-making process and the categories of information they used in problem identification and arriving at their decision. Through professional practice it was obvious that pharmacists used common sources of information that was useful for identifying medication-related issues and developing management strategies. Although this study looked only at one specific simulated encounter, it is envisaged that beyond this example, pharmacists' reasoning processed would include specific enquiries related to the patient's individual situation.

The pharmacists were engaged in dealing simultaneously with multiple tasks and problems when presented with the prescription. For example, they verbalised that they had to think about the validity and legality of the prescription, the therapeutic aspects of the medication order and integrating this with existing knowledge and patient information. What was observed is that pharmacists tended to engage in thinking processes that were involved in a specific task so that the focus of their attention was on one component of the dispensing process, before moving onto the next. The pharmacists varied in terms of where they decided to focus their attention. Some spent more time reviewing the medication order and focused their attention on clarifying the intentions of the prescriber to determine which formulation of insulin they would dispense. Others focused their attention on consulting with the patient in a process of collaborative planning about how the patient would manage the administration of their new medication.

When the pharmacists were required to consider multiple pieces of information at one time, they showed distinct patterns of cognitive processing in merging the information together and to identifying specific medication related issues. One of the main issues for the simulated patient was their increased risk of hypoglycaemia when supplying insulin in combination with existing medications. To recognise this potential clinical problem, the pharmacists demonstrated predictive reasoning (anticipating an outcome based on existing therapeutic knowledge and/or experience); and forward reasoning (obtaining new information from the prescription, the patient and the dispensing history to substantiate a hunch) to determine the potential issue.

The pharmacists used a variety of information sources as they progressed through the reasoning process. A thorough review of information provided on the prescription and in the patient's dispensing history were key in identifying discrepancies or alterations in drug, strength, dose, dosing frequency, quantity, drug formulation and drug interactions. All of the pharmacists agreed that they would be unable to determine the appropriateness of a medication order without obtaining information about the medical diagnosis but interestingly, this information is not a mandatory requirement for medication orders and is therefore not usually available to a pharmacist without consulting the patient. There is a risk with making assumptions about the indication for use of a prescribed medicine, as many drugs have multiple potential indications and specific doses and duration of use associated with each. Furthermore, an increasing number of medicines are being used beyond the scope for which they are usually recognised for use. This provides a challenge for pharmacists who are then required to elicit such information through careful medication history taking. Similarly, pathology information, such as fasting BGL and HbA1c data relevant to the simulation in this study, are examples of information not routinely available to pharmacists reviewing a medication order, yet these were identified as important for deciding whether a particular medication dose would be appropriate.

All of the pharmacists decided that the patient in the simulation would benefit from referral to other healthcare professionals (HCPs), for example a diabetes educator. While pharmacists are able to make recommendations to the patient that they pursue follow up with other HCPs, within the Australian context there are no pathways for pharmacists to formally refer to another member of the multidisciplinary team.

Additional dimensions of clinical reasoning were identified from the think aloud data which could be considered to be limitations to the study. The pharmacists reported that their decision making could have been impacted by their interaction within the unfamiliar community pharmacy environment where the simulation to place (contextual interaction). Medicine dispensing in community pharmacies relies on a number of sequential steps with familiar task orientations for the pharmacist including position of stationery, position of medications on the shelf and usual drug information resources.

Further, the spontaneous verbalisation of thoughts (concurrent think aloud) while performing the dispensing task could have disrupted the pharmacists' train of thought and therefore may have altered their decision-making process. Two pharmacists suggested that the think aloud process was disruptive but that it was unlikely to have altered the way they managed the patient. However, other pharmacists found the think aloud process to be quite natural and even beneficial, with one citing they often 'talk aloud' as an instinctive process during some medicine dispensing tasks in practice. The main influence on the reasoning process described by pharmacists was timing, in that pharmacists described usually having less time to deal with the type of task presented in the simulation. Further limitations to the study include the focus on only one simulation encounter. Thus, future work in this area could investigate decision making processes using a wider range of topics and medications.

Although the simulation scenario, simulated patient and demonstration pharmacy provide an authentic representation of a typical patient-pharmacist encounter, there were some aspects of the community pharmacy environment that were not captured during the simulation. For example, in the same consultation in a real-life pharmacy situation pharmacists are commonly engaged in multitasking activities for more than one patient and may also be exposed to a variety of disturbances such as noise and interruptions from other staff and consumers. In the simulation, the pharmacist's time was allocated purely to the specific intervention and there was less need to consider some aspects of the consultation such as privacy.

One of the key influences on the overall reasoning process described by pharmacists was generally the limited time to complete dispensing tasks. In the simulation, pharmacists were not subject to all the usual time pressures of a typical community pharmacy, for example, multiple prescriptions to handle, or interruptions such as assisting another consumer with a higher priority. However, because pharmacists recognised they would usually have limited time to deal with the type of task presented in the simulation, they followed the same principles of time management during the simulation, in the priorities they placed on their actions and decisions relating to how they chose to manage the overall consultation.

Because this is a preliminary exploratory study the findings cannot be extrapolated too broadly, however this is an important step in better understanding decision-making for a profession that continues to investigate what factors lead to medication errors in community pharmacy. The actions demonstrated by pharmacists in this study provide information about how pharmacists approach decision–making in medicine dispensing and provides opportunities for educators to use this to enhance teaching and evaluating competency.

5. Conclusions

Pharmacists are required to make decisions about the safety and appropriateness of prescription medications for large numbers of patients with diverse health needs. The reasoning skills used by pharmacists impact on patient safety and can have adverse effects on patient outcomes. All of the pharmacists in this study correctly supplied the prescription medication in the community pharmacy simulation, however, the think aloud technique uncovered a complexity of reasoning processes that led to this outcome. It is not surprising that the reasoning processes used by pharmacists align with those of other health science professions and can be defined within seven core dimensions of reasoning as relating to the review and supply of prescribed medicines. Understanding and promoting an awareness of the systematic and complex process that guide decision-making by pharmacists, could contribute to enhancement of these clinical reasoning processes. Furthermore, these findings could inform the development of a robust model to guide educational interventions to improve the training of pharmacists and the care they provide to patients.

Author Contributions: Hayley Croft, Rohan Rasiah, Conor Gilligan and Tracy Levett-Jones conceived and designed the experiment; Hayley Croft and Conor Gilligan performed the experiment; Hayley Croft analyzed the data; Hayley Croft, Rohan Rasiah, Conor Gilligan, Tracy Levett-Jones and Jennifer Schneider wrote the paper.

References

1. The Pharmacy Guild of Australia. *Dispensing Your Prescription Medicine: More than Sticking a Label on a Bottle*; The Pharmacy Guild of Australia: Canberra, Australia, 2016.
2. Croft, H.; Nesbitt, K.; Rasiah, R.; Levett-Jones, T.; Gilligan, C. Safe dispensing in community pharmacies: How to apply the SHELL model for catching errors. *Clin. Pharm.* **2017**, *9*, 214–224.
3. Philpott, L. Robots give rise to the future of pharmacy dispensing. *Aust. J. Pharm.* **2016**. Available online: www.ajp.com.au (accessed on 9 June 2016).
4. Lehnbom, E.; Oliver, K.; Baysain, M.; Westbrook, J. *Evidence Briefings on Interventions to Improve Medication Safety: Automated Dispensing Systems*; Centre for Health Systems and Safety Research: Sydney, Australia; Australian Commission on Safety and Quality in Health Care: Sydney, Australia, 2013. Available online: www.safetyandquality.gov.au (accessed on 16 September 2017).
5. Gregory, P.; Austin, Z. How do community pharmacists make decisions? Results of an exploratory qualitative study in Ontario. *Can. Pharm. J.* **2016**, *149*, 90–98. [CrossRef] [PubMed]
6. Agrawal, A. Medication errors: Prevention using information technology systems. *Br. J. Clin. Pharmacol.* **2009**, *67*, 681–686. [CrossRef] [PubMed]
7. Akhtar, S.; Rutter, P. Pharmacists thought processes in making a differential diagnosis using a gasto-intestinal case vignette. *Res. Soc. Adm. Pharm.* **2015**, *11*, 472–479. [CrossRef] [PubMed]
8. Bartels, C. Analysis of Experienced Pharmacist Clinical Decision-Making for Drug Therapy Management in the Ambulatory Care Setting. Ph.D. Thesis, University of Minnesota, Minneapolis and Saint Paul, MN, USA, 2013.
9. World Health Organisation. Human Factors in Patient Safety. In *Review of Topics and Tools*; World Health Organisation: Arlington, TX, USA, 2009.
10. Kostopoulou, O. Diagnostic errors: Psychological theories and research Implications. In *Health Care Errors and Patient Safety*; Hurwitz, B., Sheikh, A., Eds.; Wiley-Blackwell: Chichester, UK, 2009.
11. Harvey, J.; Avery, A.; Ashcroft, D.; Boyd, M.; Phipps, D.; Barber, N. Exploring safety systems for dispensing in community pharmacies: Focusing on how staff relate to organizational components. *Res. Soc. Adm. Pharm.* **2015**, *11*, 216–227. [CrossRef] [PubMed]
12. Lynskey, D.; Haigh, S.; Patel, N.; Macadam, A. Medication errors in community pharmacy. *Int. J. Pharm. Pract.* **2007**, *15*, 105–112. [CrossRef]
13. Thomas, C.; Phipps, D.; Ashcroft, D. When procedures meet practice in community pharmacies: Qualitative insights from pharmacists and pharmacy support staff. *BMJ Open.* **2016**, *6*, 1–8. [CrossRef] [PubMed]
14. Turnis, S.; Stryer, D.; Clancy, C. Practical Clinical Trials. Increasing the Value of Clinical Research for Decision Making in Clinical Health and Health Policy. *J. Am. Med. Assoc.* **2003**, *290*, 1624–1625.
15. Linn, A.; Khaw, C.; Kildea, H.; Tonkin, A. Clinical Reasoning. A guide to improving teaching and practice. *Aust. Fam. Phys.* **2012**, *41*, 18.

16. Graber, M. Metacognitive training to reduce diagnostic errors: Ready for prime time. *Acad. Med.* **2003**, *78*, 781. [CrossRef] [PubMed]

17. Levett-Jones, T.; Hoffman, K.; Dempsey, J.; Jeong, S.; Noble, D.; Norton, C.; Hickey, N. The 'five rights' of clinical reasoning: An educational model to enhance nursiong students ability to identify and manage clinically 'at risk' patients. *Nurse Educ. Today* **2009**, *30*, 515–520. [CrossRef] [PubMed]

18. Abdel-Tawab, R.; Higman, J.D.; Fichtinger, A.; Clatworthy, J.; Horne, R.; Davies, G. Development and validation of the Medication-Related Consultation Framework (MRCF). *Patient Educ. Couns.* **2011**, *83*, 451–457. [CrossRef] [PubMed]

19. American Pharmacists Association. *Principles of Practice for Pharmaceutical Care*; American Pharmacists Association: Washington, DC, USA, 2017.

20. World Health Organisation. Ensuring good dispensing practice. In *Management Sciences for Health. MDS-3: Managing Access to Medicines and Health Technologies*; Spivey, P., Ed.; World Health Organisation: Arlington, TX, USA, 2012.

21. Pharmacy Board of Australia. Guidelines for dispensing medicines. Retrieved from Australian Health Practitioner Regulation Agency. 2015. Available online: http://www.pharmacyboard.gov.au/documents/default.aspx?record=WD15%2f18499&dbid=AP&chksum=H3lV5PqPKFCPuVIkiJyUkA%3d%3d (accessed on 18 December 2017).

22. Burbach, B.; Barnason, S.; Thompson, S.A. Using "think aloud" to capture clinical reasoning during patient simulation. *Int. J. Nurs. Educ. Scholarsh.* **2015**, *12*. [CrossRef] [PubMed]

23. Forsberg, E.; Ziegert, K.; Hult, H.; Fors, U. Clinical reasoning in nursing, a think-aloud study using virtual patients—A base for an innovative assessment. *Nurse Educ. Today* **2014**, *34*, 538–542. [CrossRef] [PubMed]

24. Han, K.-J.; Kim, H.S.; Kim, M.-J.; Hong, K.-J.; Park, S.; Yun, S.-N.; Kim, K. Thinking in Clinical Nursing Practice: A Study of Critical Care Nurses' Thinking Applying the Think-Aloud, Protocol Analysis Method. *Asian Nurs. Res.* **2007**, *1*, 69–82. [CrossRef]

25. Charters, E. The Use of Think-aloud Methods in Qualitative Research: An Introduction to Think-aloud Methods. *Brock Educ.* **2003**, *12*, 68–82. [CrossRef]

26. Fonteyn, M.; Kuipers, B.; Grobe, S. A Description of Think Aloud Method and Protocol Analysis. *Qual. Health Res.* **1993**, *3*, 430–441. [CrossRef]

27. Lundgren-Laine, H.; Salantera, S. Think-Aloud Technique and Protocol Analysis in Clinical Decision-Making Research. *Qual. Health Res.* **2010**, *20*, 565–575. [CrossRef] [PubMed]

28. Edwards, I.; Jones, M. Clinical reasoning and expertise. In *Expertise in Physical Therapy Practice*; Jensen, G., Gwyer, J., Hack, L., Shepard, K., Eds.; Elsevier: Boston, MA, USA, 2007; pp. 192–213.

29. Hoffman, K. A Comparison of Decision-Making by "Expert" and "Novice" Nurses in the Clinical Setting, Monitoring Patient Haemodynamic Status Post Abdominal Aortic Aneurysm Surgery. Ph.D. Thesis, University of Technology, Sydney, Australia, 2007.

30. Alfaro-LeFevre, R. *Critical Thinking and Clinical Judgement: A Practical Approach to Outcome-Focused Thinking*, 4th ed.; Elsevier: St. Louis, MO, USA, 2009.

31. Andersen, B. Mapping the terrain of the discipline. In *Towards a Discipline of Nursing*; Gray, G., Pratt, R., Eds.; Churchill Livingstone: Melbourne, Australia, 1991; pp. 95–124.

6

Pharmacist Intervention Program at Different Rent Levels of Geriatric Healthcare

Conxita Mestres [1,*], Anna Agustí [2], Marta Hernandez [3], Laura Puerta [4] and Blanca Llagostera [3]

1   School of Health Sciences Blanquerna, University Ramon Llull, Padilla 326, 08025 Barcelona, Spain
2   Pharmacy Service, HSS Mutuam Girona, Avinguda de França 64, 17007 Girona, Spain;
    anna.agusti@mutuam.com
3   Pharmacy Service, EAR Grup Mutuam, Ausias March 39, 08010 Barcelona, Spain;
    marta.hernandez@mutuam.com (M.H.); bllagostera@mutuam.com (B.L.)
4   Pharmacy Service, HSS Mutuam Güell, Mare de Deu de la Salut 49, 08024 Barcelona, Spain;
    lpuerta@mutuam.com
*   Corresponding: concepciomm@blanquerna.url.edu

Academic Editor: Jeffrey Atkinson

Abstract: As a pharmacy service giving pharmaceutical care at different levels of health care for elderly people, we needed a standardization procedure for recording and evaluating pharmacists' interventions. Our objective was to homogenize pharmacist interventions; to know physicians' acceptance of our recommendations, as well as the most prevalent drug related problems (DRP); and the impact of the pharmacists' interventions. To achieve this goal we conducted a one year prospective study at two levels of health care: 176 nursing homes (EAR) (8828 patients) and 2 long-term and subacute care hospitals (HSS) (268 beds). Pharmacists' interventions were recorded using the American Society of Health-System Pharmacists classification as the basis. Frequency of the different DRP and the level of response and acceptance on the part of physicians was determined. The Medication Appropriateness Index (MAI) was used to evaluate the impact of the interventions on the prescription quality. Patients' mean age was 84.2 (EAR) and 80.7 (HSS), and in both cases, polypharmacy $\geq$ 9 drugs was around 63–69%. There were 4073 interventions done in EAR and 2560 in HSS. Level of response: 44% (EAR), 79% (HSS); degree of acceptance of the recommendations: 84% (EAR), 72% (HSS). Most frequent DRP: inappropriate dose, length of therapy, omissions, and financial impact. Drugs for the nervous system are those with the most DRP. MAI values/medication improved from 4.4 to 2.7 (EAR) and 3.8 to 1.7 (HSS). A normalized way of managing pharmacists' interventions for different health care levels has been established. We are on the way to increasing collaborative work with physicians and we know which DRPs are most prevalent.

Keywords: geriatrics; pharmacists' interventions; inappropriate medication; drug related problems

1. Introduction

Pharmacists have been progressively included in healthcare teams delivering integrated care. The development of pharmaceutical care [1] has permitted pharmacists to provide direct medication-related care with the aim of improving patients' quality of life. However, even though there have been great advances, they have been accomplished mostly in acute care institutions such as hospitals. These institutions have a larger staff of pharmacists that have been integrated into healthcare teams for a longer time. In other kinds of institutions, like ours, devoted to geriatric patients (long-term care, subacute care, nursing homes), there has been some improvement only recently [2].

Prescriptions for inappropriate drugs for older people are a problem with a high impact on their outcomes, due to their frailty, comorbidities, and polypharmacy. Therefore, drug-related problems (DRP) are more frequent and have a more serious impact.

Adverse drug prevalence among people between 70 and 79 years of age has been found to be 20–30% in contrast to 3–6% for ages 20–29 years old [3]. Moreover, DRP complications result in a higher rate of hospital admissions (6.6–41.3% of older patients) [4]. As a consequence, prescribing potentially unsafe medications may increase pharmacy costs, especially in countries with a higher proportion of older adults in their population [5].

The role of pharmacists in this area has been increasing and—as pointed out by different institutions such as the World Health Organization (WHO) and the American College of Clinical Pharmacy (ACCP)—pharmacists have to be a key member of the healthcare team, due to their privileged position in the review of drug treatments and their knowledge, background, and proximity to healthcare professionals and patients [6,7].

In fact, there have been some examples of the impact of pharmacists on the improvement of patients' outcomes through their interventions. However, there is not yet a consensus of how to measure these outcomes, and sometimes, results are not conclusive [2,8–10]. Our group is specialized in giving healthcare to older people at different levels: nursing homes, long-term care, home care, and subacute areas where the participation of pharmacists in integrative care is usually underdeveloped. Reviewing a document about the implementation of pharmaceutical care issued by the American Society of Hospital Pharmacy at the beginning of the 1990s [11], we found that most of the difficulties in the process are still present in our institutions. Our pharmacy service has been working to incorporate the pharmacist as a member of the care team in order to improve outcomes in our patients, but to achieve it and derive practical improvements in the outcomes of our patients, we have had to address different problems.

In a first approach, we implemented a guideline to make pharmacologic treatment revisions, and a method for recording our interventions and recommendations to nurses and physicians [12]. After achieving this, we faced other difficulties, such as the homogeneity of the information recorded, which depended on the level of healthcare where our pharmacists were working. Moreover, we wanted to evaluate the impact of our work on the improvement of inappropriate drug prescriptions.

In the present work, we report the process of homogenization of pharmacist interventions done by our pharmacy department, as well as an evaluation of this intervention depending on the type of level of care (HSS or EAR) and the impact on improvements in drug treatment.

2. Methods

2.1. Setting and Study Population

The project was undertaken at two different levels of health care managed by our institution: two long-term care and subacute care hospitals (HSS): HSS Mutuam Güell (Barcelona, Spain) (165 beds) and HSS Mutuam Girona (103 beds) and 9 teams (EARs) teams composed of a physician and 2 to 3 nurses giving healthcare support to 176 nursing homes (8828 patients) in the city of Barcelona.

The results correspond to all the pharmacist interventions performed between 1 June 2014 and 30 June 2015. All patients in these institutions were eligible to be enrolled, with the only exception of palliative patients in their last days of life.

2.2. Intervention

In the two HSS, pharmacists conducted the interventions at different moments of the patient process: admission, during the hospital stay and at discharge. In EAR, due to the small staff of pharmacists, interventions were only performed upon admission to the nursing home.

Information was obtained from different sources such as electronic prescriptions and medical records, as well as the Catalonian Health Care System electronic record (HC3).

Drug-related problems were communicated to the physician through email or telephone and recorded in a database using Microsoft Excel® 2010.

2.3. Recording of the Interventions and Outcomes

As one of our main objectives was to standardize the recording of our work, we studied different classification systems [13] of DRP. Previously [12], we used the Pharmaceutical Care Network Europe (PCNE) classification [14], but we found classification difficulties in some of our DRP. We sought a system that included the different problems that we usually find at the different healthcare levels and was easy to use in our daily work (not to increase the workload substantially). We chose the ASHP (American Society Health-System Pharmacists) classification [15] as the most appropriate system for our needs.

2.4. Measurement

Improvement in the appropriateness of drug treatments was evaluated using the MAI (Medication Appropriateness Index) [16]. The significance of the improvement of the MAI value was determined by $p < 0.0001$.

3. Results

3.1. Demographic Data

In the two HSS, pharmaceutical interventions were done for 1040 patients (48% of the patients admitted to the hospitals during the period of study). In EAR, interventions were performed on 2119 patients (72% of patients admitted to the nursing homes, during the period of study), whose demographic data are shown in Table 1.

Table 1. Demographic data of the patients.

Institution	Patients (No.)	Female (%)	Mean Age	Polypharmacy ≥ 9 Drugs	Barthel Index	Pfeiffer Index
EAR	2119	70.2	84.2 ± 7.8	69.0%	49	6
HSS	1040	58.9	80.7 ± 9.9	63.4%	45	3

EAR: Teams attending nursing homes; HSS: long-term care and subacute care hospitals. Barthel index scores: 0–20: totally dependent, 20–35: severe dependence, 40–55: moderate dependence, 60–95: mild dependence, 100: independent. Pfeiffer index score: 0–2: normal, 3–4: mild cognitive deterioration, 5–7: moderate cognitive deterioration, 8–10: significant cognitive deterioration.

In HSSs that treat patients in a more acute situation, there are fewer females and the mean age is lower. In both levels of care, Barthel values denoted a moderate impediment; Pfeiffer index values denoted a higher cognitive deterioration in EAR patients, and thus could be related to the higher mean age. Patients with dementia are mostly found in nursing homes. In both types of institutions there is a high degree of polypharmacy.

3.2. Type of Intervention Derived from DRP, Depending on the Institution

Pharmacists performed 4073 interventions in EARs (2.41 interventions/patient) and 2560 in HSS (2.46 interventions/patient). The level of response was 44% in EAR and 79% in HSS. Of the interventions/recommendations for which we obtained an answer, physicians accepted 84% (EAR) and 72% (HSS). Reasons for non-acceptance were reluctance on the part of the physician to change a treatment initiated by a specialist, or being unsure of the consequences of the change recommended by the pharmacist.

DRP that were the origin of the pharmacists' interventions were classified using the ASHP classification as a basis (Table 2).

In both types of institutions, the most frequent DRP (26.3% and 25.2%) refers to problems related to dosage and the route of administration. In order to study these problems more accurately, we made a subdivision, shown in Table 3. Inappropriate dose is one of the main problems, as it is a frequent prescription error. There are also numerous DRP in relation to the administration frequency in HSS and the excessive length of therapy in EAR.

Table 2. Interventions performed for the different DRP found, based on the ASHP classification.

Drug Related Problem	HSS		EAR	
	n = 2560		**n = 4073**	
1—Medication with no indication	353	13.7%	741	18.2%
2—Condition for which no drug is prescribed	369	14.4%	558	13.7%
3—Medication prescribed inappropriately for a particular condition	206	8.0%	485	11.9%
4—Inappropriate dose, dosage form, schedule, route of administration, or method of administration	662	26.3%	1025	25.2%
5—Therapeutic duplication	224	8.8%	174	4.3%
6—Prescribing of medication to which the patient is allergic	1	0.1%	22	0.5%
7—Actual and potential adverse drug events	59	2.3%	116	2.9%
8—Actual and potential drug-drug, drug-disease, drug-nutrient, and drug-laboratory test interactions that are clinically significant	109	4.3%	149	3.7%
9—Interference with medical therapy by social or recreational drug use	0	0.0%	0	0.0%
10—Failure to receive the full benefit of prescribed therapy	85	3.3%	220	5.4%
11—Problems arising from the financial impact of therapy	370	14.5%	409	10.0%
12—Lack of understanding of the medication	101	4.0%	72	1.8%
13—Failure of the patient to adhere to the regimen	11	0.4%	5	0.1%

EAR: Teams attending nursing homes; HSS: long-term care and subacute care hospitals.

Table 3. Different types of DRP in Category 4.

Drug Related Problem	HSS		EAR	
4.1—Inappropriate dose	208	8.1%	214	5.2%
4.2—Inappropriate dose, renal insufficiency	15	0.6%	97	2.4%
4.3—Inappropriate dose, hepatic insufficiency	0	0.0%	33	0.8%
4.4—Dosage form	38	1.5%	4	0.1%
4.5—Schedule	187	7.3%	55	1.3%
4.6—Length	101	4.0%	675	16.6%
4.7—Route of administration	101	4.0%	44	1.1%
4.8—Method of administration	12	0.5%	0	0.0%

EAR: Teams attending nursing homes; HSS: long-term care and subacute care hospitals.

In HSS, other important problems are those arising from the financial impact (14.5%), referring to situations where a more cost-effective drug could be used, a condition for which there is no medication prescribed (omissions) with 14.4%, and medications without indication (13.7%). In the first case, this is due to the fact that our patients are taking medications at home that are not included in the hospital formulary; therefore, pharmacists have to propose alternatives based on our interchange guideline. In the case of omissions, the problem usually arises from incomplete information in the clinical record of the patients at the admission. Other frequent problems are duplications, problems with the dose, and the prescription of inappropriate drugs for elderly people.

In EARs, we found 18.2% of cases of patients with medications without indication (18.2%) due to an incomplete record at admission. Omissions are also frequent (13.7%), and inappropriate drugs in geriatrics (11.9%) are also important. Problems arising from the financial impact of therapy are high (10%), as nursing homes attended by our EAR team belong to different private purveyors; and we do not have a defined formulary, but our pharmacists recommend changes for more cost-effective alternatives.

ATC most implicated in DRP in both institutions is N (nervous system) (Table 4). In EAR, it is followed by B (blood) and A (alimentary tract). In HSS, there is more dispersion with values > 10% in groups such as A, C (cardiovascular), B, and J (anti-infectives).

Table 4. ATC group of the drugs mots implicated in DRP in EARs and HSS.

ATC Group	EARs	HSS
A	13.7%	16.1%
B	17.7%	10.9%
C	9.3%	15.8%
D	0.8%	0.1%
G	4.7%	2.9%
H	1.3%	2.8%
J	1.5%	10.1%
L	0.7%	1.1%
M	5.0%	4.0%
N	41.5%	25.5%
R	2.9%	6.3%
S	1.0%	1.7%
V	0.1%	2.1%

EAR: Teams attending nursing homes; HSS: long-term care and subacute care hospitals.

3.2.1. Level of Acceptance

If we assess the degree of acceptance of the interventions, taking into account the 10 most frequent causes of the intervention (Tables 5 and 6), they range between 59.5 and 35.9% HSS, and between 57.9 and 28.5% in nursing homes.

Table 5. Acceptance degree of the most frequent DRP in HSSs.

HSS	Acceptance Degree (%)
11—Problems are arising from the financial impact of therapy	59.5
2—Condition for which no drug is prescribed	66.4
1—Medication with no indication	62.9
5—Therapeutic duplication	55.4
4.1—Inappropriate dose	65.9
3—Medication prescribed inappropriately for a particular condition	35.9
4.5—Schedule	44.4
4.6—Length	57.4
4.7—Route of administration	59.4

Table 6. Acceptance degree of the most frequent DRP in EARs.

EAR	Acceptance Degree (%)
1—Medication with no indication	44.3
4.6—Length	43.1
2—Condition for which no drug is prescribed	34.6
3—Medication prescribed inappropriately for a particular condition	57.9
11—Problems are arising from the financial impact of therapy	37.2
10—Failure to receive the full benefit of prescribed therapy	36.8
4.1—Inappropriate dose	28.5
5—Therapeutic duplication	36.8
7—Actual and potential adverse drug events	36.2

The mean MAI values per medication, after implementation by physicians of a pharmacist's recommendations in EARs decreased from 4.4 to 2.7 ($p < 0.0001$); in HSS, the values decreased from 3.8 to 1.7 ($p < 0.0001$) (Table 7).

Table 7. Mean MAI values per medication

Institution	Pre-Intervention	Post-Intervention	Min	Max	p Value
EAR	4.4	2.7	0	17	$p < 0.0001$
HSS	3.8	1.7	0	15	$p < 0.0001$

EAR: Teams attending nursing homes; HSS: long-term care and subacute care hospitals.

4. Discussion

With this project, we have been able to find a suitable classification for documenting and recording the interventions/recommendations made by our pharmacists in different types of institutions giving care to elderly people. Thanks to this, now we can review and study some of the differences found in the DRP detected as well as other problems to make improvements.

We have seen differences in levels of response by physicians between HSS and EAR. In the latter, the response is somewhat low (44%) compared to that of HSS, which was 79%. We have discussed this point with our physicians, and they state that the lack of feedback is due to workload, which makes it difficult for them to contact the pharmacist to discuss all DRPs. Curiously, we have noted that there are occasions where they have made the changes recommended by our pharmacists in the patient treatment, but they fail to communicate it to us. Other reasons for this low level of response, compared with HSS, may be that although we have been working in this area with physicians for some time, they still have not adapted this to their day-to-day the interaction with the pharmacist. Moreover, in HSS, we are working in the same building with similar schedules, making communication easier.

Our strategy has been to increase meetings with physicians and report feedback of the problems detected; this continuing information has made them more receptive and understanding of the importance of taking our recommendations into account and giving us information about what they plan to do; this is an approach that has already been described as effective in the acceptance rates [17,18]. As a consequence, we have observed that since we started the program, the level of response and acceptance is increasing (in the last semester of 2015 we had a 60% of response rate).

As for the type of DRP found, we would like to highlight that we have a high degree of problems related to dosage, schedule, and length of therapy, which we are now reviewing with physicians. Incomplete information in the records at admission (medication without a related diagnosis or indication for a drug that is not prescribed) is also to be considered. We also want to point out that a small percentage of drug omissions were detected, after informing the physician in charge. We have found these justified, because they were medications that the physicians found relatively unnecessary or not appropriate during hospitalization.

The prescription of inappropriate drugs for older people is higher in EAR than HSS. We think that a possible explanation is that in HSS we work with a formulary adjusted to the needs of our geriatric population, and in recent years, we have worked extensively with our physicians [19] on this problem. Therefore, we think that the development of formularies and interchange programs at admission in nursing homes is necessary.

In HSS, the therapeutic interchange is accepted in 59.5%; thus, we think that there is still room for a wider range of improvement. Physicians continue to be especially reluctant to change medications that patients are taking at home or that have been prescribed by specialists. In reference to the ATC group to which the drugs with more DRP belong, we have found that in all cases, the high percentage is for nervous system drugs. This is not surprising, taking into account that this is the group with more drugs prescribed, and includes drugs for dementia, analgesics, and psychoactive drugs. In HSS, we found that there are more ATC groups with high incidence of problems; for example, we have values of 10.1% for anti-infectives, versus only 1.5% in EARs. This can be explained by anti-infectives having a higher degree of prescriptions in HHS due to the fact that the patients are in a more acute situation with their illness, and infectious processes in many cases are the cause of admission. Other ATC groups with a high prevalence of problems are those related to the alimentary tract (A), especially antidiabetics and proton bomb inhibitors; cardiovascular (C), for which we have a high degree of therapeutic interchange in antihipertensives; and problems with anticoagulants (B).

On the whole, we also consider it to be very important that many of the interventions done are derived from safety problems; therefore, the work of the pharmacists increases the safety of the treatment in many ways, such as reducing the use of inappropriate drugs or detecting prescription errors.

Even though evaluating the impact of these interventions is quite complicated, we found that MAI scores per drug improved when recommendations of pharmacists were implemented by physicians. In EAR, the mean MAI value before intervention was of 4.4, and at HSS it was lower: 3.7. These values and improvements obtained (2.7 in EAR and 1.7 in HSS) are similar to those found by other authors, working with a similar population [20].

The use of the MAI score to evaluate improvements in prescriptions has many limitations. For example, it does not take into account the improvements derived from the correction of drug omissions. However, in a revision done by their designers after 20 years of use, they pointed out different studies relating high MAI scores with unscheduled ambulatory or emergency department visits, inadequate blood pressure control, or adverse drug events [21]. Taking all this into account, our main goals in the future are—besides improving physicians' response to our work—to find and implement other methods and means to evaluate the impact of pharmacists' interventions, including an economic evaluation.

5. Conclusions

- The standardization of recording pharmacists' interventions improves the management of drug related problems.
- There is still a long way to go to incorporate the pharmacist in day-to-day work with physicians in nursing homes.
- Prescriptions for non-appropriate medication for older people continue to be a recurrent DRP.
- The implication of pharmacists in medication reviews leads to a quality improvement in the prescriptions.
- It is important to give information and training to all health care professionals concerning the benefits of collaborative work with pharmacists.
- Guidelines, formularies, and interchange programs should be implemented in nursing homes.
- Knowing the most prevalent and serious DRPs allows us to focus on their prevention.

Author Contributions: Conxita Mestres, Anna Agustí, Marta Hernandez and Blanca Llagostera conceived and designed the data base, procedure and performed the interventions, their recording and analysis. Conxita Mestres wrote the paper.

References

1. American Society of Hospital Pharmacy. ASHP Statement on Pharmaceutical Care. *Am. J. Hosp. Pharm.* **1993**, *50*, 1720–1723.
2. Alldred, D.P.; Raynor, D.K.; Hughes, C.; Barber, N.; Chen, T.F.; Spoor, P. Interventions to optimise prescribing for older people in care homes. *Cochrane Database Syst. Rev.* **2013**, *2*, CD009095. Available online: http: //www.ncbi.nlm.nih.gov/pubmed/23450597 (accessed on 22 April 2017).

3.   Onder, G.; Liperoti, R.; Fialova, D.; Topinkova, E.; Tosato, M.; Danese, P.; Gallo, P.F.; Carpenter, L.; Finne-Soveri, H.; Gindin, J.; et al. Polypharmacy in nursing home in Europe: Results from the SHELTER study. *J. Gerontol. A Biol. Sci. Med. Sci.* **2012**, *67*, 698–704. [CrossRef] [PubMed]

4.   Beijer, H.J.; de Blaey, C.J. Hospitalisations caused by adverse drug reactions (ADR): A meta-analysis of observational studies. *Pharm. World Sci.* **2002**, *24*, 46–54. [CrossRef] [PubMed]

5.   Leendertse, A.J.; Van Den Bemt, P.M.L.A.; Bart Poolman, J.; Stoker, L.J.; Egberts, A.C.G.; Postma, M.J. Preventable hospital admissions related to medication (HARM): Cost analysis of the HARM study. *Value Health* **2011**, *14*, 34–40. [CrossRef] [PubMed]

6.   American College of Clinical Pharmacy. ACCP White Paper. A vision of pharmacy's future roles, responsibilities and manpower needs in the United States. *Pharmacotherapy* **2000**, *20*, 991–1022.

7.   Wiedenmayer, K.; Summers, R.S.; Mackie, C.A.; Gous, A.G.S.; Everard, M.; Tromp, D. *Developing Pharmacy Practice: A Focus on Patient Care*; International Pharmaceutical Federation, Ed.; World Health Organisation: Geneva, Switzerland, 2006.

8.   Gallagher, J.; Byrne, S.; Woods, N.; Lynch, D.; McCarthy, S. Cost-outcome description of clinical pharmacists interventions in a university teaching hospital. *BMC Health Serv. Res.* **2014**, *14*, 177. [CrossRef] [PubMed]

9.   Kopp, B.J.; Mrsan, M.; Erstad, B.L.; Duby, J.J. Cost implications of and potential adverse events prevented by interventions of a critical care pharmacist. *Am. J. Health Syst. Pharm.* **2007**, *64*, 2483–2487. [CrossRef] [PubMed]

10.   Brulhart, M.I.; Wermeille, J.P. Multidisciplinary medication review: Evaluation of a pharmaceutical care model for nursing homes. *Int. J. Clin. Pharm.* **2011**, *33*, 549–557. [CrossRef] [PubMed]

11.   American Society of Hospital Pharmacy. Implementing pharmaceutical care. *Am. J. Hosp. Pharm.* **1993**, *50*, 1585–1656.

12.   Mestres, C.; Hernandez, M.; Llagostera, B.; Espier, M.; Chandre, M. Improvement of pharmacological treatments in nursing homes: Medication review by consultant pharmacists. *Eur. J. Hosp. Pharm.* **2015**. [CrossRef]

13.   Van Mil, J.F. Drug-Related Problem Classification Systems. *Ann Pharmacother.* **2004**, *38*, 859–867. [CrossRef] [PubMed]

14.   Pharmaceutical Care Network Foundation. Classification for Drug Related Problems. V.6.2 (Revised 14-01-2010vm). 2010; pp. 1–9. Available online: http://www.pcne.org/upload/files/11_PCNE_classification_V6-2.pdf (accessed on 22 April 2017).

15.   Pharmacists AS of H-S. ASHP guidelines on a standardized method for pharmaceutical care. *Am. J. Health Syst. Pharm.* **1996**, *53*, 1713–1716.

16.   Hanlon, J.T.; Schmader, K.E.; Samsa, G.P.; Weinberger, M.; Uttech, K.M.; Lewis, I.K.; Cohen, H.J.; Feussner, J.R. A method for assessing drug therapy appropriateness. *J. Clin. Epidemiol.* **1992**, *45*, 1045–1051. [CrossRef]

17.   Tallon, M.; Barragry, J.; Allen, A.; Breslin, N.; Deasy, E.; Moloney, E.; Delaney, T.; Wall, C.; Byren, J.O.; Grimes, T. Impact of the Collaborative Pharmaceutical Care at Tallaght Hospital (PACT) model on medication appropriateness of older patients. *Eur. J. Hosp. Pharm. Sci. Pract.* **2015**, 1–6. Available online: http://ejhp.bmj.com/lookup/doi/10.1136/ejhpharm-2014-000511 (accessed on 22 April 2017).

18.   Spinewine, A.; Schmader, K.E.; Barber, N.; Hughes, C.; Lapane, K.L.; Swine, C.; Hanlon, J.T. Appropriate prescribing in elderly people: How well can it be measured and optimised? *Lancet* **2007**, *370*, 173–184. [CrossRef]

19.   Mestres, C.; Agusti, A.; Puerta, L.; Barba, M. Prescription of potentially inappropriate drugs for geriatric patients in long-term care: Improvement through pharmacist's intervention. *Eur. J. Hosp. Pharm. Sci. Pract.* **2015**, *22*, 198–201. [CrossRef]

20.   Stuijt, C.C.; Franssen, E.J.; Egberts, A.C.; Hudson, S.A. Appropriateness of prescribing among elderly patients in a Dutch residential home: Observational study of outcomes after a pharmacist-led medication review. *Drugs Aging* **2008**, *25*, 947–954. [CrossRef] [PubMed]

21.   Hanlon, J.T.; Schmader, K.E. The Medication Appropriateness Index at 20: Where it started, where it has been, and where it may be going. *Drugs Aging* **2013**, *30*, 893–900. [CrossRef] [PubMed]

7

Experiences of Pharmacy Trainees from an Interprofessional Immersion Training

Daubney Boland [1], Traci White [2] and Eve Adams [3,*]

[1] Southern New Mexico Family Medicine Residency Program, Memorial Medical Center, Las Cruces, NM 88011, USA; daubney.harper@gmail.com
[2] College of Pharmacy, University of New Mexico, Albuquerque, NM 87106, USA; tmwhite@nmsu.edu
[3] Counseling & Educational Psychology Department, New Mexico State University, Las Cruces, NM 88003, USA
[*] Correspondence: eadams@nmsu.edu

Abstract: Interprofessional education is essential in that it helps healthcare disciplines better utilize each other and provide team-based collaboration that improves patient care. Many pharmacy training programs struggle to implement interprofessional education. This purpose of the study was to examine the effect of a 30-h interprofessional training that included pharmacy students to determine if the training helped these students build valuable knowledge and skills while working alongside other health care professions. The interprofessional training included graduate-level trainees from pharmacy, behavioral health, nursing, and family medicine programs where the trainees worked within teams to build interprofessional education competencies based on the Interprofessional Education Collaborative core competencies. Sixteen pharmacy trainees participated in the training and completed pre- and post-test measures. Data were collected over a two-year period with participants completing the Team Skills Scale and the Interprofessional Attitudes Scale. Paired sample t-tests indicated that, after this training, pharmacy trainees showed significant increases in feeling better able to work in healthcare teams and valuing interprofessional practice.

Keywords: interprofessional education; interprofessional collaboration; interprofessional care; communication; team-based training; teamwork; pharmacy

1. Introduction

Pharmacists play a critical role within the healthcare team in a variety of pharmacy practice settings. More importantly, their role on the interprofessional healthcare team has become increasingly influential in terms of ensuring patient safety and good health outcomes. Pharmacist interventions improve the process of patient care and clinical outcomes through the use of medication and therapeutic management, patient counseling, and professional health education [1]. Interactions between patients, healthcare professionals, other pharmacists and support personnel require effective communication skills to ensure patient safety and good health outcomes. Poor communication between physicians and pharmacists can lead to significant medication errors; therefore, a multidisciplinary approach has become essential in providing quality clinical care [2]. Due to the complexity of healthcare delivery and increasing prevalence of chronic diseases, interprofessional education (IPE) has been implemented in health professional education to provide the knowledge, skills, and attitudes to work effectively in a multidisciplinary setting [2,3]. Interprofessional education is defined by the World Health Organization (WHO) as when "students from two or more professions learn about from and with each other to enable effective collaboration and improve health outcomes" [4]. The WHO (2010) goes on to state that by learning how to work together interprofessionally, learners are better able to work in collaborative practice with other team members.

As pharmacists are included as patient care providers on health care teams in order to evaluate complex drug regimens, it is important for the team to understand the role of the pharmacist in order to maximize the utilization of their clinical skills [5]. Team communication and integration of the pharmacist into ambulatory and hospital settings has been more successful than integrating community pharmacists into primary care; this may be due to having face-to-face time with providers within hospital settings, allowing pharmacists to communicate with other healthcare team members in person [6]. Additionally, there are often misperceptions about the role of the pharmacist, pharmacists being unclear about the roles of other healthcare professionals, lack of assertiveness by pharmacists and lack of team-based training [6]. By providing IPE during the training programs of healthcare professions, these misperceptions can lead to clarification of the impact the pharmacist can make on patient care as the medication expert on the interprofessional team. For the purpose of this article, we will discuss immersing pharmacy trainees into IPE activities with trainees of other healthcare disciplines likely to be encountered in professional practice and the impact this experience may have on their perceived skills to deliver patient-centered care utilizing a team-based approach.

Pharmacy within IPE

Pharmaceutical care is a philosophy of practice in which the patient is the primary beneficiary of the pharmacist's actions which focuses the attitudes, behaviors, commitments, concerns, ethics, functions, knowledge, responsibilities and skills of the pharmacist on the provision of medication therapy. The primary goal of pharmaceutical care is achieving precise therapeutic outcomes toward patient health and quality of life [7]. Effective patient-centered interpersonal communication skills have been taught to pharmacists through a variety of IPE methods, including didactic learning modules, standardized patients, other experiential activities and didactic-based training. Standardized patient interaction is preferred over actual patients because the standardized patient is able to actively participate in teaching and assessment in real time [8]. The Accreditation Council for Pharmacy Education (ACPE) College of Pharmaceutical Education has recognized the importance of integrating IPE into the pharmacy curriculum stating "the need for interprofessional interaction is paramount to successful treatment of patients" but this training has not been consistently standardized or implemented in pharmacy education [9]. Furthermore, a workforce shortage within various healthcare fields has complicated the ability to integrate interprofessional care in daily practice [3].

The healthcare professions involved in IPE share in the same ideology of patient-centered care and therefore creates an ideal learning environment to work together, utilizing exemplary communications skills that allow the team to work together to focus on the patient's needs [8]. Developing working relationships can be hindered by several factors including differing viewpoints on patient care, attitudes, and cultural beliefs between professions [2]. Pharmacists with experience working as part of a healthcare team have more favorable viewpoints on their role within the team structure and are less likely to see potential barriers to providing professional input due to other disciplines being overly protective of their own roles and thus not seeking that input from pharmacists [10].

2. Our Program—Interprofessional Immersion Training

The interprofessional immersion is a thirty-hour annual training developed by faculty from multiple programs including: The University of New Mexico College of Pharmacy, the Southern New Mexico Family Medicine Residency Program and several departments at New Mexico State University: The Counseling and Educational Psychology department, the School of Nursing department, the School of Social Work department, and the Anthropology department. Within these six departments, trainees are selected from each program to participate in the immersion: eight first-year family medicine residents beginning their residency, six third-year counseling psychology doctoral students beginning their primary care rotation, eight doctoral-level nurse practitioner students beginning clinical rotations, two social work students, seven pharmacy students and one clinical pharmacy resident, and five medical anthropology students who observed, facilitated focus groups, and collected qualitative data.

This program began in 2013 and recently completed its fifth iteration. For the purpose of this article, we will report the findings on the 2016 and 2017 iterations as these are the years when we really refined the training to involve more team-based experiential activities and used the same outcome measures across both years. During both iterations of this training we had 32 trainees who were placed into eight groups of four, each with representation of pharmacy, nursing, behavioral health, and a family physician resident. Medical anthropology students observed, facilitated focus groups, and collected qualitative data. The aim of this training is to bring trainees who are about to begin clinical placement in medical settings together to learn important elements of interprofessional practice that can be translated to future work environments. Faculty trainers hoped that the immersion would increase the trainees team-based attitudes, expose them to team-based skills and provide some practice of these skills during the workshop that would help them work more effectively within their future healthcare teams.

The interprofessional immersion targeted all four core competencies identified by the Interprofessional Education Collaborative (IPEC) including: values and ethics, understanding roles and responsibilities, communication, and teamwork [11]. The educational components involve interactive didactics, insight-building, team-related activities, and simulated clinical practice that address each of these competencies. The training began with an activity that allowed trainees to discuss the roles of their professions and exercises that had them identify and discuss their professional values. Then they learned about communication tools such as SBAR (Situation, Background, Assessment, Recommendation) and CUS (Concerned, Uncomfortable, Safety issue), as well as specific components from Crucial Conversations and practiced communication role-plays [12]. We utilized team-building activities throughout the training, having each member work together within their team throughout each day. The trainees then participated in multiple patient simulations where they used individual clinical and IPE skills to assess and propose treatment with a standardized patient. Teams had the opportunity to practice working together while providing simulated patient care with live actors.

Each iteration of the training had some minor variation in activities, but the core elements described above were included in the two years from which this data were collected. An Institutional Review Board approval for the research was obtained for both years and trainees completed pre and post measures, wrote in journals throughout the week, and participated in discipline-specific focus groups at the close of the training. The data presented in this article reflect the quantitative measures that were used as well as supplemental statements from students based on the qualitative data.

3. Method

3.1. Participants

Thirty-two trainees participate in this interprofessional immersion each year and this article focuses on the 16 pharmacy students who participated during the summers of 2016 and 2017. All trainees consented to participate in research. A demographics questionnaire was completed in addition to several questionnaires that were administered to the participants immediately before and after the immersion experience. The training was held at New Mexico State University (NMSU) in Las Cruces, New Mexico, which is located approximately 3 h south of the only college of pharmacy in New Mexico, the University of New Mexico (UNM) College of Pharmacy. Students were recruited to participate if they were completing an Introductory Pharmacy Practice Experience (IPPE) or Advanced Pharmacy Practice Experience (APPE) within the area or were taking the course for elective credit. This training is not mandatory for this pharmacy program, however, faculty and preceptors for the pharmacy program highly encourage their students to participate and they have been successful in recruitment of new students each year.

For the 2016 cohort, the average age was 25, two identified as Asian, three as White/Non-Hispanic, and three as Hispanic. For the 2017 cohort the mean age was 25, with a range from 23 to 34. There were three male and five female, four participants identified as Hispanic, three reported being White/Non-Hispanic, and one identified as Biracial. Additionally, in the 2017 cohort, six of the eight pharmacy trainees reported planning to work in a primary care setting and within a rural community.

3.2. Measures

Team Skills. The Team Skills Scale (TSS) is a self-reporting measure used to assess participants' self-assessment of their interprofessional team skills [13]. The measures consist of 17 items and uses a five-point Likert-scale, with (1) being poor and (5) being excellent. While it was originally developed to have three subscales: interprofessional skills, discipline-specific skills, and geriatric skills, it has since been used for its total score on team skills [14]. High scores on the TSS indicate that the participant reports a stronger ability to work within teams. Previous studies using the TSS total score found high internal consistency when completed by student and graduate health professionals (e.g., a Cronbach's alpha of 0.95) [15]. For this study, the pre- and post-test alphas for the TSS were 0.82 and 0.91, respectively.

Interprofessional Attitudes. The Interprofessional Attitudes Scale (IPAS) is a self-report measure used to assess the attitudes of individuals as they relate to the interprofessional education competencies [16]. The IPAS is a 27 item instrument that uses a five-point Likert scale ranging from (1) strongly disagree to (5) strongly agree. There are five subscales: (1) Teamwork, Roles and Responsibilities; (2) Patient-Centeredness; (3) Interprofessional Biases; (4) Diversity and Ethics; and (5) Community-Centeredness. These attitudes are only measured at the subscale level so there is no total score. Higher scores on each subscale indicate a greater espousal of the attitude related to that particular domain of interprofessionalism. Because the focus of this study's interprofessional immersion did not include community-based healthcare or diversity in healthcare, we did not include these subscales in our hypotheses. Additionally, we were only interested in one item of the Interprofessional Biases subscale (Item #15, "Health professionals/students from other disciplines have prejudices or make assumptions about me because of the discipline I am studying"), so we did not use the entire Biases subscale. In the instrument development study of the IPAS, the internal consistency alphas for the subscales ranged from 0.62 to 0.92. For this study, the pre- and post-test alphas for the Teamwork subscale were 0.88 and 0.70, respectively and on the Patient Centeredness subscale they were 0.90 and 0.96.

Supplemental Data. In addition to quantitative data, qualitative data were collected in the form of journals. Each student kept a journal throughout the training and responded to specific questions pertaining to IPE such as, "what was the most surprising thing you learned about another profession today; what stands out to you most about your experience with patient simulations today in terms of working with your team; compare your experience with patient simulations from yesterday and today." Due to the limited scope of this article, qualitative statements from students will be used as a supplement to the quantitative findings.

3.3. Hypotheses and Data Analysis

Using the statistical software program SPSS, paired sample *t*-tests were conducted to analyze the quantitative data collected in the form of the two self-report measures. Our hypotheses were that there would be a significant increase from pre-test to post-test in participants' self-reported team skills on the TSS and in positive attitudes on the teamwork, roles, and responsibilities subscale of the IPAS. In order to assess for a general placebo effect, where participants would respond more favorably on all items at the time of post-test; we hypothesized that there would be no change on the Patient-Centeredness subscale of the IPAS because the immersion focus was on team-skills. There should be no reason for Patient-Centeredness to increase, except due to a general placebo effect. While we could have utilized the entire Biases subscale, we were particularly interested in item #15 of this IPAS subscale, which states, "Health professionals/students from other disciplines have prejudices or make assumptions about me because of the discipline I am studying." If the immersion was successful in creating an appreciation of all the healthcare team professions, then we hypothesized that there would be no increase on this item. In other words, a successful interprofessional immersion minimally should not increase any professional biases so as to make trainees feel more alienated or judged by the trainees in other professions after having interacted with each other during the immersion.

From a qualitative viewpoint, reflections in student journals were reviewed to evaluate how the pharmacy students identified with their role on the team and their perceived abilities to participate in future interprofessional collaborations due to a better understanding of team-based care.

4. Results

A significant difference was found in pharmacy trainees' reported team skills [t (15) = −7.26, p = 0.001] as evidenced by an increase in TSS scores from pre-test (M = 3.51, SD = 0.38) to post-test (M = 4.30, SD = 0.43). Similarly, there was a significant increase in the pharmacy trainees reported attitudes indicating that they valued working within a healthcare team [t (15) = −3.18, p = 0.006] with the pre-test IPAS teamwork scores being lower (M = 4.41, SD = 0.45, than the post-test scores (M = 4.75, SD = 0.29). See Table 1 for the t-test results.

Table 1. Paired-sample t-test results for interprofessional immersion variables.

Variable	Before Immersion Pre-Test (n = 16)		After Immersion Post-Test (n = 16)		
	M	SD	M	SD	t
Team Skills Scale	3.51	0.38	4.30	0.43	−7.26 ***
IPAS Teamwork	4.41	0.45	4.75	0.29	−3.18 **
IPAS Patient-Centered	4.76	0.37	4.75	0.46	0.09
IPAS Item #15	3.38	1.15	3.38	1.15	0.00

Note: TSS = Team Skills Scale (potential range of scores 1–5); IPAS = Interprofessional Attitudes Scale (potential range of scores 1–5); Item 15: "Health professionals/students from other disciplines have prejudices or make assumptions about me because of the discipline I am studying" (potential range of scores 1–5); ** p < 0.01, *** p < 0.001.

Regarding our exploration of the null hypothesis that there would be no significant differences between pre- and post-test scores on the patient-centeredness subscale of the IPAS and Item #15 of the Bias subscale of the IPAS (i.e., perceptions of other professions being biased about one's own profession), the null hypothesis was supported. There was no significant difference on the participants' attitudes about being patient-centered [t (15) = 0.09, p = 0.933], with pre-test scores (M = 4.76, SD = 0.37) being virtually the same as the post-test scores (M = 4.75, SD = 0.46). Similarly, there was no significant difference on Item 15 [t (15) = 0.00, p = 1.00] with pre-test scores regarding perceptions of professional bias (M = 3.38, SD = 1.15) being exactly the same as the post-test scores (M = 3.38, SD = 1.15).

In regards to the journals, there were comments that reflected changes in the perception of working within healthcare teams. Practicing together helped reduce hierarchy often experienced in healthcare. One pharmacy student reflected,

> "During this week hierarchy was not an issue. My interprofessional team was very mindful of the importance of each team members' contributions. Having this mindset enabled for trust and positive relations to form from the beginning. From my experience outside of this week, healthcare is very 'hierarchical,' which complicates patient care."

Another pharmacy student reflected,

> "Everyone was able to step back and accommodate to the needs of the team we all worked very well together and were able to see our strengths and weaknesses and build on them to improve teamwork."

Pharmacy trainees also reflected on how their perceptions of working within teams had changed as a result of this training. In regards to an ability to work as a team, one of the pharmacy trainees reflected,

> "I think fully understanding what each discipline is an expert on and their role and then seeing them as tools rather than a challenge to your patient care process will have a very positive impact on patient care. It is going to be very interesting to see the future outcomes of health professionals who are trained as a team from the beginning of their education."

Another student reflected on how working within a team was both surprising and helped her be better in her own role. The pharmacy trainee stated,

> "Working with my team in today's simulation had the opposite effect of what I was expecting. I had previously thought teamwork and being put on the spot in front of other healthcare providers would be more nerve racking than an individual patient encounter, but surprisingly it was less stressful and the combined brain power proved to provide better, more encompassing care and was actually enjoyable for me."

This pharmacy student reflected on how the experience helped him feel more comfortable in his role within the team and affirmed that team-based care can be an effective way to practice. He stated,

> "I felt that I fit very well in my role as a pharmacy student with my team. I think that I complement their focuses very well and make a great impact with medication and lifestyle management. They asked a lot of good questions that helped me think more about my assessment. I also think we all did not overstep boundaries and didn't try to talk over one another and didn't belittle one another either. I feel that I appreciate the roles of the team members [much] more after today."

Lastly, a family medicine physician resident made this journal reflection regarding the importance of knowing one's team members and their roles as well as the importance of having a shared goal.

> "Working in a team involves many 'moving parts.' It would never work unless each team member buys into the team and the team shares a common goal. My team has bonded really well and has learned a lot about each other. This helped us greatly during the simulation. It is not enough to just know your role in the team, but you must also know others' roles as well."

5. Conclusions

Results on the Team Skills Scale (TSS), the Interprofessional Attitudes Scale (IPAS), and comments in their journals highlight that this interprofessional training produced some positive change in pharmacy trainees' perceptions about their ability and desire to work on interprofessional healthcare teams. The results provide empirical support that even a relatively brief interprofessional training can produce changes in pharmacy students' perspectives in working within healthcare teams, both in terms of their self-efficacy regarding their team-based skills and in their attitudes about the importance of team-based care. This is consistent with previous studies utilizing the Team Skills Scale (TSS) and qualitative responses to interprofessional training with pharmacy professionals [14]. Robben et al. reported significantly higher perceptions of team skills after their interprofessional training, as well as students described increased awareness/appreciation of the lenses and functions of other professions.

While there were a small number of participants, the differences in pre- and post-test scores were significant enough to be detected. In particular, the average score for participants' self-report of their team skills on the TSS at pre-test was mid-way between "Good" and "Very Good", whereas the average post-test score was mid-way between "Very Good" and "Excellent." Regarding attitudes about teamwork on the IPAS the participants were closer to "Agree" at the pre-test and then closer to "Strongly Agree" at post-test. While there was no control group, it is important to note that other subscales (i.e., patient-centeredness) did not change from pre- to post-test. In a controlled trial evaluation where pre-licensed health service students received either 11 hours of interprofessional training or their discipline's normal curriculum, Darlow et al. reported significantly heightened mean differences on the TSS in the intervention group versus the control group [17]. The authors feel that this may be due to the fact that the trainees already possessed strong values and attributes of patient-centeredness. This could also be due to the fact that pharmaceutical care aims to be patient-centered and this is already delivered throughout the pharmacy curriculum. The authors hypothesized that there would be not significant differences from pre- to post-test in this particular area. This support of the null hypothesis highlights the importance of tying interprofessional skill improvement to improved patient care when engaging pharmacy trainees in IPE. Some research points to mixed findings around changes in health service students' attitudes in response to shorter interprofessional trainings (e.g., three-day training vs. one-year), with some medical students reporting no attitude change towards interprofessional teamwork in shorter trainings and heighted positive attitudes in longer trainings [18,19]. However, in this study it is more likely that pharmacy students' patient centeredness remained constant, regardless of length of training, evidenced by journal entries highlighting how students felt they could work more effectively and comfortably within healthcare teams.

Pharmacy journal entries highlighted how students felt they could work more effectively and comfortably within healthcare teams and how doing so would improve the quality of the healthcare for patients. This qualitative theme complements our TSS and IPAS results, in which pharmacy trainees reported increased team skills and increased attitudinal valuation of working on an interprofessional healthcare team. A study utilizing the IPAS has reported that students' perceptions of overall interprofessional competence increases significantly after IPE trainings, and that as perceptions of competence increased, attitudes toward teamwork also become more positive [20].

Additionally, we were specifically interested in assessing if the immersion training had a negative effect on the pharmacy trainees' perceptions of how pharmacy was viewed by trainees in other healthcare professions. The results of paired sample t-test on Item 15 of the IPAS indicated that pharmacy trainees neither agreed nor disagreed with this statement at both pre- and post-test. Thus, this brief immersion did not create more negative biases about the other healthcare professions. Ideally, participants should ultimately disagree with this statement, feeling that the trainees of other professions have positive perceptions of their own discipline. This finding suggests that when planning interprofessional immersion trainings the faculty should directly address any biases in debriefings with trainees to determine if there might be specific activities that would help address this concern. For example, at the end of an immersion it might be important to have trainees from each of the healthcare professions sharing specifically positive perceptions they now have about other professions as a result of interacting in the team-based activities.

A recent study by Peeters et al. suggests that delivering interprofessional education focused in smaller groups within a larger classroom-based course was helpful for students to achieve learning objectives based on IPEC competencies and student satisfaction with the course [21]. Our study adds to the IPE literature because it demonstrates the positive impact of a briefer training IPE experience, delivered in small group, team-based activities with four healthcare disciplines. More research is needed to determine what active ingredients of IPE trainings are most effective in creating the increases in self-efficacy related to team skills, as well as more positive attitudes about team-based work. For example, in our interprofessional immersion, we provided many real-world examples of team-based care as the faculty trainers work in teams in their daily professional practices and model these relationships and communication skills with fellow faculty throughout the course. Future research could leave this component out of the interprofessional immersion to see if this negatively impacted the change in scores from pre- to post-test.

A limitation of the current study is that the outcomes measures did not directly assess changes in communication styles or habits, nor the trainees' ability to work in his or her specific work-setting. The trainers hope that the skills learned will transfer to other work settings and that through practice these skills will be more comfortable and likely to be utilized. Pecukonis argues that it can be difficult to translate interprofessional education into practice [22]. By providing this training at the start of the trainees' clinical experiences in interprofessional settings, we hope they will be able to apply these team skills immediately in their clinical setting. To gather empirical support for this goal, future research needs to incorporate an assessment of the participants' team-based skills as well as gather longitudinal data from participants. In order to enhance our understanding of the specific team-based skills learned during our training, our faculty hopes to analyze data collected from video recordings of trainees working together during patient simulations as well as collect data from past graduates that participated in this interprofessional training. There is little research on IPE that assesses actual skills observed by independent raters, particularly in "real-world" settings.

The trainees in our study varied in their years of pharmacy education, ranging from completing their first year of pharmacy school to beginning practice as a pharmacy resident. This variation may have affected participants' scores on the TSS and IPAS due to variance in knowledge, skills and/or confidence levels. Although the training emphasized a focus on team-based skills and communication rather than professional knowledge-based skills, these differences in training level may impact participants' self-reporting of team-based skills and attitudes. With larger sample sizes, it will be possible to examine the impact of participants' training level. The research on IPE has not determined when is the optimal time for such training to occur.

There is great importance in building interprofessional education skills to help reduce medical errors, increase communication, provide better patient care and reduce provider burn-out. One way to enhance these skills is through specific training surrounding the interprofessional education competencies. This study provides evidence that brief, team-based learning can be an effective modality for learning these skills, building trainees' confidence in being able to work within healthcare teams, and creating a greater appreciation for this type of healthcare delivery.

Author Contributions: D.B. completed the IRB for this study, conceived and developed framework for this manuscript, and contributed to the largest amount of writing; T.W. contributed to the literature review and relevant literature within the area of pharmacy; E.A. analyzed data and provided thorough edits for the manuscript. All faculty involved in the training contributed to the development of the interprofessional immersion and the assessment tools used for data collection.

Acknowledgments: The authors would like to thank all of the many individuals and organizations that have worked together to put on this interprofessional training each year, with a special thanks to the Southern New Mexico Family Medicine Residency Program, the Counseling & Educational Psychology Department at New Mexico State University (NMSU), the NMSU School of Nursing, and the University of New Mexico College of Pharmacy.

References

1. Nikansah, N.; Mostovetsky, O.; Yu, C.; Chheng, T.; Beney, J.; Bond, C.M.; Bero, L. Effect of outpatient pharmacists' non-dispensing roles on patient outcomes and prescribing patterns. *Cochrane Database Syst. Rev.* **2010**, *7*, 7. [CrossRef] [PubMed]
2. Gallagher, R.M.; Gallagher, H.C. Improving the working relationship between doctors and pharmacists: Is inter-professional education the answer? *Adv. Health Sci. Educ.* **2012**, *17*, 247–257. [CrossRef] [PubMed]
3. Page, R.L.; Hume, A.L.; Trujillo, J.M.; Leader, W.G.; Vardeny, O.; Neuhauser, M.M.; Dang, D.; Nesbit, S.; Cohen, L.J. Interprofessional education: Principles and application a framework for clinical pharmacy. *Pharmacother. J. Hum. Pharmacol. Drug Ther.* **2009**, *29*, 879. [CrossRef]
4. World Health Organization. *Framework for Action on Interprofessional Education and Collaborative Practice*; WHO: Geneva, Switzerland, 2010. Available online: http://www.who.int/hrh/resources/framework_action/en (accessed on 17 March 2018).
5. Farrell, B.; Ward, N.; Dore, N.; Russell, G.; Geneau, R.; Evans, S. Working in interprofessional primary health care teams: what do pharmacists do? *Res. Soc. Adm. Pharm.* **2013**, *9*, 288–301. [CrossRef] [PubMed]

6. Jorgenson, D.; Dalton, D.; Farrell, B.; Tsuyuki, R.; Dolovich, L. Guidelines for pharmacists integrating into primary care teams. *Can. Pharm. J.* **2013**, *6*, 342–352. [CrossRef] [PubMed]

7. Hepler, C.D.; Strand, L.M. Opportunities and responsibilities in pharmaceutical care. *Am. J. Health-Syst. Pharm.* **1990**, *47*, 533–543.

8. Hess, R.; Hagemeier, N.E.; Blackwelder, R.; Rose, D.; Ansari, N.; Branham, T. Teaching communication skills to medical and pharmacy students through a blended learning course. *Am. J. Pharm. Educ.* **2016**, *80*, 1–10. [CrossRef] [PubMed]

9. Accreditation Council for Pharmacy Education. Accreditation Standards and Key Elements for the Professional Program in Pharmacy Leading to the Doctor of Pharmacy Degree "Standards 2016". February 2015. Available online: https://www.acpe-accredit.org/pdf/Standards2016FINAL.pdf (accessed on 17 March 2018).

10. Dobson, R.; Henry, C.; Taylor, J.; Zello, G.; Lachaine, J.; Forbes, D.; Keegan, D. Interprofessional health care teams: Attitudes and environmental factors associated with participation by community pharmacists. *J. Interprof. Care* **2006**, *20*, 119–132. [CrossRef] [PubMed]

11. Interprofessional Education Collaborative (IPEC) Expert Panel. *Core Competencies for Interprofessional Collaborative Practice: Report of an Expert Panel*; IPEC: Washington, DC, USA, 2011.

12. Patterson, K. *Crucial Conversations: Tools for Talking When Stakes Are High*; McGraw-Hill: New York, NY, USA, 2012.

13. Hyer, K.; Heinemann, G.D.; Fulmer, T. Team Skills Scale. In *Team Performance in Health Care: Assessment and Development*; Heinemann, G.D., Zeiss, A.M., Eds.; Plenum: New York, NY, USA, 2002; pp. 159–163.

14. Robben, S.; Perry, M.; van Nieuwenhuijzen, L.; van Achterberg, T.; Rikkert, M.O.; Schers, H.; Heinen, M.; Melis, R. Impact of interprofessional education on collaboration attitudes, skills, and behavior among primary care professionals. *J. Contin. Educ. Health* **2012**, *32*, 196–204. [CrossRef] [PubMed]

15. Fulmer, T.; Hyer, K.; Flaherty, E.; Mezey, M.; Whitelaw, N.; Jacobs, M.O.; Luchi, R.; Hansen, J.C.; Evans, D.A.; Cassel, C.; et al. Geriatric interdisciplinary team training program evaluation results. *J. Aging Health* **2005**, *17*, 443–470. [CrossRef] [PubMed]

16. Norris, J.; Carpenter, J.G.; Eaton, J.; Guo, J.W.; Lassche, M.; Pelt, M.A.; Blumenthal, D.K. The development and validation of the interprofessional attitudes scale: Assessing the interprofessional attitudes of students in the health professions. *Acad. Med. J. Assoc. Am. Med. Coll.* **2015**, *90*, 1394–1400. [CrossRef] [PubMed]

17. Darlow, B.; Coleman, K.; McKinlay, E.; Donovan, S.; Beckingsale, L.; Gray, B.; Neser, H.; Perry, M.; Stanley, J.; Pullon, S. The positive impact of interprofessional education: A controlled trial to evaluate a programme for health professional students. *BMC Med. Educ.* **2015**, *15*. [CrossRef] [PubMed]

18. Park, J.; Hawkins, M.; Hamlin, E.; Hawkins, W.; Bamdas, J. Developing positive attitudes toward interprofessional collaboration among students in the health care professions. *Educ. Gerontol.* **2014**, *40*, 894–908. [CrossRef]

19. Shrader, S.; Griggs, C. Multiple interprofessional education activities delivered longitudinally within a required clinical assessment course. *Am. J. Pharm. Educ.* **2014**, *12*. [CrossRef] [PubMed]

20. Coiro, M.J.; Preis, J. Increases in graduate students' interprofessional competence associated with clinical training activities. *Health Interprof. Pract.* **2018**, *3*. [CrossRef]

21. Peeters, M.J.; Sexton, M.; Metz, A.E.; Hasbrouck, C.S. A team-based interprofessional education course for first-year health professions students. *Curr. Pharm. Teach. Learn.* **2017**, *9*, 1099–1110. [CrossRef] [PubMed]

22. Pecukonis, E. Interprofessional education: A theoretical orientation incorporating professional-centrism and social identity theory. *J. Law Med. Ethics* **2014**, *42*, 60–64. [CrossRef] [PubMed]

8

Determinants of Hospital Pharmacists' Job Satisfaction in Romanian Hospitals

Magdalena Iorga [1,*], Corina Dondaș [2], Camelia Soponaru [3] and Ioan Antofie [4]

[1] Department of Behavioral Sciences, University of Medicine and Pharmacy "Grigore T. Popa", Iasi 700115, Romania

[2] Department of Career Counseling, University of Medicine and Pharmacy "Grigore T. Popa", Iasi 700115, Romania; dondascorina@gmail.com

[3] Department of Psychology, University "Alexandru Ioan Cuza", Iasi 700506, Romania; puzdriac@yahoo.com

[4] Department of Hospital Pharmacy, C.F. Hospital, Cluj-Napoca 599597, Romania; ioanantofie@ymail.com

* Correspondence: magdalena.iorga@umfiasi.ro

Abstract: *Aim*: The purpose of this study is to identify the level of job satisfaction among hospital pharmacists in Romania in relation to environmental, socio-demographic, and individual factors. *Material and Methods*: Seventy-eight hospital pharmacists were included in the research. The Job Satisfaction Scale was used to measure the level of satisfaction with their current jobs, and the TAS-20 was used to evaluate emotional experience and awareness. Additionally, 12 items were formulated in order to identify the reasons for dissatisfaction with jobs, such as budget, number of working hours, legislation, relationships with colleagues, hospital departments, or stakeholders. Data were analyzed using IBM SPSS Statistics version 23. *Results*: The analyses of the data revealed a low level of satisfaction regarding the pay–promotion subscale, a high level of satisfaction with the management–interpersonal relationship dimension, and a high level of satisfaction regarding the organization–communication subscale. Seventy-four percent of subjects are dissatisfied about the annual budget, and 86.3% are not at all satisfied with present legislation. *Conclusions*: These results are important for hospital pharmacists and hospital management in order to focus on health policies, management, and environmental issues, with the purpose of increasing the level of satisfaction among hospital pharmacists.

Keywords: hospital pharmacists; job satisfaction; personality traits

---

1. Introduction

Job satisfaction is an important factor for increasing a person's involvement in the workplace, and also for motivation [1]. It represents a combination of positive or negative feelings that workers have towards their work, and the perceived relationships between a person's expectations and the actual results. Satisfaction with work is closely linked to that individual's behavior in the workplace [2–5].

The interest in studying job satisfaction has a two-fold purpose: Identifying the various factors that may increase the pharmacists' workplace satisfaction, and, implicitly, patients' satisfaction, as well as improving the quality of the services provided [6–9]. When compared to the general population, older data show that pharmacists may be slightly less satisfied with their specific jobs than the general population [7].

Over the decades, the profession of hospital pharmacist interacted closely with other medical health care professionals in hospitals; hence, the importance of pharmacists in a multidisciplinary team has increased [8]. As part of a team providing health services, pharmacists are involved in accomplishing various tasks and in making decisions that have an impact on a patient's quality of life.

Thus, job satisfaction level may actively influence employees' motivation to get involved in hospital activities [10–12].

Kerschen et al. [13] reported that hospital pharmacists obtained mean satisfaction scores, and some studies identified that the primary factor in employee retention is employee job satisfaction [14,15]. Among professionals in the same pharmaceutical department, pharmacists appeared to be more satisfied than support personnel [7]. Job positioning and skill use repeatedly appeared to be related to pharmacist job satisfaction [15].

Factors that influence job satisfaction are related to a burnout work pattern [16], work environment, external pressures (commercials), and sector of practice [17–19]. Some studies have shown that hospital pharmacists are more satisfied when compared to community pharmacists, who are more pressured by the number of working hours, by a poor relationship with physicians, or by the lack of promotion opportunities [20]. Job dissatisfaction impacts job performance, resulting in an increased number of errors [21,22].

The levels of job satisfaction among hospital pharmacists was identified by studies revealing different scores. For example, 77% of hospital pharmacists were satisfied with their jobs in Australia [23], 67% in India [24], and 67.3% in the United States of America (USA) [25].

Previous studies showed that socio-demographic factors have an influence on pharmacist job satisfaction. For example, a study performed by Majd et al. [26] showed that younger pharmacists were significantly less satisfied with their incomes compared to older pharmacists, while other studies [27] reported that men were less satisfied compared to women. Additionally, there are studies that found a positive relationship between job factors and a hospital pharmacist's level of job satisfaction. Different studies showed that gender and job position influence overall job satisfaction to a significant degree [28]. When it comes to motivation factors, pharmacists ranked recognition, promotion, job satisfaction, job feedback, autonomy, and task significance among the most influential motivators to pharmacists. Pharmacists' superiors considered financial rewards to be more important than non-financial incentives and benefits [29]. In a previous study [30] targeting forensic physicians, it was found that alexithymia is negatively correlated with one of the factors of job satisfaction, namely, organization and communication skills, and since alexithymia is metaphorically considered an "emotional numbness", determination as to whether it has an influence on pharmacists, as well as whether it affects their job satisfaction level, is wanted.

Several studies have been conducted on hospital pharmacists' satisfaction, but this topic has not been analyzed in Romania thus far. In Romania, private or public hospitals comprise hospital pharmacists and clinical pharmacists. The former administers the pharmacy department; they deal with the supply and delivery of medicines for hospital departments and of subsidized drugs. The latter, which consists of clinician pharmacists, must be assigned to a medical or surgical clinic: They advise physicians concerning doses and they contribute to the personalized medicine programs of all patients.

Six university pharmacy schools and two departments of pharmacy within medical schools, providing medico-pharmaceutical education, are accredited by the Romanian Ministry of Education. The standard curriculum is about five years in length, including six months of internship training, in country or abroad. From a legal point of view, Romania conforms to European Union (EU) directives regarding education and mutual recognition of diplomas for pharmacists [31,32].

The number of pharmacists (76.3 for 100,000 inhabitants) is lower in Romania, as compared to the European Union average of 82.8, but is similar to that of Eastern European countries [32,33]. There are approximately 5200 pharmacies in the country, and each is mandated to have at least one pharmacist. Each of the 450 hospitals has a pharmacy where one to three hospital pharmacists usually work [33]. The College of Pharmacists is the national association with which all of the pharmacists should register, as noted by specific legislation. One-hundred and sixty pharmacists that are working in hospitals are also registered in The National Association of Hospital Pharmacists in Romania (ANFSR), and their salaries are paid by hospital pharmacies. The right to free practice is granted by the College of Pharmacists, and pharmacists may follow specialized postgraduate training courses.

The graduation process is assured by a residency exam in general pharmacy. However, in the period of 2004–2017, this exam was not organized. The only residency exams that were organized in the last 13 years were for clinical pharmacy and for laboratory pharmacy. Currently, hospital pharmacists (ANFSR), supported by the College of Pharmacists, are struggling to establish, with the Health Minister, the promotion of new laws for the benefit of hospital pharmacists, as well as the quality of pharmaceuticals in hospitals.

The annual budget that hospital pharmacists have to manage is limited by hospital decisions. A study analyzing the transition period and the impact on health policies in Romania found that health spending increased significantly between 2001 and 2007. This trend continued in the following years, due to the high level of expenditures for both hospital services and pharmaceuticals; for example, most of expenditures that were registered in 2005, for instance, were payments of debts pertaining to the previous year [34].

Thus, promotion and budget could be two main important sources of dissatisfaction among hospital pharmacists. The goal of this study is to evaluate the level of job satisfaction among hospital pharmacists in Romania, and to identify the influence of socio-demographic, environmental, or personality constructs, such as alexithymia on work satisfaction. The present study is the first one of its kind conducted in Romania, and its findings are important because they will join those obtained by studies conducted in other countries. The similarities and differences in the tasks of hospital pharmacists in different countries lead to diverse levels of satisfaction with work. Some of them are related to personality factors, but others are determined by national health policies or by the transition process.

2. Material and Methods

The present research was part of a broader study that was approved by the National Association of Hospital Pharmacists in Romania (ANFSR). Seventy-eight subjects, out of 160 pharmacists registered with ANFSR (a rate of 48.75%), answered questionnaires. The subjects worked in public hospitals, in 20 out of the 42 counties in Romania (covering more than half of the country's territory). Informed consent and a document including personal data were obtained before the questionnaires were completed. Subjects were informed about the confidentiality of personal data, as well as the research objectives.

In order to identify problems related to job satisfaction among pharmacists working in public hospitals, and to evaluate the level of satisfaction with their jobs, the following instruments were applied:

(a) a fill-in form, including socio-demographic characteristics (age, gender, department, work experience in years, years of work at the present institution, quality of head pharmacist);

(b) an open-ended questionnaire with 12 items, regarding job-related opinions and regarding relationships with colleagues, staff, and stakeholders; and,

(c) two psychological tools to evaluate pharmacists' level of alexithymia and the level of satisfaction with their jobs (Toronto Alexithymia Scale and Job Satisfaction Scale).

The Job Satisfaction Scale—JSS [35]—consists of 32 items representing three factors that were related to job satisfaction: Pay–promotions (14 items), management–interpersonal relationships (eight items), organization–communication (10 items), and overall job satisfaction. The questionnaire was adapted from the "Job Satisfaction Survey", proposed by P.E. Spector in 1997, a tool with 36 items evaluating nine aspects of job satisfaction: Payment, promotion, supervision, secondary benefits, potential rewards, regulations, co-workers, the nature of work, and communication. The adapted version of this scale, containing 32 items, was applied to a population of 566 subjects with the following internal consistency coefficients: Payment and promotion, 0.820; leadership and interpersonal relationships, 0.760; and organizational and communication, 0.738; the Cronbach's alpha coefficient for the total score was 0.872.

The Toronto Alexithymia Scale—TAS-20 [36] is a personality construct, called "emotional blindness". It refers to trouble in identifying and describing emotions and the tendency to minimize emotional experience and focus attention externally. It was used for this research to identify the difficulties with emotional processing and emotional awareness. It is a questionnaire that demonstrates a good internal consistency (Cronbach's alpha = 0.81) and test–retest reliability (0.77, $p < 0.001$), adequate levels of convergent, and concurrent validity in other studies [37]. The authors found it to be stable and replicable across clinical and nonclinical populations. In the present study, hospital pharmacists had to rate answers on a Likert–type scale (1 = strongly disagree to 5 = strongly agree). A total of 20 items targeted three domains: Difficulty describing feelings, difficulty identifying feelings, and externally oriented thinking. The total score for alexithymia was calculated as the sum of these three subscales. A score lower than or equal to 51 meant that subjects did not have alexithymia; a score between 52 and 60 was equal to borderline alexithymia, and subjects with a total score higher than or equal to 61 were characterized by alexithymia.

The obtained data were processed using IBM SPSS Statistics version 23 (IBM Japan, Tokyo, Japan). Mean and standard deviation were used for descriptive analyses of data, the t-test for independent samples, and one-way ANOVA for comparative analysis, in addition, Pearson and Spearman correlations were used to point out the relationships between variables.

3. Results and Discussions

3.1. Descriptive Analysis

Instruments: For the three dimensions of the JSS score, the Cronbach's alpha scores were: 0.710 for pay–promotions, 0.679 for management–interpersonal relationships, and 0.796 for organization–communication. The Cronbach's alpha total score for job satisfaction was 0.834. For TAS-20, Cronbach's alpha scores obtained for all the three dimensions were: 0.438, 0.783, and 0.523, respectively. The total score for alexithymia was 0.738, suggesting a good internal consistency. The low score for Cronbach's alpha concerning the first domain of TAS was probably due to two causes: The number of variables that are not normally distributed, and the existence of lower and higher scores that contribute to the medium level of the total score. For this reason, the results referring to this domain should be cautiously considered as conclusions.

Socio-demographic data: Seventy women (89.7%) and eight men (10.3%) were included in the research, with 59 (75.6%) being heads of hospital pharmaceutical departments (mean age 45.57 ± 10.12, with a minimum age of 25 and a maximum age of 61). In total, 47 pharmacists (60.3%) were married or in a relationship, and 52 of them (67.5%) had children; 31 subjects (39.7) reported as being single. The duration of experience in the pharmaceutical field in years is M = 19.07 ± 11.23 (with a minimum of one and a maximum of 37 years of work). The period of employment at their current jobs was 10.81 ± 9.78 (with a minimum of one and a maximum of 33 years), the number of working hours per week was 37.51 ± 3.96 (with a minimum of 35 and a maximum of 50 h/week).

Job-related data: Twelve items were formulated. Seven items focused on identifying the relationship between the pharmacist and other members of hospital staff (managers, medical directors, sales managers, pharmaceutical company representatives). They had to answer on a Likert-type of scale from 1 (never) to 5 (always). The frequency of answers to these items is presented in Table 1.

The most frequent conflictual relationships are those with staff working in the purchasing department, and with pharmaceutical company representatives. In what concerns their relationships with the latter, conflicts may be explained by the fact that medical warehouses no longer supply hospitals with medication if its unpaid bills exceed three to six months. The purchasing department is in charge of concluding framework agreements and subsequent contracts, and is also responsible for maintaining connections with medical warehouses. Therefore, it is the intermediary link between the hospital pharmacy and the medical warehouse; however, a pharmacist, in fact, has little power when it comes to accelerating the process of delivering medications to a patient. Therefore, the results may reflect the awareness of the pharmacist's inability to categorically influence the process of delivering drugs to beneficiaries.

Table 1. The frequency of answers for items I1–I7.

	Items Do You Have Conflicts with …	Never	Sometimes	Often	Most of the Time	Always
I1	The purchasing department	38.7%	46.7%	8%	6.7%	0%
I2	Hospital general manager	55.3%	34.2%	6.6%	2.6%	1.3%
I3	Hospital medical manager	66.7%	32%	0%	1.3%	0%
I4	Heads of clinical departments	48%	49.3%	2.7%	0%	0%
I5	Physicians	50.7%	46.7%	1.3%	1.3%	0%
I6	Pharmaceutical companies	28.9%	60.5%	7.9%	1.3%	1.3%
I7	Colleagues at the pharmacy	79.2%	18.1%	1.4%	1.4%	0%

Five other items questioned hospital pharmacists' opinions regarding: Item (8) current legislation; item (9) budget; item (10) working time; item (11) relationships with colleagues; and, item (12) reasons for conflicts with peers. Most hospital pharmacists ($N = 63$, 86.3%) declared that they were not at all satisfied with the present legislation. The responses to the item questioning the pharmacists' opinions regarding working time revealed that 60 of them (83.3%) were satisfied with their working hours/week, and only 12 of them (16.7%) were not satisfied with their weekly schedules. When compared to other healthcare personnel working at a hospital, pharmacists are not frequently obligated to have extra working hours.

Hospital pharmacists were asked if they were satisfied with the relationships with their colleagues from the pharmaceutical department. Seventy-one subjects (95.9%) claimed that they were satisfied, and only three of them (4.1%) reported not being satisfied with the relationships with their colleagues. Among the reasons that were mentioned as causes of conflicts between pharmacists, the questioned subjects mentioned communication ($N = 35$, 52.2%), subordinated relationships ($N = 8$, 11.9%), job-related tasks ($N = 20$, 29.9%), and job description ($N = 4$, 6%).

Regarding pharmacists' contentment with the annual budget, the frequency of their responses showed that only 19 (26%) were satisfied with the financial budget at their disposal, and 54 (74%) were discontent with it. The results showed that the most stringent problem at work was related to budget. In Romania, an allotted budget refers to the sum of money that is allocated by hospitals for medicine. A pharmacist has to manage this sum to ensure that a hospital has the minimum amount of medicines needed. Prior to the constitution of the Health Insurance House, funds for medicines used to come from a separate budget line; the money currently arrives in one large payment, which the manager distributes as they see fit, and purchasing medicine is not always a priority.

Psychological data: The result for TAS-20 (total score = 44.89) showed that pharmacists had a low level of alexithymia ($N = 55$, 74.3% non-alexithymia, $N = 4$, 18.9% with borderline alexithymia, and $N = 5$, 6.8% with alexithymia). Detailed results for all three dimensions, and for alexithymia and job satisfaction subscales, are presented in Table 2.

Table 2. Results for Job Satisfaction Scale and Toronto Alexithymia Scale.

Instruments	Domains	Mean ± Standard Deviation
JSS	Payment–promotion	3.38 ± 0.65
	Management–interpersonal relationship	4.33 ± 0.66
	Organization–communication	4.41 ± 0.70
	Total score	3.92 ± 0.55
TAS-20	Difficulty describing feelings	12.97 ± 5.48
	Difficulty identifying feelings	13.90 ± 5.18
	Externally oriented thinking	18.01 ± 4.27
	Total score	44.89 ± 11.56

For JSS, the obtained data showed that, regarding pay–promotion, hospital pharmacists showed a low level of satisfaction; for management–interpersonal relationships the score proved a very high level of satisfaction; and for organization–communication, hospital pharmacists had a high level of satisfaction. The histograms for all three dimensions of job satisfaction are presented in Figures 1–3.

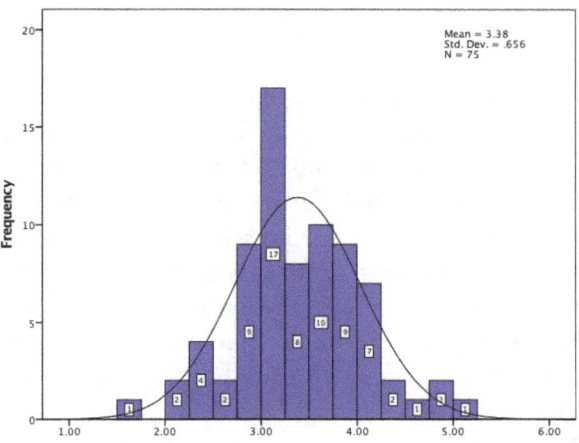

Figure 1. Payment and promotion.

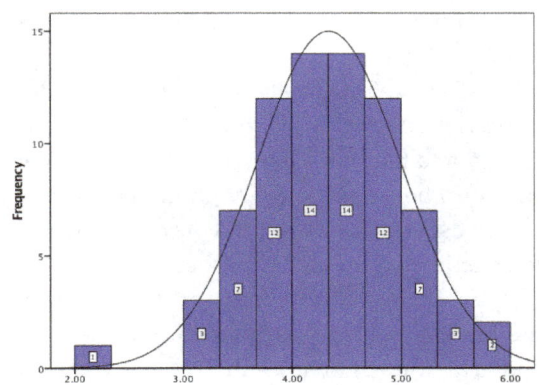

Figure 2. Management and interpersonal relationships.

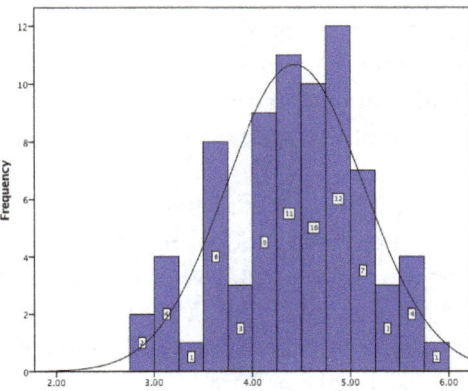

Figure 3. Communication and organization.

The results that were obtained in the three subscales of job satisfaction emphasized the fact that the greatest level of discontent was related to promotion possibilities and pay level. In Romania, promotion is based on a medical residency exam and training. In general practice pharmacy, no residency exam has been organized since 2004, as was highlighted in the Introduction. Therefore, promotion occurs within the pharmacy, and the chances of getting a promotion are minimal. Nevertheless, upon analyzing an individual's right to improve and develop at the workplace, we considered that the currently-implemented conditions of the hospital pharmacist position are in violation of the constitutional right to develop at work.

3.2. Correlation Analysis

In order to choose an appropriate statistical procedure, the normality of the data distribution with a sample Kolmogorov–Smirnov test was tested. For the alexithymia construct, it was found that two dimensions are not normally distributed (difficulty describing feelings and difficulty identifying feelings), while the third component (externally oriented thinking) and the total score of alexithymia had a normal score distribution. For JSS, all of the dimensions and total scores are normally distributed.

For the socio-demographic variables (age, total number of years in the pharmaceutical field, working years in the hospital, and the number of working hours per week), it was found that they are not normally distributed. Pearson correlations were used for the variables that were normally distributed, and, for variables that were not normally distributed, Spearman correlations were applied. The correlation analyses between variables that were considered were not, in general, statistically significant. The only significant correlations were negative, namely those between the management–interpersonal relationship dimensions (JSS), with externally-oriented thinking ($R = -0.272$ *, $p = 0.021$) and total score for alexithymia ($R = -0.241$ *, $p = 0.042$). The results showed that the more externally-oriented thinking a person/alexithymic is, the less satisfied they are regarding management–interpersonal relationships.

This third dimension of TAS-20 refers to an individual's tendency to focus their attention externally. Management and interpersonal relationships refer to satisfaction with their relationships with colleagues and superiors, and to a tendency to avoid conflicts. It seems that a person who focuses on external events is more prone to being sensitive to them, and are less satisfied with events and relationships. This explanation is also valid for the total alexithymia score.

No correlations were identified between age, experience, number of working hours, or the other two subscales of TAS-20, and satisfaction with the pay–promotion or organization–communication sub-dimension of the JSS. The findings of this study are at odds with the results obtained by other studies (age and sex did not have an impact on job satisfaction of pharmacists) [26–28].

3.3. Comparative Analysis

In order to perform a comparative analysis, a t-test for independent variables was used and one-way ANOVA was used for the variables with more than two levels. The comparative analysis considering the independent variables of age (25–40, 41–55, 56–65 years old), level (pharmacist, specialist, or hospital primary pharmacist), administrative tasks (pharmacist or head pharmacist), satisfaction with the annual budget, colleagues, legislation, or work time revealed no significant differences.

The only significant statistical difference that was obtained was between pharmacists that were satisfied with the annual budget and those who were not. Subjects who reported being more satisfied with the financial budget were more satisfied with management–interpersonal relationships ($M_{satisfied} = 4.53$, $M_{dissatisfied} = 4.19$; $t (68) = 2.037$, $p = 0.046$) and organization–communication ($M_{satisfied} = 4.63$, $M_{dissatisfied} = 4.26$; $t (68) = 2.071$, $p = 0.042$), and with their job—total job satisfaction ($M_{satisfied} = 4.07$, $M_{dissatisfied} = 3.80$; $t (68) = 2.025$, $p = 0.047$). No significant difference was identified when considering the levels of alexithymia and job satisfaction.

The present research showed that the low level of satisfaction was related to the pay and promotion dimension. External motivation factors influence job satisfaction, given that some studies have found recognition, promotion, and pay to be important factors for work satisfaction [27]. These findings were congruent with results from the literature. In a study by Popa and Bazgan, two types of factors were identified as being responsible for the level of job satisfaction: Extrinsic factors deriving from the organizational context (salary, policies practiced in the organization, working conditions, autonomy and control, job security, interpersonal relations), and intrinsic factors, related to personal experience and to the relationship with the work environment (recognition by others, responsibility for own work and others' work, advancement, personal fulfilment) [38].

The findings of this study showed that some variables, such as age, level (pharmacist, specialist, or hospital primary pharmacist), administrative tasks (pharmacist or head pharmacist), satisfaction with the annual budget, the relationship with their colleagues, legislation, or work time revealed no significant differences.

The results were consistent with the findings of other studies, which found that gender, job positions, education levels, the size and location of hospitals, and work experience were not significant factors in determining job satisfaction. As some studies have shown, job-related predictors of job satisfaction are skill use (as the most important factor in evaluating their ideal job) and recognition [37,39].

Payment and promotion should be related to a method of acknowledgement, as well as to the possibility of professional development and promotion, which is not encouraged by the present Romanian legislation. Recognition is also related to the job tasks of hospital pharmacists in Romania: Hospital pharmacists are not part of the medical team, and they are not involved in medical decisions. Access to a patient's medical data chart is not always allowed for pharmacists, and only in a small number of medical cases do physicians seek their advice regarding drug administration. In this situation, a hospital pharmacist cannot determine whether a medical treatment is appropriate for the needs or conditions of a patient.

Hospital pharmacists are not always involved in the elaboration of medical guidelines; their involvement in therapeutic acts being limited. The restricted participation in the provision of healthcare has, on the other hand, a bright side. Hospital pharmacists are not held liable for professional errors, ethical dilemmas, or malpractice issues. When compared to other medical specialties in the country, hospital pharmacists have higher scores for job satisfaction than forensic physicians or obstetrics and gynecological physicians in the country [30].

3.4. Strengths and Limitations of the Study

The strength of the present study is provided by the results referring to a medical specialty scarcely featured in the scientific literature. Results of studies targeting hospital pharmacists' job satisfaction are missing in Romania, and the present study is the first that is developed in the country. The results are representative, when considering the fact that the number of hospital pharmacists working in public institutions is relatively small.

The first limitation is due to the small number of male subjects, and a significant comparative analysis was not statistically relevant; the second limitation is related to national policies and legislation that is applied in this medical field, which have an important impact on the level of satisfaction among hospital pharmacists in Romania. Finally, another limitation is due to the poor Cronbach's alpha score for the first domain of TAS-20, which is why the results should be considered cautiously.

4. Conclusions

Hospital pharmacists in Romania obtained a low level of satisfaction with respect to payment and promotion dimensions, as well as a very high level of satisfaction for the management–interpersonal dimension, and a high level of satisfaction for the organization–communication dimension of job satisfaction. Most hospital pharmacists are discontent regarding the annual budget, the present legislation, and the relationships with staff working in the purchasing department and pharmaceutical company representatives. Since individual characteristics or alexithymia do not influence the level of job satisfaction, the results are important for health policy-makers in order for them to find ways to increase job satisfaction among hospital pharmacists in Romania, by focusing on professional issues and environmental factors, as well as on health policies.

Acknowledgments: This research was funded by research Grant No. 1/08.06.2016, offered by the National Association of Hospital Pharmacists in Romania (ANFSR).

Author Contributions: M.I. conceived and designed the experiments; I.A. and C.S. performed the experiments; and M.I. and C.D. analyzed the data and wrote the paper. The responses to reviewers' comments were jointly addressed by M.I., C.D., C.S. and I.A. All authors read and approved the final version of the manuscript.

References

1. Lau, W.M.; Pang, J.; Chui, W. Job satisfaction and the association with involvement in clinical activities among hospital pharmacists in Hong Kong. *Int. J. Pharm. Pract.* **2011**, *19*, 253–263. [CrossRef] [PubMed]

2. Mobley, W.H.; Locke, E.A. The relationship of value importance to satisfaction. *Organ. Behav. Hum. Perform.* **1970**, *5*, 463–483. [CrossRef]

3. Davis, K.; Nestrom, J.W. *Human Behavior at Work: Organizational Behavior*, 7th ed.; McGraw Hill: New York, NY, USA, 1985; Volume 109.

4. Munyewende, P.O.; Rispel, L.C.; Chirwa, T. Positive practice environments influence job satisfaction of primary health care clinic nursing managers in two South African provinces. *Hum. Res. Health* **2014**, *12*, 27. [CrossRef] [PubMed]

5. Aziri, B. Job Satisfaction: A Literature Review. *Manag. Res. Pract.* **2011**, *3*, 77–86.

6. Noel, M.W.; Hammel, R.J.; Bootman, J.L. Job satisfaction among hospital pharmacy personnel. *Am. J. Health-Syst. Pharm.* **1982**, *39*, 600–606.

7. Chui, M.A.; Look, K.A.; Mott, D.A. The association of subjective workload dimensions on quality of care and pharmacist quality of work life. *Res. Soc. Adm. Pharm.* **2014**, *10*, 328–340. [CrossRef] [PubMed]

8. Mak, V.S.; Clark, A.; March, G.; Gilbert, A.L. The Australian pharmacist workforce: Employment status, practice profile and job satisfaction. *Aust. Health Rev.* **2013**, *37*, 127–130. [CrossRef] [PubMed]

9. Ahmad, A.; Atique, S.; Balkrishnan, R.; Patel, I. Pharmacy profession in India: Current scenario and Recommendations. *Ind. J. Pharm. Edu. Res.* **2014**, *48*, 12–15.

10. Hale, A.; Coombes, I.; Stokes, J.; Aitken, S.; Clark, F.; Nissen, L. Patient satisfaction from two studies of collaborative doctor–pharmacist prescribing in Australia. *Health Expect.* **2016**, *19*, 49–61. [CrossRef] [PubMed]

11. Kahn, W.A.; Heaphy, E.D. Relational contexts of personal engagement at work. In *Employee Engagement in Theory and Practice*; Routledge: Abingdon-on-Thames, UK, 2014; pp. 82–96.

12. Kumar, P.; Mehra, A.; Inder, D.; Sharma, N. Organizational commitment and intrinsic motivation of regular and contractual primary health care providers. *J. Fam. Med. Prim. Care* **2016**, *5*, 94. [CrossRef] [PubMed]

13. Kerschen, A.M.; Armstrong, E.P.; Hillman, T.N. Job satisfaction among staff, clinical, and integrated hospital pharmacists. *J. Pharm. Pract.* **2006**, *19*, 306–312. [CrossRef]

14. Baum, A. Stress, intrusive imagery, and chronic distress. *Health Psychol.* **1990**, *9*, 653–675. [CrossRef] [PubMed]

15. Suleiman, A.K. Stress and job satisfaction among pharmacists in Riyadh, Saudi Arabia. *Saudi J. Med. Med. Sci.* **2015**, *3*, 213. [CrossRef]

16. Robers, P.A. Job satisfaction among US pharmacists. *Am. J. Health-Syst. Pharm.* **1983**, *40*, 391–399.

17. Higuchi, Y.; Inagaki, M.; Koyama, T.; Kitamura, Y.; Sendo, T.; Fujimori, M.; Uchitomi, Y.; Yamada, N. A cross-sectional study of psychological distress, burnout, and the associated risk factors in hospital pharmacists in Japan. *BMC Public Health* **2016**, *16*, 534. [CrossRef] [PubMed]

18. Schafheutle, E.I.; Seston, E.M.; Hassell, K. Factors Influencing Pharmacist Performance: A review of the peer-reviewed literature. *Health Policy* **2011**, *102*, 178–192. [CrossRef] [PubMed]

19. Moghada, M.J.F.; Peiravian, F.; Naderi, A.; Rajabzadeh, A.; Rasekh, H.R. An analysis of job satisfaction among Iranian pharmacists through various job characteristics. *Iran. J. Pharm. Res. IJPR* **2014**, *13*, 1087–1096.

20. Hassell, K.; Seston, E.; Shann, P. Measuring job satisfaction of UK pharmacists: A pilot study. *Int. J. Pharm. Pract.* **2007**, *15*, 259–264. [CrossRef]

21. Al Khalidi, D.; Wazaify, M. Assessment of pharmacists' job satisfaction and job related stress in Amman. *Int. J. Clin. Pharm.* **2013**, *35*, 821–828. [CrossRef] [PubMed]

22. Bond, C.A.; Raehl, C.L. Pharmacists' assessment of dispensing errors: Risk factors, practice sites, professional functions, and satisfaction. *Pharmacother* **2001**, *21*, 614–626. [CrossRef]

23. Nichols, P.; Copeland, T.S.; Craib, I.A.; Hopkins, P.; Bruce, D.G. Learning from error: Identifying contributory causes of medication errors in an Australian hospital. *Med. J. Aust.* **2008**, *188*, 276–279.

24. Ahmad, A.; Patel, I. Job satisfaction among Indian pharmacists. *J. Pharm. Bioallied Sci.* **2013**, *5*, 326. [CrossRef] [PubMed]

25. Mott, D.A.; Doucette, W.R.; Gaither, C.A.; Pedersen, C.A.; Schommer, J.C. Pharmacists' attitudes toward worklife: Results from a national survey of pharmacists. *J. Am. Pharm. Assoc.* **2004**, *44*, 326–336. [CrossRef]

26. Majd, M.; Hashemian, F.; YounesiSisi, F.; Jalal, M.; Majd, Z. Quality of Life and Job Satisfaction of Dispensing Pharmacists Practicing in Tehran Private-sector Pharmacies. *Iran. J. Pharm. Res.* **2012**, *11*, 1039–1044. [PubMed]

27. McHugh, P.P. Pharmacists' attitudes regarding quality of worklife. *J. Am. Pharm. Assoc.* **1999**, *39*, 667–676. [CrossRef]

28. Nyame-Myreku, M.N. *Determinants of Job Satisfaction Among Hospital Pharmacists and Their Intent to Leave Using Herzberg's Two-Factor Theory*; Capella University, ProQuest Dissertations Publishing: Minneapolis, MN, USA, 2012.

29. Benslimane, N.; Khalifa, M. Evaluating Pharmacists' Motivation and Job Satisfaction Factors in Saudi Hospitals. In *Unifying the Applications and Foundations of Biomedical and Health Informatics*; IOS Press: Amsterdam, the Netherlands, 2016; pp. 201–204.

30. Iorga, M.; Dondas, C.; Ioan, B.G.; Toader, E. Job Satisfaction among Forensic Physicians in Romania. *Revista de Cercetare si Interventie Sociala* **2017**, *56*, 5–18.

31. Vlădescu, C.; Scîntee, G.; Olsavszky, V.; Allin, S.; Mladovsky, P. Romania: Health system review. *Health Syst. Trans.* **2008**, *10*, 1–172.

32. Vermeulen, L.C.; Moles, R.J.; Collins, J.C.; Gray, A.; Sheikh, A.L.; Surugue, J.; Ranjit, E. Revision of the International Pharmaceutical Federation's Basel Statements on the future of hospital pharmacy: From Basel to Bangkok. *Am. J. Health-Syst. Pharm.* **2016**, *73*, 1077–1086. [CrossRef] [PubMed]

33. Rechel, B.; Lessof, S.; Busse, R.; McKee, M.; Figueras, J.; Mossialos, E.; van Ginneken, E. A Framework for Health System Comparisons: The Health Systems in Transition (HiT). In *Series of the European Observatory on Health Systems and Policies*; WHO: Copenhagen, Denmark, 2016.

34. Vlădescu, C.; Scîntee, S.G.; Olsavszky, V.; Hernández-Quevedo, C.; Sagan, A. Romania: Health system review. *Health Syst. Trans.* **2016**, *18*, 1–170.

35. Stoica-Constantin, A.; Constantin, T. *Conflict, Change, and Organizational Health*; Editura Universității Alexandru Ioan Cuza: Iași, Romania, 2009.

36. Bagby, R.M.; Parker, J.D.; Taylor, G.J. The twenty-item Toronto Alexithymia Scale—I. Item selection and cross-validation of the factor structure. *J. Psychosom. Res.* **1994**, *38*, 23–32. [PubMed]

37. Sansgiry, S.S.; Ngo, C. Factors affecting job satisfaction among hospital pharmacists. *Hosp. Pharm.* **2003**, *38*, 1037–1046.

38. Popa, D.; Bazgan, M. Job Satisfaction and Performance in the Context of the Romanian Educational Reform. *J. Eng. Stud. Res.* **2011**, *17*, 79–84.

39. Liu, C.S.; White, L. Key determinants of hospital pharmacy staff's job satisfaction. *Res. Soc. Admin. Pharm.* **2011**, *7*, 51–63. [CrossRef] [PubMed]

9

Simulation as a Central Feature of an Elective Course: Does Simulated Bedside Care Impact Learning?

Michael C. Thomas * and **Peter J. Hughes**

McWhorter School of Pharmacy, Samford University, Birmingham, AL 35229, USA; pjhughes@samford.edu
* Correspondence: mthoma13@samford.edu

Abstract: A three-credit, simulation-based, emergency medicine elective course was designed and offered to doctor of pharmacy students for two years. The primary objective was to determine if there was a difference in exam performance stratified by student simulation experience, namely either as an active observer or as part of bedside clinical care. The secondary objective was to report student satisfaction. Examination performance for simulation-based questions was compared based on the student role (evaluator versus clinical) using the Student's t-test. Summary responses from Likert scale-based student satisfaction responses were collected. A total of 24 students took the course: 12 in each offering. Performance was similar whether the student was assigned to the evaluation team or the clinical team for all of the comparisons (mid-term and final 2015 and 2016, all p-values > 0.05). Students were very satisfied with the course. Of the 19 questions assessing the qualitative aspects of the course, all of the students agreed or strongly agreed to 17 statements, and all of the students were neutral, agreed, or strongly agreed to the remaining two statements. Direct participation and active observation in simulation-based experiences appear to be equally valuable in the learning process, as evidenced by examination performance.

Keywords: simulation; emergency medicine; pharmacy practice

1. Introduction

High-fidelity simulation has been used to imitate a behavior or process as part of training in military, aviation, and medical professions [1]. Its use in schools/colleges of pharmacy appears to be common; however, the extent within individual curricula is variable [2]. Many reports detail either a single simulation activity or a limited number of simulation activities [3–6]. Results from a systematic review of 109 medical simulation studies identified 12 features that lead to effective learning: feedback, repetitive practice, curriculum integration, increasing difficulty, adaptability to various learning styles, a variety of clinical problems, a controlled learning environment, individualized learning, clearly defined outcomes, and the degree of realism [7]. These best practices were included as the framework in the design of an elective course.

The sole professional pharmacy degree in the Unites States is the doctor of pharmacy (PharmD). Doctor of pharmacy degree programs must be accredited by the Accreditation Council for Pharmacy Education by meeting minimum standards in the professional curriculum [8]. Coursework for PharmD students is commonly completed in four years after students complete their prerequisite coursework. The practice of pharmacy is complex. According to outcomes published by the Center for the Advancement of Pharmacy Education, pharmacists need to be learners, caregivers, managers, promoters, providers, problem solvers, educators, advocates, collaborators, includers, communicators, self-aware, leaders, innovators, and professionals [9]. Similarly, thought leaders were asked to predict the future importance of a number of areas of pharmacy practice. Competencies that were predicted to increase in importance included patient care, using information technology, critical thinking and problem solving, communication, and contributing to patient care teams [10]. Becoming a professional begins with the white coat ceremony for most doctor of pharmacy students in the United States [11]. If pharmacy students are inculcated into the profession after donning the white coat, they should begin to think and act like professionals well before entering their advanced pharmacy practice experiences (APPE). This attitude was summarized in an editorial response written by a student when he called for institutions to provide an environment that helps students grow professionally [12]. However, students need ample opportunity to practice, receive correction, and improve in a safe environment.

Over the last decade, emergency pharmacy practice expanded in the United States, with recent data indicating that 16.4% of hospitals were assigning a pharmacist to the emergency department (ED) [13]. The practice of pharmacy in emergency departments within the United States has been recently described. Based on this nationwide survey of pharmacists in the United States, ED-based pharmacists dedicate a significant amount of time on direct patient care activities related to medication management and time-dependent emergencies such as cardiac arrest, stroke, or trauma [14]. Similarly, opportunities for pharmacy students completing APPEs in this area are offered by most schools/colleges of pharmacy, commonly as electives [15]. However, pharmacy students are unlikely to be exposed to specialized clinical areas such as emergency medicine before their APPEs. With appropriate facilities and expertise, students can experience unique areas of practice in a safe and controlled environment. The present course was purposely designed to blend both didactic and simulation-based learning. This manuscript describes the design of the course, the effect of simulation on examination performance, and student perceptions over a two-year period. This project received institutional review board approval. All of the subjects who took the class opted into the data analysis, and signed an informed consent to be included in the analysis. The main objective of this investigation was to determine if there was a difference in the examination performance for students participating in simulation activities at the bedside versus those who actively observed and evaluated bedside activities. An additional objective was to determine student perception of the course and associated activities using course and supplemental questions.

2. Materials and Methods

The elective course was called Topics in Emergency Medicine, a Simulated Approach. It was designed to give students the opportunity to expand their experiences and practice pharmacy in a simulated hospital setting that included both clinical and operational pharmacy experiences. It was offered and capped at 12 students in the spring semester of the second professional year in a doctor of pharmacy program. Bedside simulation activities were conducted using the simulation suite housed in the college of pharmacy building. The simulation suite contained a high-fidelity mannequin (iStan, CAE Healthcare, Sarasota, FL, USA) and was made to look like a hospital room (Figure 1a). It had a fully functioning hospital bed, emergency cart (simulated medications, airway devices, intravenous fluids, etc.), suction canister, and associated furniture. On a separate floor in the building, there was a mock pharmacy that can be used to simulate retail or hospital pharmacy activities. The mock pharmacy was equipped with a laminar flow hood, multiple computer terminals, and simulated drugs (Figure 1b,c). A third tool that was used for simulation activities was live video streaming technology (LearningSpace, CAE Heatlhcare, Sarasota, FL, USA). Multiple cameras were located in each simulation area, offering several viewpoints. There was the capability to record and live-stream any of the audio and video feeds using any computer with Internet access. Live video technology was used in this course to allow students the ability to evaluate simulation activities in an adjacent room in real time without disrupting the clinical team (Figure 1d).

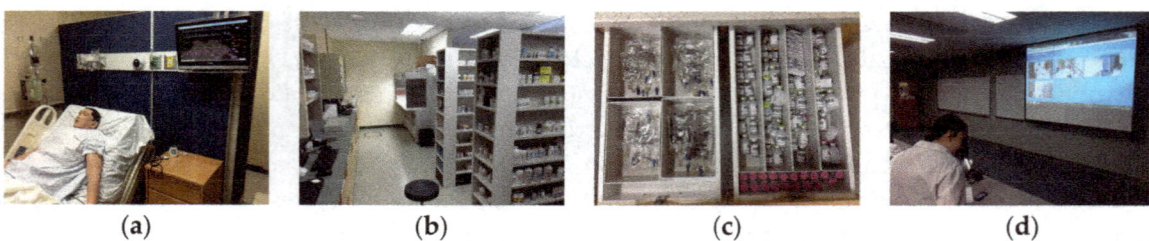

(a)   **(b)**   **(c)**   **(d)**

Figure 1. Images showing key elements of the simulated environment: (**a**) Simulation suite showing high-fidelity mannequin; (**b**) Mock pharmacy; (**c**) Simulated medications; (**d**) Classroom showing live video feed of simulation.

Both didactic and simulation-based educational strategies were used for each week of this three-credit elective. Topics were chosen by the instructor based on their ability to design simulation activities, and when pharmacotherapy principles were essential for the care of patients in an emergency setting. Each week, a new disease state or condition was covered in a 75-min lecture-based class. After about three weeks of fundamental material, specific clinical content was introduced. Topics included: basic life support, advanced cardiovascular life support, anaphylaxis, electrolyte emergencies, hypertensive emergency, venous thromboembolism, seizures, acute ischemic stroke, acute toxicology, and rapid sequence intubation with post-sedation management. The lectures served as the foundational knowledge that students would need in the simulation experiences. The next 75-min class period was devoted to simulation experiences. At the beginning of the semester, the instructor assigned each student to one of two teams. On simulation days, the class would report to either the mock pharmacy or the simulation area based on their assigned team. Each team had 35 min in each area every week. The teams would switch and report to the other area (mock pharmacy or simulation area).

Although the main focus of the course was related to emergency pharmacy practice, students were also given the opportunity to experience the operational aspects of a mock hospital pharmacy. When the course was designed, the instructor wanted learners in the course to experience a full sense of realism whenever possible. Using the mock pharmacy allowed expanded realism, decreased group size in the simulation suite, and allowed the practice of previously learned skills such as making parenteral compounds. For example, if a medication was needed in the simulation suite, a verbal order would need to be called in to the inpatient mock pharmacy, and subsequently the medication would be prepared, checked, and delivered to the bedside. These steps of the medication use processes are important for pharmacy practice in the hospital environment. They allowed students in the mock pharmacy to exercise practical skills while increasing a sense of realism. As students reported to their assigned area, they would learn their assigned role for the day. There were six defined roles in the mock pharmacy. These were designed so that students would have a variety of rotating experiences. Each role had an associated letter labeled: A, a, B, b, C, c. The roles and responsibilities were reviewed prior to the first simulation experience, and the definitions of each role were included on printed instructions located in the mock pharmacy. The responsibility of each role was as follows: 'A' received telephone orders, entered the orders into the pharmacy order entry system (Neehr Perfect), and answered the drug information question. The role of 'a' was to help the 'A' with the drug information question, verify the appropriate entry of the medication order, and print any labels that were needed for the telephone order. There were two roles (B, b) focused on parenteral medications. One was responsible for cleaning the laminar flow hood, and they were responsible for preparation of parenteral products. The other role was responsible for checking a pre-arranged intravenous (IV) batch. This was typically five to six products that contained two to three planted mistakes. Any mistakes identified required the student making parenteral products to prepare the correct product. The final two roles (C, c) were focused on the entry and verification of admission orders. Printed orders were provided, and medication orders were entered into the pharmacy order entry system with subsequent verification. All six roles were intentionally designed to provide students with practical experiences in inpatient pharmacy environments. Since the course had multi-week simulations, each student had experience in each role.

The teams in the mock pharmacy use operational pharmacy notes to track the completion of their tasks (Figure 2). This template is where they documented the answer to their drug information question, how many errors they found in the IV batch, the results of their peer-to-peer order entry, and a space to communicate any issues that may still be confusing to members of the team.

Operational Pharmacy Note

Names   Date:_____
A:_____
a:_____
B:_____
b:_____
C:_____
c:_____

☐ Drug Information Question in Folder

Answer to Drug Information Question:_____
_____
_____
_____
_____

☐ STAT Order Transcribed on Form 0923 PHYSICIAN ORDERS and placed in
      folder
Database used as a reference for STAT order _____
   ☐ Order entered into VistA
   ☐ Verified by "a"
   ☐ Time from receipt of order to drug leaving the pharmacy (min:sec)_____

Instructions for preparation of STAT order (e.g., amount of drug, diluent, etc...)_____
_____
_____

Number of errors with IV batch requiring remaking_____

Description of each error (be specific)_____
_____
_____
_____
_____

Number of Admission Orders Entered_____

Number of Admission Orders Verified_____

Number of Errors Found by "c" on Admission Orders_____

What confusion remains?_____
_____
_____
_____

Figure 2. Operational pharmacy note template.

The other team was further split into two groups of three, and reported to the simulation area. One group entered a classroom adjacent to the simulation suite, and was responsible for evaluating and debriefing the clinical team that was taking care of the patient. If students were on the clinical team one week, they would be on the evaluation team the following week, and vice versa. This allowed an equal distribution of experiences. They had several camera views projected onto a large screen of the team interacting with the high-fidelity mannequin in addition to a feed that showed the vital signs and waveforms (e.g., an electrocardiogram lead) of the mannequin. The debrief team used a form that was designed for this class to guide the debrief of the clinical team on five domains (verbal expression, non-verbal expression, response to the patient, degree of focus, logic, coherence, and overall performance), and provide feedback on areas of strength (+) and areas of improvement (delta) for each domain (Figure 3).

Debrief Worksheet

Date:

Debrief Team:

Debrief Team Leader:

Simulation Team:

	Positive	Delta
Verbal Expression		
Non-Verbal Expression		
Response to the Patient		
Degree of Focus, Logic, Coherence		
Overall		

Figure 3. Debrief worksheet.

The three students who were assigned to the simulation suite had limited or no information about the patient before entering the room. However, students were aware that the main problem would be from the previous class's didactic material. When they entered the room, they needed to gather information from multiple sources. Information may come from an actor playing the part of a family member in the room, the patient, the medical chart, or a combination of these elements. During the 15-min simulation, students needed to synthesize the important information that was necessary to make decisions (focused physical exam, allergies, home medications, etc.). If the patient required immediate treatment, including pharmacotherapy, it was the students' responsibility to order it from the mock pharmacy (if not in the crash cart) or administer it to the patient (if it was in the crash cart) with appropriate reassessment. At the end of 15 min, the simulation was terminated, and the clinical team had 15 min to compose a clinical progress note. During this time, the debrief team (those watching from the adjacent room) also used this time to discuss their observations and complete the debrief form. After 15 min, the debrief team entered the simulation suite and guided a discussion about the team's performance, including positive elements and opportunities for improvement. Similar to the mock pharmacy experience, the roles of students rotated from week to week, and each student had multiple experiences with each role throughout the semester.

During simulation days, the main role of the instructor was facilitator. Due to the time-sensitive nature of each activity, the instructor would provide time cues or delegate time cues as appropriate. However, every effort was made to avoid entering the simulation room until the time was up with the high-fidelity mannequin in order to preserve authenticity. The instructor would stop into the mock pharmacy and ensure there were not any questions or technology issues. Oftentimes, students would ask about procedural issues that they may face as a pharmacist in a hospital setting. While the debrief team watched the simulation, the instructor could probe the small group for questions on how the simulation group was doing with communication, therapeutic decision making, acting on critical vital signs, or similar lines of questioning. All of the simulation events were recorded, archived, and available to the instructor for review.

3. Results

This investigation focused on two areas of assessment. The first was performance on examination questions stratified by student role in the simulation (evaluation team or clinical team), and the second was student satisfaction with the course.

Performance in this course was evaluated through assignment completion, participation, and examination performance. A total of 55% of the course grade was group performance, and 45% was based on individual efforts. Group efforts were graded through assessing clinical (25%) and operational pharmacy notes (25%) against a grading rubric. Additionally, groups were assessed on their debrief note and discussion with the clinical team (5%) Individually, students were assessed for professionalism and participation (10%) and performance on two written examinations, a mid-term (17.5%) and comprehensive final examination (17.5%). The examinations were paper-based and included fill-in-the-blank, multiple choice, and matching. The questions covered material from simulations and the didactic portion of the course.

Twenty-four students were enrolled in the course: 12 in each semester it was offered. One student in the second offering of the course was unable to finish, but did complete the mid-term examination and associated course activities.

The course design allowed students to equally experience simulation at the bedside and being part of the debrief team. Examination questions were written based on learning objectives for the didactic portion of the course. Some learning objectives were reinforced during the bedside simulation activities. Content on examinations could be derived solely from the didactic lecture or, when it was also experienced, in the simulation suite. Using the simulation objectives, the instructor determined whether every question on mid-term and final examinations addressed experiences in the simulation. Since students were either on the clinical team or evaluation team for every simulation, this allowed for a comparison of exam performance on questions directly addressed by their role in the simulation experiences (Table 1). Using the Student's t-test, clinical and evaluation teams performed similarly on mid-term and final examinations over two years. The amount of each examination that was directly attributed to simulation objectives was: 25 out of 50 (50%) for the mid-term in 2015; 57 out of 77 (74%) for the final in 2015; 19 out of 52 (37%) for the mid-term in 2016; and 37 out of 77 (48%) for the final in 2016.

Table 1. Average performance on examination questions linked to simulation objectives.

Examination	Clinical Team (Mean ± SD)	Evaluation Team (Mean ± SD)	p-Value
Mid-term 2015 ($n = 12$)	67.5 ± 13.5%	71.6 ± 12.1%	0.30
Final 2015 ($n = 12$)	84.6 ± 6.3%	82.0 ± 6.2%	0.24
Mid-term 2016 ($n = 12$)	76.6 ± 11.5%	68.4 ± 12.9%	0.12
Final 2016 ($n = 11$)	72.7 ± 7.6%	73.2 ± 5.2%	0.45

SD = standard deviation.

Feedback on the class was sought from students using a standard course evaluation instrument and a supplementary set of questions specific to this course. These evaluations were administered during the last week of each semester according to guidelines established at the college of pharmacy.

Each question or domain was assessed on a five-point Likert scale (Strongly Disagree, Agree, Neither Agree or Disagree, Agree, Strongly Agree). Students were also free to submit open-ended comments.

Students rated a total of 21 evaluative statements. The course was very well received. All of the students agreed or strongly agreed to 19 of the statements, and 95% agreed or strongly agreed to the two remaining statements. No statement received a score of less than neutral. The complete results are shown in Table 2. The course evaluation instrument generated 71 total comments. The majority of comments were positive ($n = 68$; 94%), and were categorized into seven categories: Enjoyable ($n = 23$), Challenging ($n = 10$), Effective/Beneficial ($n = 10$), Teamwork ($n = 2$), Realism ($n = 8$), and Learning ($n = 15$). The comments that were related to improvement opportunities included two that felt increased time for simulation would be beneficial, and one desired a different pharmacy order entry system.

Table 2. Course evaluation responses by students.

Statement	SD %	D %	N %	A %	SA %
The course objectives were well covered ($n = 22$)	0	0	0	9.1	90.9
The course expectations were met ($n = 22$)	0	0	0	9.1	90.9
The course challenged me intellectually ($n = 22$)	0	0	0	4.5	95.5
The course concepts were presented in an organized manner ($n = 22$)	0	0	0	13.6	86.4
Instructional material(s) increased my understanding ($n = 22$)	0	0	0	4.5	95.5
The course assignments were interesting and stimulating ($n = 22$)	0	0	0	4.5	95.5
The course helped me to develop stronger critical thinking skills ($n = 22$)	0	0	4.5	9.1	86.4
This course helped me develop skills I can use on APPE rotations in hospital settings ($n = 20$)	0	0	0	5	95
The simulation days helped me apply what I learned in the classroom ($n = 20$)	0	0	0	10	90
Bedside simulation using the high-fidelity simulation man (iStan) was valuable to my learning ($n = 20$)	0	0	0	5	95
Order entry in the mock pharmacy was valuable to my learning ($n = 20$)	0	0	5	30	65
Making intravenous admixtures was valuable to my learning ($n = 20$)	0	0	0	10	90
Checking order entry was valuable to my learning ($n = 20$)	0	0	0	20	80
Checking intravenous admixtures was valuable to my learning ($n = 20$)	0	0	0	20	80
Receiving and transcribing a telephone order was valuable to my learning ($n = 20$)	0	0	0	20	80
The course improved my ability to self-assess ($n = 20$)	0	0	0	25	75
The course improved my confidence in making intravenous admixtures ($n = 20$)	0	0	0	25	75
The course improved my communication skills amongst team members ($n = 20$)	0	0	0	20	80
The course improved my ability to effectively communicate with patients in the acute care setting ($n = 20$)	0	0	0	25	75
The simulation and mock pharmacy experiences felt realistic	0	0	0	15	85
Considering the content covered in the course, I would be able to positively contribute to the care of a real patient	0	0	0	15	85

SD = Strongly disagree; D = disagree; N = Neutral; A = Agree; SA = Strongly Agree; APPE: advanced pharmacy practice experiences.

4. Discussion

In this novel simulation-based emergency medicine elective course, performance on objective examination questions did not differ based on participation in bedside simulation activities on the clinical team or active observation through participation on the evaluation team. Additionally, the course was well received, and students felt that the experiences prepared them for authentic patient care activities. This course is unique in educating pharmacy learners in emergency medicine because it provided repeat simulation experiences over the entire semester. This repetitive element is a core feature that leads to effective learning using simulation [7]. Only one other example was found in the pharmacy education literature of repetitive simulation activities [16].

Students were exposed to eight to 10 simulation activities. For about half of the activities, students were active observers of the clinical team in the simulation suite, and for the other half of the activities, the students were active participants as part of the clinical team. Simulation-based learning activities allow students to practice taking care of patients in safe environments where mistakes become teachable moments instead of medical errors. Simulation-based activities help students practice skills such as communication and physical assessment while integrating clinical aspects of care.

There is an ongoing debate as to the "practice readiness" of doctor of pharmacy graduates [17,18]. It likely depends on the area of pharmacy practice; however, students learn more through active learning than passive methods [19]. Active learning requires an application of knowledge and skills, and helps students apply information to future situations [20]. Few studies have been conducted to compare simulation-based activities to traditional instruction. However, one study of simulation-based activities was shown to be superior to problem-based learning in a group of fourth-year medical students [21]. Although the design of this course did not allow the measurement of distinct methods of teaching, it did allow for a comparison based on experiences within the course (clinical team versus evaluation team). The results showed that during simulation experiences, active observation or participation produced a similar performance on examination questions. It should be noted that all of the students received the same didactic lecture material, and all of the exam questions were directed toward the attainment of didactic learning objectives. By virtue of the course design, some of these objectives were reinforced during simulation-based activities. The results are reassuring, because taking part in both teams (observer or participant) was deemed important to the design of the course. In other investigations, it was not clear whether simulation improved examination performance. For example, a recent study of doctor of pharmacy students showed that performance on a written examination was no different if students took part in classroom lecture or a high-fidelity simulation for teaching advanced cardiac life support [20]. Other studies have shown improvement in pre-knowledge and post-knowledge [4,16,22].

In regards to student perceptions of the course, the results were very positive, and are consistent with other reports of student perceptions of learning and the effectiveness of simulation-based activities [3,6,11,23,24]. All of the students agreed or strongly agreed with the statement: "This course helped me develop skills I can use on APPE rotations in hospital settings". Similarly, all of the students selected agree or strongly agree to the statement: "Considering the content covered in the course, I would be able to positively contribute to the care of a real patient". Both of these lend support for a step toward practice readiness.

This course provided weekly opportunities for students to apply material learned in the classroom and test their understanding in settings that they will encounter in a hospital-based practice. They were challenged to provide formative feedback to their peers and work under tight time constraints to get all of the work done. Over the semester, they became more efficient and adept at each of the assigned tasks. Observationally, they seemed to treat the mannequin as a real patient. Students conducted themselves in a professional manner while at the bedside. One element that was likely underestimated at the genesis of the course was the importance of communication as a central feature. Over time, the teams improved their ability to gather information from the patient, the chart, and the patient monitor. Students improved internal communication, and worked more efficiently and effectively as a team. The clinical team received both praise and criticism from the debrief team, which shaped and improved communication and decision making in the simulation suite. The debrief teams demonstrated interpersonal communication skills as they filled out the debrief worksheet, and decided what elements to include. Finally, they communicated their findings with respect. Students actively watching the simulation had the luxury of talking without disrupting the simulation. It also afforded opportunities for the instructor to capitalize on teachable moments while in the room observing the simulation.

Although not directly assessed on examinations, the experiences in the mock pharmacy provided realistic experiences. The operational pharmacy teams rotated their roles, and each student had experiences that were similar to an inpatient hospital pharmacy. They worked to support the care of the patient in the simulation suite by taking a telephone order, properly labeling the product, and delivering it to the bedside in a short amount of time. The focus during each simulation experience was less about the right decision, and more about the process and learning from mistakes. When common misconceptions arose, these were reviewed during the didactic class time.

The qualities represented in this course are especially important since the publication and endorsement of the core entrustable professional activities (EPAs) for new pharmacy graduates [25]. The explicit nature of these activities is to set a baseline or standard for performance tasks that new graduates should be able to complete upon graduation from a doctor of pharmacy program. Specifically, the activities utilized in this elective course satisfied five of the six EPA domains (i.e., patient care provider domain, population health promoter domain, information master domain, and practice manager domain) [25]. Activities were not built into this course to satisfy the interprofessional team member domain, although this domain is a logical next step for the evolution of a course of this nature. Undergirding all of the core EPA domains are the tenets of professionalism, self-awareness, and communication, which are all skills or traits upon which students enrolled in this elective course depended for successful completion [25].

An essential aspect of this course was the use of a high-fidelity simulation mannequin. While this may be a perceived barrier, many colleges and schools have access to this technology. A survey conducted in 2013 reported that of the 88 responding schools, 30 had their own high-fidelity mannequin, and 47 had access to a formal simulation center [2]. For any simulation experience to be effective, sufficient planning is necessary to develop a sense of realism. Cases must be well designed knowing the capabilities of the equipment and personnel. For this course, cases were developed by a single instructor and reviewed with the simulation manager before each simulation activity. The simulation manager served as the voice of the patient and controlled physiologic responses as the disease was treated or not treated by students during the simulation. The instructor for the course could communicate with the simulation manager during the case using text messaging if there were obvious mistakes requiring dynamic adjustments to the case. For example, if students failed to provide epinephrine to a patient with anaphylaxis in a timely fashion, the patient's clinical condition would be programmed to deteriorate. Over the semester, cases became more complex, and required a chart with some elements at the bedside. For example, a 12-lead electrocardiogram was printed and put at the bedside for the pulmonary embolism case. Other times, there would be a focused physical exam note by the emergency physician noting his or her findings. This was because some things cannot be easily simulated, such as the results of a fundoscopic exam, or findings from the skin such as tenting, dry mucous membranes, or diaphoresis. When lab results were important, these were also placed on the bedside chart. A patient name band was also created using standard address labels affixed to colored paper and wrapped around the wrist. It contained the name of the patient and their date of birth.

To increase realism in the operational pharmacy, basic supplies were purchased. These included syringes, needles, alcohol pads, intravenous piggyback solutions in various sizes, and cleaning supplies for the laminar flow hood. Fortunately, there was a working laminar flow hood where parenteral products could be made in the mock pharmacy. This helped to increase realism; however, the activity could also be done on a workbench, and a flat surface could be defined as the laminar flow hood. Since simulated drugs can be expensive, every attempt was made to reuse supplies. For example, empty vials were used for the batch, and base solutions were continuously reused. Standard address labels containing drug names and concentrations were affixed to 10 mL of sterile water or 0.9% sodium chloride vials so that virtually any drug could be made available. Each week, about six to eight vials were used with the associated syringes and needles. To maintain realism, when compounding parenteral products, students would only use new vials, needles, and syringes.

There are several limitations to this investigation. First, there was some heterogeneity with respect to content delivery and testing from the first to second year. This was based on continuous improvement efforts and course refinement. However, the framework of the course remained unchanged, it was taught by a single instructor, and data analysis was conducted based on the experiences of each cohort. Secondly, the number of students was relatively small, and the investigation was conducted at a single institution.

It should be noted that implementing a course such as this could be very time consuming, especially during the planning phases. If details are not worked out, realism soon fades, and student confidence in the design may suffer. Checklists worked well to mitigate this potential challenge.

5. Conclusions

Performance on objective examination questions did not differ based on participation in bedside simulation activities or evaluating the clinical team. The course was very well received, and students felt that it prepared them for APPE experiences in the hospital setting, and to ultimately take care of patients.

Author Contributions: M.C.T. conceived and designed the study, analyzed the data, and drafted preliminary findings. M.C.T. and P.J.H. wrote and revised the paper.

Acknowledgments: This course was offered at Western New England University College of Pharmacy. The author would like to thank Benjamin Hogan and Thomas Moore for their help during the conduct and planning each simulation session as well as the students who participated in the course.

References

1. Bradley, P. The history of simulation in medical education and possible future directions. *Med. Educ.* **2006**, *40*, 254–262. [CrossRef] [PubMed]
2. Vyas, D.; Bray, B.S.; Wilson, M.N. Use of simulation-based teaching methodologies in US colleges and schools of pharmacy. *Am. J. Pharm. Educ.* **2013**, *77*, 53. [CrossRef] [PubMed]
3. Robinson, J.D.; Bray, B.S.; Willson, M.N.; Weeks, D.L. Using human patient simulation to prepare student pharmacists to manage medical emergencies in an ambulatory setting. *Am. J. Pharm. Educ.* **2011**, *75*, 3. [CrossRef] [PubMed]
4. Seybert, A.L.; Barton, C.M. Simulation-based learning to teach blood pressure assessment to doctor of pharmacy students. *Am. J. Pharm. Educ.* **2007**, *71*, 48. [CrossRef] [PubMed]
5. Davis, L.E.; Storjohann, T.D.; Spiegel, J.J.; Beiber, K.M.; Barletta, J.F. High-fidelity simulation for advanced cardiac life support training. *Am. J. Pharm. Educ.* **2013**, *77*, 59. [CrossRef] [PubMed]
6. Mieure, K.D.; Vincent, W.R., III; Cox, M.R.; Jonas, M.D. A high-fidelity simulation mannequin to introduce pharmacy students to advanced cardiovascular life support. *Am. J. Pharm. Educ.* **2010**, *74*, 22. [CrossRef] [PubMed]
7. Issenberg, S.B.; McGahie, W.C.; Petrusa, E.R.; Gordon, D.L.; Scalese, R.J. Features and uses of high-fidelity medical simulations that lead to effective learning: A BEME systematic review. *Med. Teach.* **2005**, *27*, 10–28. [CrossRef] [PubMed]
8. Accreditation Council for Pharmacy Education. Accreditation Standards and Key Elements for the Professional Program Leading to the Doctor of Pharmacy Degree ("Standards 2016"). Available online: www.acpe-accredit.org (accessed on 25 April 2018).
9. Medina, M.S.; Plaza, C.M.; Stowe, C.D.; Robinson, E.T.; DeLander, G.; Beck, D.E.; Melchert, R.B.; Supernaw, R.B.; Roche, V.F.; Gleason, B.L.; et al. Center for the advancement of pharmacy education 2013 educational outcomes. *Am. J. Pharm. Educ.* **2013**, *77*, 162. [CrossRef] [PubMed]
10. Beardsley, R.S.; Zorek, J.A.; Zellmer, W.A.; Vlasses, P.H. Results of the pre-conference survey: ACPE invitational conference on advancing quality in pharmacy education. *Am. J. Pharm. Educ.* **2013**, *77*, 46. [CrossRef] [PubMed]
11. Brown, D.L.; Ferrill, M.J.; Pankaskie, M.C. White coat ceremonies in US schools of pharmacy. *Ann. Pharmacother.* **2003**, *37*, 1414–1419. [CrossRef] [PubMed]
12. Karpen, S. Academic entitlement: A student's perspective. *Am. J. Pharm. Educ.* **2014**, *78*, 44. [CrossRef] [PubMed]
13. Pedersen, C.A.; Schneider, P.J.; Scheckelhoff, D.J. ASHP national survey of pharmacy practice in hospital settings: Prescribing and transcribing-2013. *Am. J. Health-Syst. Pharm.* **2014**, *71*, 924–942. [CrossRef] [PubMed]

14.   Thomas, M.C.; Acquisto, N.M.; Shirk, M.B.; Patanwala, A.E. A national survey of emergency pharmacy practice in the United States. *Am. J. Health-Syst. Pharm.* **2016**, *73*, 386–394. [CrossRef] [PubMed]

15.   Thomas, M.C.; Sun, S. Advanced pharmacy practice experiences for pharmacy students in emergency department settings. *Curr. Pharm. Teach. Learn.* **2015**, *7*, 378–381. [CrossRef]

16.   Seybert, A.; Kane-Gill, S.L. Elective course in acute care using online learning and patient simulation. *Am. J. Pharm. Educ.* **2011**, *75*, 54. [CrossRef] [PubMed]

17.   Murphy, J.E. Practice-readiness of US pharmacy graduates to provide direct patient care. *Pharmacotherapy* **2015**, *35*, 1091–1095. [CrossRef] [PubMed]

18.   Robinson, D.; Speede, M. Is post-graduate training essential for practice readiness? *Pharmacotherapy* **2015**, *35*, 1096–1099. [CrossRef] [PubMed]

19.   Deslauriers, L.; Schelew, E.; Wieman, C. Improved learning in a large-enrollment physics class. *Science* **2011**, *332*, 862–864. [CrossRef] [PubMed]

20.   Gleason, B.L.; Peeters, M.J.; Resman-Targoff, B.H.; Karr, S.; McBane, S.; Kelley, K.; Thomas, T.; Denetclaw, T.H. An active-learning strategies primer for achieving ability-based educational outcomes. *Am. J. Pharm. Educ.* **2011**, *75*, 186. [CrossRef] [PubMed]

21.   Steadman, R.H.; Coates, W.C.; Huang, Y.M.; Matevosian, R.; Larmon, B.R.; McCullough, L.; Ariel, D. Simulation-based training is superior to problem-based learning for the acquisition of critical assessment and management skills. *Crit. Care Med.* **2006**, *34*, 151–157. [CrossRef] [PubMed]

22.   Ray, S.M.; Wylie, D.R.; Rowe, A.S.; Heidel, E.; Franks, A.S. Pharmacy student knowledge retention after completing either a simulated or written patient case. *Am. J. Pharm. Educ.* **2012**, *76*, 86. [CrossRef] [PubMed]

23.   Seybert, A.L.; Laughlin, K.K.; Benedict, N.J.; Barton, C.M.; Rea, R.S. Pharmacy student response to patient-simulation mannequins to teach performance-based pharmacotherapeutics. *Am. J. Pharm. Educ.* **2006**, *70*, 48. [CrossRef] [PubMed]

24.   Fernandez, R.; Parker, D.; Kalus, J.S.; Miller, D.; Compton, S. Using a human patient simulation mannequin to teach interdisciplinary team skills to pharmacy students. *Am. J. Pharm. Educ.* **2007**, *71*, 51. [CrossRef] [PubMed]

25.   Haines, S.T.; Pittenger, A.L.; Stolte, S.K.; Plaza, C.M.; Gleason, B.L.; Kantorovich, A.; McCollum, M.; Trujillo, J.M.; Copeland, D.A.; Lacroix, M.M.; et al. Core entrustable professional activities for new pharmacy graduates. *Am. J. Pharm. Educ.* **2017**, *81*, S2. [PubMed]

10

Pharmacy Practice and Education in the Czech Republic [†]

Petr Nachtigal [1], Tomáš Šimůnek [1] and Jeffrey Atkinson [2,*]

[1]   Faculty of Pharmacy, Charles University, Akademika Heyrovského 1203,
     Hradec Králové 500 05, Czech Republic; Petr.Nachtigal@faf.cuni.cz (P.N.); Tomas.Simunek@faf.cuni.cz (T.Š.)
[2]   Pharmacolor Consultants Nancy, 12 rue de Versigny, 54600 Villers, France
*   Correspondence: jeffrey.atkinson@univ-lorraine.fr
†   Website of the Pharmacy faculty of the Charles University: www.faf.cuni.cz.

Academic Editor: Antonio Sanchez-Pozo

Abstract: The PHARMINE ("Pharmacy Education in Europe") project studied the organisation of pharmacy education, practice and legislation in the European Union (EU) with the objectives of evaluating to what degree harmonisation had taken place with the EU, and producing documents on each individual EU member state. Part of this work was in the form of a survey of pharmacy education, practice, and legislation in the various member states. We will publish the individual member state surveys as reference documents. This paper presents the results of the PHARMINE survey on pharmacy education, training, and practice in the Czech Republic. Czech community pharmacies sell and provide advice on Rx and Over-the-counter (OTC) medicines; they also provide diagnostic services (e.g., blood pressure measurement). Pharmacists (*lékárník* in Czech) study for five years and graduate with a *Magister* (Mgr., equivalent to M.Pharm.) degree. The Mgr. diploma is the only requirement for registration as a pharmacist. Pharmacists can own and manage community pharmacies, or work as responsible pharmacists in pharmacies. All practising pharmacists must be registered with the Czech Chamber of Pharmacists. The ownership of a community pharmacy is not restricted to members of the pharmacy profession; the majority of pharmacies are organised into various pharmacy chains. There are two universities providing higher education in pharmacy in the Czech Republic: the Faculty of Pharmacy in Hradec Kralove, Charles University, which was established in 1969, and the Faculty of Pharmacy of the University of Veterinary and Pharmaceutical Sciences in Brno, which was established in 1991. The pharmacy curriculum is organized as a seamless, fully integrated, five-year master degree course. There is a six-month traineeship supervised by the university, which usually takes place during the fifth year. Thus, the pharmacy curriculum is organised in accordance with the EU directive on sectoral professions that lays down the imperatives for pharmacy education, training, and practice in the various member states of the EU. Currently, no specialisation courses are available at the university level. Specialisation is organised in the form of postgraduate, continuing professional development by the Czech Chamber of Pharmacists, and delivered by the Institute of Postgraduate Education for Health Professions.

Keywords: pharmacy; education; practice; Czech Republic

1. Introduction

The PHARMINE ("Pharmacy Education in Europe") consortium surveyed the state of pharmacy education and practice in the member states of the EU, including the Czech Republic, in 2012, with an update in 2017. The methodology used in the PHARMINE study and the principal results obtained have already been published [1].

The PHARMINE consortium was interested in general practice and education, and in specialisation in pharmacy education for hospital and industrial pharmacy practice. Pharmacy education, training, and practice in the EU are unique in that they fall under two jurisdictions. As for other sectoral professions such as medicine, the European Commission issues directives on the education and training for the sectoral profession of pharmacy [2]. This directive lays down the broad imperatives for education and practice in the EU. An EU directive is a legal act that requires member states to achieve a particular result (in this case, the harmonisation of pharmacy training and practice) without dictating the means of achieving that result. Directives leave the 28 member states with an amount of leeway as to the exact laws and rules to be adopted. Member states may also embrace legislation on specific national practices, such as those relating to specialisation, as well as the ownership and management of community pharmacies.

The situation in Europe is further developed by the Bologna agreement on the harmonisation of the various European degree courses, and student and staff exchange [3]. The Bologna agreement, signed by the education ministers of the governments of the 48 members of the European Higher Education Area (which includes the 28 EU member states), proposes a bachelor (three years) plus master (two years) degree structure for all of the degrees, including pharmacy. This agreement is in opposition to the EU directive that stipulates a five-year "tunnel" degree structure for pharmacy, i.e., a degree course that has no possibility for intermediate entry or exit, for example, after a three-year bachelor period. Another aspect of the Bologna process is the development of tools to promote exchange, such as the European Credit Transfer and Accumulation System (ECTS), which provides credits to students for defined learning outcomes and their associated workload. Another tool is the Diploma Supplement, which provides a description of the nature, level, context, content, and status of the studies that were successfully completed by the student. These systems allow students to study for several months in another university in another EU member state and—importantly—to validate such studies carried out in their host university by their home university. This paper looks at how this system has developed in Czech universities.

The PHARMINE report also dealt with other personnel working in pharmacies, such as assistant pharmacists; their education, training, and responsibilities were surveyed.

In the light of the context described above, it is particularly interesting to examine how this affects pharmacy education and practice in a country—in this instance, the Czech Republic—that recently joined (in 2004) the EU.

Regarding the general health situation in the Czech Republic compared to the EU, life expectancy at birth (see Table 1) in the Czech Republic is only slightly lower than the EU average of 79.4 years, as is healthy life expectancy (EU average 70.2 years). However, it is worth noting that the expenditure on health is 33% lower than the EU average ($3611 per capita). As seen above, health expenditure is mainly in the public sector ($2013) rather than in the private sector ($69).

Table 1. Health statistics for the Czech Republic [4,5].

Total Population	10, 543, 000
Life expectancy at birth m/f/both sexes (years)	75.9/81.7/78.8
Healthy life expectancy at birth (years)	69.4
Total expenditure on health per capita	2434 $

2. Design

Information was obtained from various sources who replied to a questionnaire on pharmacy practice (community, hospital, and industrial), pharmacy organisation and legislation, pharmacy education and training, and finally the impact of the adoption of the Bologna declaration and the EU directive on the sectoral practice of pharmacy. The latter included information on the organisation of the degree course with or without the existence of a bachelor/master structure, and also on the effect of ECTS and the Erasmus programme on student and staff exchange [6].

The information is presented in the form of tables in order to facilitate legibility. This form of presentation was developed in association with this journal's editorial direction, and has been described in detail in a previous publication [7]. This presentation will ease: the consultation of these country profiles by students and staff envisaging exchange programmes with other member states, research on pharmacy education and practice in the EU, and other matters.

Much of the information for the Czech Republic was provided by the Ministry of Health of the Czech Republic [8].

3. Evaluation and Assessment

3.1. Organisation of the Activities of Pharmacists, Professional Bodies

Table 2 provides details of the numbers and activities of community pharmacists and pharmacies in the Czech Republic. Items such as competences are expounded upon in the "comments" column.

Table 2. Numbers and activities of community pharmacists and pharmacies [9], Appendix A.

Item	Numbers	Comments
Pharmacists	6000	1757 Inhabitants/Pharmacist
Pharmacies	2420 (+251 sub units)	Pharmacists/pharmacy: 2.2 Inhabitants/pharmacy: 3947
Competences and roles of community pharmacists		1. Supplying prescription and OTC medicines and medical devices, 2. Giving advice on medicines and lifestyle, 3. Compounding of medicines, 4. Keeping records (registration) of narcotic drugs, 5. Ordering of medicines, 6. Services to nursing and care homes, 7. Blood pressure and glycaemia monitoring, 8. Patient counselling service—individual consultations of drug-related problems, 9. Supplying prescriptions for wards in health care facilities, 10. Reporting of adverse drug reactions (ADR) to governmental authorities.
Is ownership of a community pharmacy limited to pharmacists?	No	Any physical or juridical person has legal right to own a public pharmacy [10].
Rules on geographical distribution of pharmacies?	No	There are no governmental restrictions on the geographical distribution of community pharmacies as a function of population density.
Are drugs and health care products available to the general public by channels other than pharmacies?	Yes	The following can deliver some health care products: (i) Veterinary doctors, (ii) Shops selling medical devices, (iii) Medical emergency teams, (iv) Hospitals

The data in Table 2 shows that compared with the EU linear regression estimation (for definition and calculation, see Atkinson and Rombaut, reference [1]), the ratio of the actual number of community pharmacists in the Czech Republic (/population) compared with the linear regression estimation for the Czech Republic = 0.84. Thus, the number of pharmacists per population is close to the EU norm. The same comparison for community pharmacies produces a ratio of 0.77.

The activities and occupations of pharmacists in the Czech Republic are similar to those of community pharmacists in other EU member states [1].

Table 3 provides details of the numbers and activities of assistant pharmacists in the Czech Republic.

Table 3. Numbers and activities of assistant pharmacists.

Item	Numbers	Comments
Are persons other than pharmacists involved in community practice?	Yes	In addition to pharmacists, assistant pharmacists are also considered to be professional pharmacy staff.
Their titles and number(s)	4600	In Czech, they are designated as "*Diplomovaný Specialista*" (DiS).
Organisations providing and validating education and training of assistant pharmacists		Education is provided by Medical Colleges and Secondary Medical Schools. Education is validated by passing the final exam, which is called the *Absolutorium*.
Duration of studies (years)	3 years	
Subject areas		English or German, Latin, Information and Communication Technologies, Chemistry and Biochemistry, Psychology and Communication, Health Education, Anatomy and Physiology, Microbiology and Hygiene, Human Nutrition, Pharmaceutical Botany, Analysis of Drugs, Pharmacology, Compounding of Medicines, Laboratory Technology, First Aid, Pathophysiology and Pathology, Pharmacognosy, Pharmaceutical Chemistry, Basics of Radiology, Pharmacy Practice, Public Health Care, Dispensing, Medical Devices, Practical Training.
Competences and roles		1. Supplying OTC drugs, 2. Medical devices and other health products, 3. Compounding of medicines.

The legislation of the Czech Republic recognises assistant pharmacists as health care professionals. Although their education and training is in the form of a three-year course, it cannot be compared with a "B. Pharm.", as defined by the Bologna declaration (see above).

Table 4 provides details of the numbers and activities of hospital pharmacists in the Czech Republic.

Table 4. Numbers and activities of hospital pharmacists.

Item	Numbers	Comments
Does such a function exist?	Yes	The legislation covers: - the area of state-owned hospitals (and hospital pharmacies) - list of pharmaceutical specializations including hospital pharmacy - specialisation curricula, including hospital pharmacy
Number of hospital pharmacists	430	
Number of hospital pharmacies	93	
Competences and roles of hospital pharmacists		1. Supplying of prescription medicines for wards and outpatient clinics 2. Clinical pharmacy consulting, 3. Compounding of medicines for wards and outpatients, 4. Production of patient-specific medicines (e.g., cytotoxic preparations, all-in-one sterile bags), 5. Supplying of specialised individual medical devices for patients and medical materials for wards, 6. Supplying and check of raw materials for the pharmacy and specialised laboratories of the hospital, 7. Supplying and evidence of narcotic drugs, 8. Adverse effects reporting, 9. Participation in clinical drug evaluation (safety and efficacy), 10. Patient counselling service—individual consultations of drug-related problems, 11. Information service for healthcare professionals.

The number of hospital pharmacists is low when compared with the EU average. The ratio of the actual number compared with the linear regression estimation = 0.40, (for definition and calculation, see Atkinson and Rombaut, reference [1]). The ratio for hospital pharmacies compared with the EU average is 0.59.

Table 5 provides details of the numbers and activities of industrial pharmacists and pharmacists in other sectors, in the Czech Republic.

Table 5. Numbers and activities of industrial pharmacists and pharmacists in other sectors.

Item	Numbers	Comments
Industrial Pharmacy and Pharmacists		
Number of pharmaceutical companies with production, R&D, and distribution	228	There are 228 licensed distributors in the Czech Republic. There are no reliable sources to divide the producers and distributors according to the mentioned groups.
Companies producing generic drugs only		Zentiva (https://www.zentiva.com/) Teva Pharmaceutical Industries Ltd. (http://www.tevapharm.com/)
Number of pharmacists working in industry	15	These are only the persons registered with the Czech Chamber of Pharmacists. There are possibly many more, but this number is not known, since they need not be registered with the Czech Chamber of Pharmacists.
Competences and roles		1. Preclinical drug evaluation (safety and efficacy), 2. Clinical drug evaluation (safety and efficacy), 3. Research, 4. Technology, 5. Management, 6. Marketing, Control, 7. Production, 8. Development, 9. Business.
Pharmacists Working in Other Sectors		
Number of pharmacists working in other sectors	43	These are only the persons registered with the Czech Chamber of Pharmacists. There are possibly many more, but this number is not known, since they need not be registered with the Czech Chamber of Pharmacists.
Sectors in which pharmacists are employed		1. Armed forces, 2. Secondary school education and training, 3. Universities, 4. National health services, 5. SUKL (State Institution of Drug Control: registration of drugs—www.sukl.cz), 6. IKEM (Institute of Clinical and Experimental Medicine—clinical trials—www.ikem.cz), 7. Laboratories (research, production, control, development), 8. Distribution, 9. Sales management and marketing.
Competences and roles in other sectors		Education and Training, Research, Management, Control, Production, Consulting, Drug evaluation and registration.

Industrial pharmacists in the Czech Republic have similar practices and duties to those in other EU countries [1]. As the numbers of industrial pharmacists were not available for most of the European countries, a comparison with the EU average is not possible.

Table 6 provides information on professional associations for pharmacists in the Czech Republic.

Table 6. Professional associations for pharmacists in the Czech Republic.

Item		Comments
Registration of pharmacists	Yes	Registration with the Czech Chamber of Pharmacists (http://www.lekarnici.cz/) is compulsory for all practising pharmacists. The Czech Chamber of Pharmacists is an independent, non-political, autonomous professional organisation responsible for the interests, professionalism, ethics, and honour of the pharmaceutical profession. The law prescribes obligatory membership in the Chamber for all pharmacists practising in pharmacies in the Czech Republic. The Czech Chamber of Pharmacists: 1. Ensures that its members exercise their profession in conformity with the highest professional standards, as well as with the principles of medical ethics and within the law; 2. Serves as the guarantor of professionalism on the part of its members and certifies the fulfilment of the requirements for the practice of medicine; 3. Reviews and defends the rights of the professional; 4. Defends the professional honour of its members; 5. Maintains the register of its members. The Chamber is entitled to: 1. Participate in negotiations concerning the price lists for pharmaceuticals; 2. Take part in competition proceedings to fill leading positions in the health care sector; 3. Establish requirements for practice by its members; 4. Investigate malpractice complaints filed against its members; 5. Issue opinions on the conditions and forms of the Continuing Education of Pharmacists; 6. Participate in specialisation exams. For more information, see the web site: http://www.lekarnici.cz.
Creation of pharmacies and control of territorial distribution	Yes	Territorial distribution of pharmacies is not regulated. Any physical or juridical person has the legal right to open a new pharmacy, but it must receive a licence from the regional District Office.
Ethical and other aspects of professional conduct	Yes	The ethical code of the Czech Chamber of Pharmacists is valid since 2005 (http://www.lekarnici.cz/).
Quality assurance and validation of university courses	Yes	A representative of the Czech Chamber of Pharmacists is a member of the Scientific Council of the Faculty of Pharmacy that approves any changes in the pharmacy curricula.

References to the various legislative and other documents [9] concerning pharmacy regulations and practice are found in the appendix.

3.2. Pharmacy Faculties, Students, and Courses

Table 7 provides details of pharmacy higher education institutions (HEIs), staff, and students in the Czech Republic.

Table 7. Pharmacy higher education institutions (HEIs), staff, and students in the Czech Republic.

Item	Number	Comments
Number of pharmacy HEIs in the Czech Republic	2	The two HEIs are: 1. Charles University, Faculty of Pharmacy in Hradec Králové (FPCU) (www.faf.cuni.cz) 2. The University of Veterinary and Pharmaceutical Sciences Brno, Faculty of Pharmacy (FPVPU) (http://faf.vfu.cz/).
Public pharmacy HEIs	2	There are no private pharmacy HEIs in the Czech Republic.

Table 7. *Cont.*

Item	Number	Comments
Faculty attachment		The faculties of pharmacy are independent bodies.
Do HEIs offer B and M degrees?	No	Only a master degree; a bachelor degree does not exist.
Teaching staff		
Staff (nationals)	190	
Professionals from outside the HEIs	7 (academic)	Staff from Slovakia. There are also 50 staff consisting of: community and hospital pharmacists involved in traineeship, management persons from pharmaceutical industry, psychologists, and economic experts.
Students		
Graduates that become registered pharmacists	200	The data are from the academic year 2014/15. Information about the admission procedure is available at: http://www.faf.cuni.cz/studium/prijimaci_rizeni/bakalarske_ magisterske/20112012/Stranky/default/aspx. Twenty-five to 30% of students drop out during the five years of study, and 90% of those who graduate become registered pharmacists (the remaining 10% do not work in pharmacies and need not be registered with the Czech Chamber of Pharmacists).
Number of places on entry following secondary school	300	
Number of applicants for each entry place	1130	Data from the academic year 2014/15. 4.2 applicants per place.
Number of EU international students	350	Main origins: 210 from Slovakia, who do not have to learn Czech since the Slovak and Czech languages are very similar; 27 from Greece.
Number of non-EU international students	26	Kosovo, Kazakhstan, Russian federation, Iran, Iraq, Saudi Arabia, Egypt, Zimbabwe, United Arab Emirates, Vietnam, Belarus, Uzbekistan.
Entry requirements following secondary school		
Specific national entrance examination for pharmacy	Yes	Written tests in biology and chemistry.
Fees per year		
For home and EU students		No tuition fee for courses in Czech. 7600 € for courses in English
For non EU students		7600 € for courses in English

The education website [11] provides information on the educational system in the Czech Republic as well as study and educational opportunities not only in the Czech Republic but throughout Europe. It also provides links to the legislation regulating education in the Czech Republic (the current wording of the School Act, Higher Education Act, Act on Pedagogical Workers and the White Book, etc.), various documents from the area of education and training; publications from the area of the school system, and selected documents relating to international activities.

It is to be noted that courses are given in Czech and English [12].
Table 8 provides details of the specialisation electives in pharmacy HEIs in the Czech Republic.

Table 8. Specialisation electives in pharmacy HEIs.

Item		Comments
Do HEIs Provide Specialised Courses?	No	

Specialisation provided by other organisations?	Postgraduate	Specialisation training for hospital pharmacy
		Hospital pharmacy specialisation training lasts four years; it includes
		
		- four-year practice in pharmacy with at least two years in hospital pharmacy
		- Several theoretical courses focused on pharmacotherapy, legislation, hospital pharmacy technologies, etc.
		- Practical training at accredited hospital pharmacies (compounding, sterile preparations, cytotoxic compounding and handling, quality assurance)
		- Each aspirant must:
		
		   - pass two tests during training
		   - submit a thesis (within the scope of hospital pharmacy)
		   - pass the board examination to obtain the specialisation diploma in hospital pharmacy.

Table 9 provides details of past and present changes in pharmacy education and training in the Czech Republic.

Table 9. Past and present changes in education and training in the Czech Republic pharmacy HEIs.

Item		Comments
Have there been any major changes since 1999?	Yes	Transfer to Bologna credit transfer system, also known as the European Credit Transfer and Accumulation System (ECTS) [3] and the introduction of six months of practical training in the fifth year.
Are any major changes envisaged before 2019?	Yes	As and if required by the directives of the EU.

3.3. Teaching and Learning Methods

Table 10 provides details of student hours by the learning method (for further details on the definitions of the different methods, see Atkinson and Rombaut, reference [1]).

Table 10. Student hours by learning method.

Method	Year 1	Year 2	Year 3	Year 4	Year 5	Total
Lecture	364	350	322	378	0	1502
Tutorial	84	182	157	140	0	560
Practical	280	252	196	98	0	597
Project	0	0	0	168	252	420
Community traineeship	40	0	0	0	960	1000
Industrial/academic traineeship	0	80	0	0	0	80
Electives						
Choice	112	56	84	0	0	252
Optional	0	0	84	64	0	148
Total	**880**	**920**	**840**	**848**	**1212**	**4559**

Formal lectures constitute 30% of student hours. Similar percentages are devoted to traineeship and to project work; the latter two take place mainly in the fourth and fifth years of studies. This suggests that student exchange would be easier in these later years, as there would be less need for exact coordination in the timing of deliverance of given subject matters (in lecture, practicals or tutorials) between the host and the home university as in the first three years.

3.4. Subject Areas

Table 11 provides details of student hours by subject area (for further details on the definitions of the subject areas, see Atkinson and Rombaut, reference [1]).

Table 11. Student hours by subject area.

Subject Area	Year 1	Year 2	Year 3	Year 4	Year 5	Total
CHEMSCI	168	308	42	56	0	574
PHYSMATH	168	0	14	0	0	182
BIOLSCI	168	98	0	0	0	266
PHARMTECH	0	0	406	336	0	742
MEDISCI	56	280	196	126	0	658
LAWSOC	140	28	112	182	0	462
GENERIC	196	168	28	168	0	560
TRAINEESHIP	0	0	0	0	856	856
Total	896	882	798	868	856	4300

CHEMSOC: chemical sciences; PHYSMATH: physical and mathematical sciences; BIOLSCI: biological sciences; PHARMTECH: pharmaceutical technology; MEDISCI: medicinal sciences; LAWSOC: law and social sciences; GENERIC: generic competences.

Taking the MEDISCI/CHEMSCI ratio as an indicator [13] of the nature of the M. Pharm. degree course (ratio = 658/574 = 1.1), it appears that the course is balanced compared with EU courses that are more "chemical science" e.g., Germany (ratio = 0.7), or more "medicinal science" e.g., Ireland (ratio = 2.6). Generic activities and traineeship make up $((650 + 856)/4300) \times 100 = 38\%$ of student hours.

3.5. Impact of the Bologna Principles [3]

Table 12 provides details regarding the various ways in which the Bologna declaration impacts on the pharmacy HEIs of the Czech Republic.

Table 12. Ways in which the Bologna declaration impacts on the Czech Republic pharmacy HEIs.

Item		Comments
"Comparable degrees with diploma supplement"	Yes	
"Two main cycles (B and M) with entry and exit at B level"	No	There is a five-year "tunnel" degree structure.
"European Credit Transfer System (ECTS) system of credits with links to life-long learning (LLL)"	Yes	The ECTS system of credits was introduced in 2006/2007.
"Addressing obstacles to mobility"	Partial	We offer a parallel pharmacy study programme in English for incoming international students. Incoming Erasmus students receive certain financial support from the Czech Ministry of Education to cover part of their expenses for accommodation. Outgoing Erasmus students receive about 350 € per month financial support from the Czech Ministry of Education.
"Application of European QA"	Yes	The study programmes are regularly accredited by the Accreditation Commission of the Czech Republic, which is a full member of the European Association for Quality Assurance in Higher Education (ENQA) [14].

Table 12. *Cont.*

Item	Comments
European dimension	The Faculty of Pharmacy, Charles University, has an agreement on co-supervision of PhD courses with the Faculty of Pharmacy, University of Coimbra, Portugal.
ERASMUS staff exchange to Prague from elsewhere	Staff months: 1 Portugal, Italy, Poland, Lithuania.
ERASMUS staff exchange from Prague to other HEIs	Staff months: 2. Poland, Spain, Italy, Slovenia.
ERASMUS student exchange to Prague from elsewhere	Student months: 140 Portugal, Spain, Poland, Italy, Slovakia, Germany.
ERASMUS student exchange from Prague to other HEIs	Student months: 170 Germany, Sweden, Slovenia, Italy, Portugal, Finland, Great Britain, Austria, Spain, Estonia.

Data in the above table are in exchange months per year. They show that there is substantial student exchange, and thus that application of Bologna principles such as ECTS works.

3.6. Impact of EU Directive 2013/55/EC [2]

Table 13 provides details regarding the various ways in which the EU directive impacts on pharmacy education and training in the Czech Republic.

Table 13. Ways in which the elements of the EC directive (left column) impact on Czech Republic pharmacy HEIs.

Item	Comments
"Evidence of formal qualifications as a pharmacist shall attest to training of at least five years' duration..."	The curriculum fulfils the EU requirements.
"...four years of full-time theoretical and practical training at a university or at a higher institute of a level recognised as equivalent, or under the supervision of a university;"	The curriculum fulfils the EU requirements.
"...six-month traineeship in a pharmacy that is open to the public or in a hospital, under the supervision of that hospital's pharmaceutical department."	We would prefer a compulsory period of four months in community or hospital pharmacy for all students, plus two months either in industry (for those that plan to work in industry after graduation) or an additional two months in a pharmacy for those planning to work in a pharmacy.

The Czech Republic mainly conforms to the different aspects of the EU directive, with notably a five-year tunnel degree. Aspects of the Bologna agreement such as the ECTS and the Diploma Supplement are present.

4. Discussion and Conclusions

Regarding the state of pharmacy in the Czech Republic compared with the EU, in many aspects, the activities and occupations of Czech pharmacists are attuned to those in other EU member states, in spite of the fact that the Czech Republic only recently (2004) joined the EU. The numbers of pharmacists in relation to the population are lower than the EU norm. Assistant pharmacists are officially recognised; they undergo a three-year training period. This cannot, however, be assimilated to a bachelor degree in pharmacy.

As in most other EU member states, the profession of hospital pharmacist exists, although this is not recognised by the EU directive. Hospital pharmacists receive their training following graduation, but such training is not organised by the university. Again, as in most EU countries, the Czech pharmacy chamber deals with specific problems relating to the organisation and ethics of practice. The chamber has also an advisory role concerning university courses for pharmacy.

There are two pharmacy HEIs in Hradec Králové and Brno. There is a substantial foreign student intake, especially from Slovakia, and courses are given in Czech and English. Czech pharmacy faculties utilise the ECTS to promote student exchange. These are valid throughout the EHEA. The course is balanced amongst three main elements: lectures, project work, and a pre-graduate traineeship. The course also strikes a balance between medicinal and chemical subjects.

Acknowledgments: With the support of the Lifelong Learning Program of the European Union (142078-LLP-1-2008-BE-ERASMUS-ECDSP).

Author Contributions: Petr Nachtigal and Tomáš Šimůnek provided all the data and information and helped in the revisions of the manuscript; Jeffrey Atkinson wrote the first manuscript and dealt with revisions.

References

1. Atkinson, J.; Rombaut, B. The 2011 PHARMINE report on pharmacy and pharmacy education in the European Union. *Pharm. Pract.* **2011**, *9*, 169–187. [CrossRef]

2. The European Commission Directive 2013/55/EU on Education and Training for Sectoral Practice Such as That of Pharmacy. Available online: http://eur-lex.europa.eu/legal-content/FR/TXT/?uri=celex: 32013L0055 (accessed on 7 July 2017).

3. The European Higher Education Area (EHEA)—Bologna Agreement of Harmonisation of European University Degree Courses. Available online: http://www.ehea.info/ (accessed on 7 July 2017).

4. World Health Organisation. World Health Statistics 2016: Monitoring health for the SDGs. Available online: http://www.who.int/gho/publications/world_health_statistics/2016/Annex_B/en/ (accessed on 7 July 2017).

5. OECD The Organisation for Economic Co-Operation and Development, Health Expenditure and Financing. Available online: http://stats.oecd.org/Index.aspx?DataSetCode=SHA (accessed on 7 July 2017).

6. Erasmus Plus Programme for Student and Staff Exchange in the EU. Available online: https://info.erasmusplus.fr/ (accessed on 7 July 2017).

7. Atkinson, J. The Country Profiles of the PHARMINE Survey of European Higher Educational Institutions Delivering Pharmacy Education and Training. *Pharmacy* **2017**, *3*, 34. Available online: http://www.mdpi.com/2226--4787/5/3/34 (accessed on 7 July 2017). [CrossRef] [PubMed]

8. The Ministry of Health of the Czech Republic. Available online: http://www.mzcr.cz/En/ (accessed on 7 July 2017).

9. Links to All Important Czech Laws Relevant to All Aspects of Pharmacy Can Be Found at the Website. Available online: http://www.lekarnici.cz/ (accessed on 7 July 2017).

10. The Czech Republic Public Administration Portal: Health Care. Available online: http://portal.gov.cz/portal/eng/health-care.html (accessed on 7 July 2017).

11. The Czech Republic Education Website. Available online: http://app.edu.cz/portal/page?_pageid=33, 274837&_dad=portal&_schema=PORTAL (accessed on 7 July 2017).

12. The Pharmacy Curriculum in English. Available online: http://www.faf.cuni.cz/Study/Undergraduate/Pharmacy/Study-plan/ (accessed on 7 July 2017).

13. Atkinson, J.; De Paepe, K.; Sánchez Pozo, A.; Rekkas, D.; Volmer, D.; Hirvonen, J.; Bozic, B.; Skowron, A.; Mircioiu, C.; Marcincal, A.; et al. Does the Subject Content of the Pharmacy Degree Course Influence the Community Pharmacist's Views on Competencies for Practice? *Pharmacy* **2015**, *3*, 137–153. [CrossRef] [PubMed]

14. The European Association for Quality Assurance in Higher Education (ENQA). Available online: http://www.enqa.eu/ (accessed on 7 July 2017).

11

Quality of Life and Medication Adherence of Independently Living Older Adults Enrolled in a Pharmacist-Based Medication Management Program

Christopher Harlow [1], Catherine Hanna [2], Lynne Eckmann [3], Yevgeniya Gokun [4], Faika Zanjani [5], Karen Blumenschein [6,*] and Holly Divine [6]

[1] St. Matthews Community Pharmacy, Louisville, KY 40207, USA; cpharlow@gmail.com
[2] American Pharmacy Services Corporation, Frankfort, KY 40601, USA; channa@apscnet.com
[3] Wheeler Pharmacy, Home Connection, Lexington, KY 40507, USA; eckmann8@aol.com
[4] General Dynamics Information Technology, Little Rock, AR 72205, USA; jane.gokun@gdit.com
[5] Department of Behavioral and Community Health, University of Maryland School of Public Health, College Park, MD 20742, USA; fzanjani@umd.edu
[6] Department of Pharmacy Practice and Science, University of Kentucky College of Pharmacy Lexington, KY 40536, USA; holly.divine@uky.edu
*   Correspondence: KBLUM1@uky.edu

Academic Editors: Karen B. Farris and Antoinette B. Coe

Abstract: This study sought to understand the medication adherence and quality of life (QOL) of recipients of a pharmacist-based medication management program among independently living older adults. Using a cross-sectional, quasi-experimental study design, we compared older adults enrolled in the program to older adults not enrolled in the program. Data were collected via face-to-face interviews in independent-living facilities and in participants' homes. Independently living older adults who were enrolled in the medication management program ($n = 38$) were compared to older adults not enrolled in the program (control group ($n = 41$)). All participants were asked to complete questionnaires on health-related quality of life (QOL, using the SF-36) and medication adherence (using the four-item Morisky scale). The medication management program recipients reported significantly more prescribed medications ($p < 0.0001$) and were more likely to report living alone ($p = 0.01$) than the control group. The medication management program recipients had a significantly lower SF-36 physical functioning score ($p = 0.03$) compared to the control group, although other SF-36 domains and self-reported medication adherence were similar between the groups. Despite taking more medications and more commonly living alone, independent living older adults enrolled in a pharmacist-based medication management program had similar QOL and self-reported medication adherence when compared to older adults not enrolled in the program. This study provides initial evidence for the characteristics of older adults receiving a pharmacist-based medication management program, which may contribute to prolonged independent living and positive health outcomes.

Keywords: pharmacist roles; adherence; older adults; medication management; quality of life; medication use

1. Introduction

Community pharmacists generally see patients with chronic medical conditions at least monthly, at the time medications are refilled. This regular interaction places pharmacists in a unique position to monitor and manage medications for older adults. Furthermore, extensive training in pharmacotherapy and patient communication uniquely prepares pharmacists to play a vital role in minimizing medication-related problems. Pharmacist interventions can improve patient drug knowledge and adherence [1]; however, little is known about the population that participates in pharmacist interventions, and this is especially true in the older adult population.

A systematic review evaluating pharmacist interventions to optimize medication use in nursing home settings provided equivocal results [2]. Reviews assessing pharmacist interventions with older patients to improve health outcomes, QOL, adherence, and cost-effective care also provide mixed findings and suggest further research is needed [3,4]. Despite findings from these systematic reviews, it is clear that regular interaction and medication management provide pharmacists with the opportunity to circumvent many drug therapy problems in older adults, thereby easing patient, family, and caregiver burden. Drug therapy problems can be categorized into seven areas: unnecessary drug therapy, need of additional drug therapy, ineffective drug therapy, too low a dosage, too high a dosage, adverse drug reactions, and non-compliance [5]. Polypharmacy and drug therapy problems have been linked with poor health outcomes. For example, patients who have more medications in their home are more likely to have increased severity of their illnesses and are at higher risk for therapeutic duplications [6].

Humanistic parameters, such as quality of life, have been evaluated as predictors of outcomes in the older population. Health-related quality of life surveys, such as the Short Form (SF)-12 and SF-36, have been shown to be independent predictors of hospitalization and mortality [7]. These self-reported surveys provide specific feedback on patients' physical and mental performance; a decline in these performances has been linked to a change in health status and predicts future adverse events [8].

Medication non-adherence has also been associated with poor health outcomes including disease progression and increased costs [9]. Research has demonstrated that a comprehensive program provided by pharmacists, including blister-packed medications, is associated with substantial improvements in medication adherence among older adults resulting in meaningful improvements in health [10]. Estimates of non-adherence in the older adult vary from 40% to 75%, and there are still many unanswered questions as to the most effective pharmacist-based intervention for promoting medication adherence [11].

Unfortunately, a non-invasive "gold standard" for measuring adherence is unavailable. A recent study in the United Kingdom compared three common methods for measuring adherence (electronic monitoring, pill counts, and self-report) in older adults and found substantial differences between the three methods. The use of pill counts and self-reported surveys tended to correlate better with adherence rates than prescription-bottle caps equipped with an electronic monitor that recorded when the bottles were opened. However, the inconsistency with the electronic record in the study has been postulated to be related to the varying patterns of bottle opening versus the number of pills taken out [12].

The objective of this study was to understand the medication adherence and quality of life of recipients that participate in a pharmacist-based medication management program. The ultimate goal of the service described in this study is to prolong independent living and improve overall health status for older adults.

2. Materials and Methods

2.1. Description of the Pharmacist-Based Medication Management Service

The pharmacist-based medication management program studied was developed specifically for independently living older adults residing either in independent living facilities or within their own home. The program is offered by a local community pharmacy. The program origins date back to the late 1980s, when a former consultant pharmacist observed that patients residing in independent and assisted living beds at a Central Kentucky nursing facility would benefit from pharmacist consultations and adherence-based services. Originally, services were only offered to residents at that one facility; however, over time, the program grew to include patients living in other facilities, and patients living in their own homes. The program was designed to allow a pharmacist to manage, monitor, and optimize medication therapy with the goal of prolonging independent living in the older patient. A key component of the program is the direct, individualized care and time devoted to each patient. Patients are referred to the program from a variety of sources ranging from self-referral to healthcare practitioner recommendation. Patients or caregivers, as well as practitioners, most often learn of the service through word-of-mouth marketing or through previous experience with the service and call the pharmacy themselves to initiate the enrollment process. Most often, these referrals are precipitated by an adverse medication event or hospitalization.

The pharmacist-based medication management program consists of three primary components: assessment, prescription organization, and weekly support/medication dispensing. When the patient is first enrolled, initial home-based assessments are conducted to obtain baseline information for the pharmacist to better understand the patient's specific needs. These assessments include demographic information, medication comprehension, cognitive assessments, and fall-risk assessments. This information is documented in a chart that is kept in the pharmacy, and information is updated after each weekly visit. Once the patient is enrolled into the program, all of their prescription and non-prescription medications are organized, stored at the pharmacy, and managed by a clinical pharmacist. Each week, a 7-day supply of the patient's routine medications is prepared and delivered to the patient's home by a pharmacy technician or pharmacist. The patient's routine medications are dispensed in a weekly medication organizer; "as needed" medications are maintained separately. Refills are also managed through the medication management service. The pharmacist obtains prescriber authorization for refills prior to the supply of medication being depleted. If the patient has a change in a medication (for example, an increase or decrease in dose) or is started on a new medication during the week, the pharmacist on-call will be notified to dispense the medication and update the medication organizer for the patient.

During the weekly visit, the pharmacist reviews the previous week's medication organizer for missed doses and documents each missed dose in the patient's chart. The pharmacist follows up with the patient or caregiver regarding patterns for missed doses and intervenes as appropriate. The pharmacist also monitors patients for other medication-related problems including adverse drug reactions, drug–drug interactions, and falls.

Other services provided to each patient include counseling on all new or changed prescription orders, ensuring the weekly medication organizers are stored in appropriate areas of the home, an up-to-date medication list, and ongoing medication review. The clinical pharmacist is on-call 24 h per day and maintains a constant line of communication between the prescriber, the patient, and caregivers.

2.2. Study Design and Population

To understand the recipients of the pharmacist-based medication management program a cross-sectional, quasi-experimental study of independently living older adults residing in central Kentucky was conducted during January and February of 2011. The study included the program recipients (intervention group), consisting of patients currently enrolled in the pharmacist-based medication management program, and a control group that was recruited for comparison. Intervention patients resided within their own home, or within independent-living facilities. The control group, living in a similar situation as the intervention group, was recruited from independently living older adults residing at three independent living facilities in the same central Kentucky town. Participants over the age of 60 and living independently were eligible for inclusion. Exclusion criteria were severe cognitive impairment (indicated by a lack of understanding of the research design and purpose of their participation) and an inability to read or write English fluently.

The control group was recruited at three independent-living facilities in central Kentucky using flyers approved by the University of Kentucky Institutional Review Board. Control participants were asked to attend a group session for participation. The group session consisted of a description of the research, an explanation of why the participants were being asked to participate, and completion of the questionnaires. Group sessions lasted approximately 20 min. Participants were asked to complete demographic, medication adherence, and quality of life measurements. The control group completed their questionnaires and returned them to the primary investigator at the end of the live session. Intervention participants were interviewed on an individual basis in their homes. All study participants were reimbursed $15 for their time to participate. The study was approved by the University of Kentucky Institutional Review Board, and informed consent was obtained from each participant prior to participation.

2.3. Measurements

A single "snap-shot" assessment of the quality of life and medication adherence was evaluated for both program participants and the control group. In this project, health-related quality of life was measured with the SF-36v2 Health Survey [13]. The SF-36v2 consists of 36 items to construct eight health domains. The domains include physical functioning (PF), role physical (RP), bodily pain (BP), general health (GH), vitality (VT), social functioning (SF), role emotional (RE), and mental health (MH). These domains are further summarized into a physical component score (PCS) and a mental component score (MCS), which have been standardized to the United States population (mean score 50; standard deviation (SD) 10). Higher scores indicate better functioning.

Medication adherence was measured with the self-reported 4-item Morisky Scale [14], which consists of four questions assessing medication-taking behavior, as listed in Figure 1. An answer of yes to zero questions indicates high adherence behavior, answering yes to one or two questions indicates medium adherence behavior, and answering yes to three or four questions indicates low adherence behavior [14]. Medication adherence for the intervention group was also objectively measured by conducting a retrospective chart review for a total of six weeks of data. The adherence rate was calculated as a percent of medication doses actually taken divided by number of medication doses prescribed.

Do you ever forget to take your medicine?	Yes	No
Are you careless at times about taking your medicine?	Yes	No
When you feel better do you sometimes stop taking your medicine?	Yes	No
Sometimes if you feel worse when you take your medicine, do you stop taking it?	Yes	No

Figure 1. 4-item Morisky scale questions [14].

Data Analysis

Continuous variables were summarized with the use of means and SDs, or medians and interquartile range (IQR) for non-normally distributed data. The SF-36v2 data were not normally distributed, so the differences between the intervention and control groups were compared using the Wilcoxon rank-sum test. Categorical variables were summarized using descriptive statistics (counts, percentages) and compared with chi-square tests or, when appropriate, Fisher's exact test.

3. Results

3.1. Subjects

A total of 79 independently living older adults participated in the study. Figure 2 shows the participant recruitment flowchart. The intervention group included 38 participants and the control group included 41 participants. At the time of the study, 55 individuals were enrolled in the medication management program; 12 were excluded from the study due to severe cognitive impairment, and 5 declined participation. Three group sessions were conducted to recruit control participants. A total of 44 control participants were identified; 3 were excluded from the study due to severe cognitive impairment.

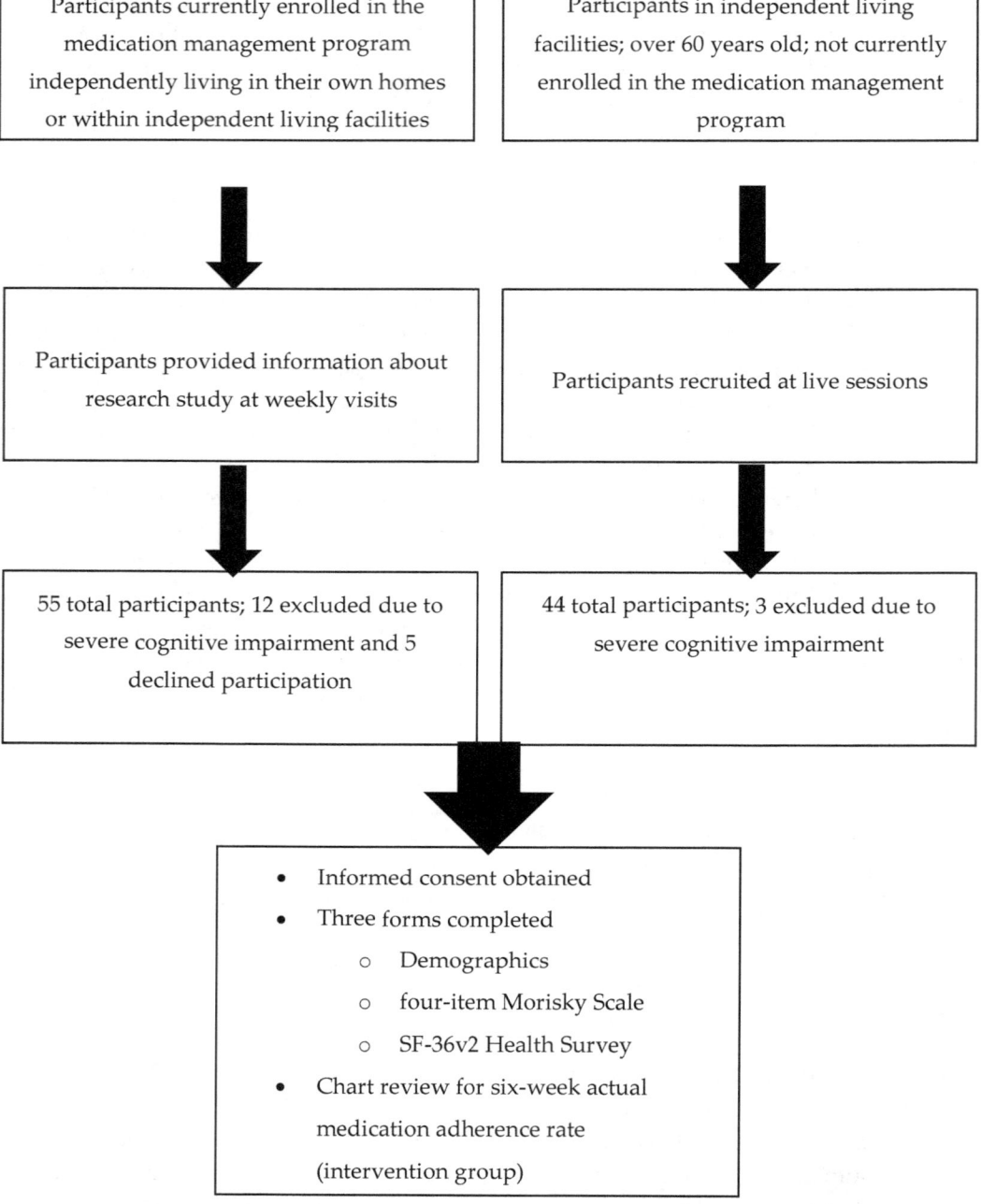

Figure 2. Subject Recruitment.

Characteristics of the intervention and control groups are presented in Table 1. The median age for the intervention group was slightly higher compared to the control group (87 vs. 84, respectively), but this difference was not statistically significant ($p = 0.07$). Overall, the characteristics of the two study groups were similar except for the number of routine medications, number of persons living in household, and annual income. The intervention group was using significantly more regularly scheduled medications (10 vs. 5 in the control group, $p < 0.0001$), was more likely to live alone (78.9% vs. 48.8% in the control group, $p = 0.01$), and had a significantly higher annual household income ($p = 0.001$).

Table 1. Characteristics of the intervention and control groups.

	Intervention Group (*n* = 38)	Control Group (*n* = 41)	*p* Value
Median Age (IQR)	87 (83–89)	84 (77–88)	0.07
Sex, Females (%)	29 (76.3%)	27 (65.9%)	0.45
Highest level of education			
Some college or less	21 (55.3%)	15 (36.6%)	0.22
Bachelor's degree or equivalent	9 (23.7%)	16 (39.0%)	
Masters degree or higher	8 (21.0%)	10 (24.4%)	
Median number of regularly scheduled medications (including prescription, over-the-counter, and herbal products) (IQR)	10 (8–13)	5 (4–8)	<0.0001
Median number of disease states (IQR)	3.5 (2–5)	3 (2–5)	0.17
Trouble reading due to vision	14 (36.8%)	11 (26.8%)	0.34
Number of subjects with at least one hospital or emergency department visit in past 6 months	16 (42.1%)	15 (36.6%)	0.62
Median number of visits to hospital or emergency department in past 6 months (if greater than zero) (IQR)	1.5 (1–2.5)	1 (1–2)	0.20
Number of subjects with at least one fall in past 6 months	13 (34.2%)	14 (34.1%)	>0.90
Median number of falls in past 6 months (if greater than zero) (IQR)	1 (1–3)	1 (1–2)	0.50
Duration of time in current home			
0–12 months	11 (28.9%)	8 (19.5%)	0.33
1–3 years	10 (26.3%)	17 (41.5%)	
4 or more years	17 (44.7%)	16 (39%)	
Number of people living in current household			
1 person	30 (78.9%)	20 (48.8%)	0.01
2 persons	8 (21.1%)	21 (51.2%)	
Annual household income			
0–$25,000	8 (21.1%)	12 (29.2%)	
$25,001–$50,000	6 (15.7%)	17 (41.5%)	0.0014
$50,001–$100,000	3 (7.9%)	8 (19.5%)	
Greater than $100,000	13 (34.2%)	2 (4.9%)	
Not specified	8 (21.1%)	2 (4.9%)	

3.2. Medication Adherence

In the intervention group, 60.5% reported a high adherence rate, while 43.9% of the control group reported a high adherence rate using the self-reported four-item Morisky Scale (Figure 3), although the difference was not statistically significant (*p* = 0.21). The intervention group had a median objective medical chart adherence rate of 99% (range of 88% to 100%) during the six-week retrospective chart review (Table 2).

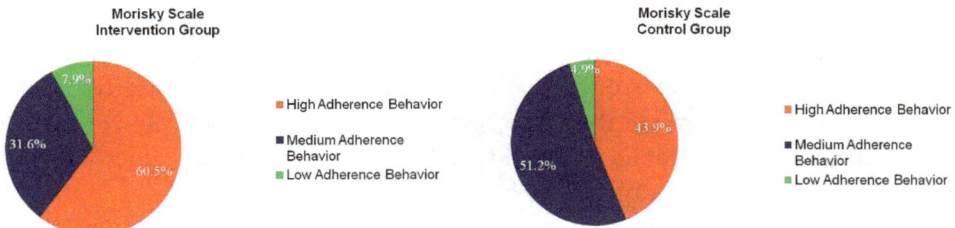

Figure 3. Adherence.

Table 2. Six-week objective medication adherence rate (%) for the intervention group (n = 33) *.

Mean (SD)	98 (0.03)
Median (Range)	99 (88–100)

* Five subjects were excluded from the retrospective chart review due to lack of six-week adherence information.

3.3. Quality of Life

With the exception of PF, there was no difference between the two groups in the eight domains of the SF-36 (Table 3). The intervention group had a significantly lower median PF compared to the control group (p = 0.03).

Table 3. SF-36v2 norm-based scores.

	Intervention (n = 38)	Control (n = 41)	p Value
Physical Component Summary (PCS)	41.77 (11.31)	45.37 (8.80)	0.12
Mental Component Summary (MCS)	55.85 (48.34–59.76)	54.67 (50.12–60.17)	0.97
Physical Functioning (PF)	36.49 (26.92–47.97)	46.06 (38.40–49.89)	0.03
Role-Physical (RP)	39.19 (32.46–54.91)	45.93 (39.19–52.66)	0.06
Bodily Pain (BP)	51.51 (42.64–62.00)	50.71 (42.64–55.55)	0.69
General Health (GH)	53.19 (43.68–57.94)	53.19 (46.05–55.56)	0.97
Vitality (VT)	52.60 (40.72–55.57)	52.60 (49.63–58.54)	0.15
Social Functioning (SF)	54.84 (37.27–57.34)	52.33 (47.31–57.34)	0.64
Role Emotional (RE)	54.43 (38.76–56.17)	52.69 (42.24–56.17)	0.97
Mental Health (MH)	53.48 (48.25–58.72)	56.10 (53.48–58.72)	0.36

Data are expressed as median (with IQR) except PCS, which is reported with mean and standard deviation; p-values were based on non-parametric analyses except PCS, for which a two-sample t-test was appropriate.

4. Discussion

This evaluation of medication adherence and quality of life for independently living older adults participating in a pharmacist-based medication management program found that participants had similar QOL and self-reported medication adherence when compared to independent-living older adults not enrolled in the program, despite participants taking more prescribed medications and more commonly living alone. As previously described, medication adherence and quality of life have been shown to predict health outcomes in the older adult [1,6–11]. Adverse health outcomes result in a functional decline and a loss of independence in older adults. Interventions to improve health outcomes may reduce the risk of this loss [15,16]. Study findings demonstrate that various levels of independent living exist in the older population. It is concluded that assumptions about patient ability to manage their medications based on their level of relative "independence" should be made cautiously in the health care community.

In this study of independently living older adults, findings indicated that medication management program recipients reported being prescribed significantly more medications and were more likely to live alone. From the literature, it is well understood that taking more medications can add to the frailty and poor health outcomes of older adults. Moreover, living alone has been shown to be an independent predictor of frailty and decline in activities of daily living in older patients [17].

The physical functioning was significantly lower in the pharmacy program recipients, indicating a lower functionality level of independent living. All other QOL indicators were similar between the two groups. Thus, medication management program recipients have relatively similar QOL compared to other independently living older adults, but are prescribed more medications and have lower levels of physical functioning.

Literature documents the strong positive correlation between high rates of medication adherence and positive health outcomes [9,10,18–20]. Although this study did not find a difference in self-reported medication adherence, the pharmacy program participants had a documented chart medication adherence rate exceeding 90%.

As stated previously, patients are referred to medication management programs from a variety of sources, often as a result of an adverse medication event or hospitalization. Early implementation of an effective pharmacist-based medication management program could help address adverse medication-related issues and potentially prolong independent living. To improve care for the independently living older adult, it is essential to recognize the negative outcomes of suboptimal medication management. Although not directly assessed in this study, prolonged independence for the older adult reduces overall healthcare costs by preventing or delaying institutionalization. The findings of this study suggest that further evaluation of pharmacist-based medication management programs for older adults is warranted to assess potential causal relationships as well as patient, family, and caregiver perceived value of such programs. Healthcare providers should be more proactive in identifying older adults who require assistance with managing their medications and refer to pharmacists who specialize in comprehensive medication management to maintain independent living among this population.

One important limitation of this study was the difference in the recruitment process between the two groups. Participants in the intervention group were already enrolled in the medication management program possibly because they were at a higher risk for losing their independence. The research session was conducted in their home during a regular medication management program visit due to feasibility of administering the surveys. Participants in the control group attended a live session outside their home producing a different environment for completing the research questionnaires. Another limitation of the study was the cross-sectional design, which evaluated a snapshot of self-reported adherence and quality of life. Lack of baseline measures for program participants precludes an assessment of impact. Future research should study participants over time to evaluate the true impact of the medication management program on medication adherence and quality of life using a longitudinal, clinical trial design.

5. Conclusions

This study provides initial evidence for characterizing older adults receiving a pharmacist-based medication management program. Individuals enrolled in the medication management program had comparable quality of life and self-reported adherence to control participants, even though the program recipients were taking more medications and were more likely to live alone.

Acknowledgments: The authors thank Amy Burke, University of Kentucky College of Pharmacy Department of Pharmacy Practice and Science for data entry and review. This work was supported in part by the American Pharmacists Association Foundation Knowlton Center for Pharmacist-Based Health Solutions.

Author Contributions: Christopher Harlow, Catherine Hanna, Lynne Eckmann, Faika Zanjani, Karen Blumenschein, and Holly Divine jointly conceived the idea and design of the project; Christopher Harlow and Lynne Eckmann implemented the project and collected the data; Yevgeniya Gokun analyzed the data; Christopher Harlow, Karen Blumenschein, and Holly Divine wrote the manuscript. All authors reviewed and approved the manuscript.

References

1. Holland, R.; Desborough, J.; Goodyer, L.; Hall, S.; Wright, D.; Loke, Y.K. Does pharmacist-led medication review help to reduce hospital admissions and deaths in older people? A systematic review and meta-analysis. *Br. J. Clin. Pharmacol.* **2007**, *65*, 303–316. [CrossRef] [PubMed]
2. Verrue, C.L.R.; Petrovic, M.; Mehuys, E.; Remon, J.P.; Stichele, R.V. Pharmacists interventions for optimization of medication use in nursing homes. A systematic review. *Drugs Aging* **2009**, *26*, 37–49. [CrossRef] [PubMed]
3. Spinewine, A.; Fialova, D.; Byrne, S. The role of the pharmacist in optimizing pharmacotherapy in older people. *Drugs Aging* **2012**, *29*, 495–510. [CrossRef] [PubMed]

4. George, J.; Elliott, R.A.; Stewart, D.C. A systematic review of interventions to improve medication taking in elderly patients prescribed multiple medications. *Drugs Aging* **2008**, *25*, 307–324. [CrossRef] [PubMed]

5. Cipolle, R.J.; Strand, L.M.; Morley, P.C. *Pharmaceutical Care Practice: The Clinician's Guide*, 2nd ed.; McGraw-Hill: New York, NY, USA, 2004.

6. Sorensen, L.; Stokes, J.A.; Purdie, D.M.; Woodward, M.; Roberts, M.S. Medication management at home: Medication-related risk factors associated with poor health outcomes. *Age Ageing* **2005**, *34*, 626–632. [CrossRef] [PubMed]

7. Dorr, D.A.; Jones, S.S.; Burns, L.; Donnelly, S.M.; Brunker, C.P.; Wilcox, A.; Clayton, P.D. Use of health-related, quality of life metrics to predict mortality and hospitalizations in community-dwelling seniors. *J. Am. Geriatr. Soci.* **2006**, *54*, 667–673. [CrossRef] [PubMed]

8. Fan, V.S.; Au, D.H.; McDonell, M.B.; Fihn, S.D. Intraindividual change in SF-36 in ambulatory clinic primary care patients predicted mortality and hospitalizations. *J. Clin. Epidemiol.* **2004**, *57*, 277–283. [CrossRef] [PubMed]

9. Sokol, M.C.; McGuigan, K.A.; Verbrugge, R.R.; Epstein, R.S. Impact of medication adherence on hospitalization risk and healthcare cost. *Med. Care* **2005**, *43*, 521–530. [CrossRef] [PubMed]

10. Lee, J.K.; Grace, K.A.; Taylor, A.J. Effect of a pharmacy care program on medication adherence and persistence, blood pressure, and low-density lipoprotein cholesterol: A randomized controlled trial. *J. Am. Med. Assoc.* **2006**, *296*, 2563–2571. [CrossRef] [PubMed]

11. Doggrell, S.A. Adherence to medicines in the older-aged with chronic conditions: Does intervention by an allied health professional help? *Drugs Aging* **2010**, *27*, 239–254. [CrossRef] [PubMed]

12. Smith, H.; Hankins, M.; Hodson, A.; George, C. Measuring the adherence to medication of elderly patients with heart failure: Is there a gold standard? *Int. J. Cardiol.* **2009**, *145*, 122–123. [CrossRef] [PubMed]

13. Ware, J.E.; Kosinski, M.; Dewey, J.E. *How to Score Version 2 of the SF-36® Health Survey*; Quality Metric Incorporated: Lincoln, RI, USA, 2000.

14. Morisky, D.E.; Green, L.W.; Levine, D.M. Concurrent and predictive validity of a self-reported measure of medication adherence. *Med. Care* **1986**, *24*, 67–74. [CrossRef] [PubMed]

15. Aminzadeh, F.; Dalziel, W.B. Older adults in the emergency department: A systematic review of patterns of use, adverse health outcomes, and effectiveness of interventions. *Ann. Emerg. Med.* **2002**, *39*, 238–247. [CrossRef] [PubMed]

16. Armstrong, J.J.; Stolee, P.; Hirdes, J.P.; Poss, J.W. Examining three frailty conceptualizations in their ability to predict negative outcomes for home-care clients. *Age Ageing* **2010**, *39*, 755–758. [CrossRef] [PubMed]

17. Freiheit, E.A.; Hogan, D.B.; Eliasziw, M.; Meekes, M.F.; Ghali, W.A.; Partlo, L.A.; Maxwell, C.J. Development of a frailty index for patients with coronary artery disease. *J. Am. Geriatr. Soc.* **2010**, *58*, 1526–1531. [CrossRef] [PubMed]

18. Rose, A.J.; Glickman, M.E.; D'Amore, M.M.; Orner, M.B.; Berlowitz, D.; Kressin, N.R. Effects of daily adherence to antihypertensive medication on blood pressure control. *J. Clin. Hypertens.* **2011**, *13*, 416–421. [CrossRef] [PubMed]

19. Baroletti, S.; Dell'Orfano, H. Medication adherence in cardiovascular disease. *Circulation* **2010**, *121*, 1455–1458. [CrossRef] [PubMed]

20. Zedler, B.K.; Joyce, A.; Murrelle, L.; Kakad, P.; Harpe, S.E. A pharmacoepidemiologic analysis of the impact of calendar packaging on adherence to self-administered medications for long-term use. *Clin. Ther.* **2011**, *33*, 581–597. [CrossRef] [PubMed]

12

Clinical Pharmacy Education in Japan: Using Simulated Patients in Laboratory-Based Communication-Skills Training before Clinical Practice

Rie Kubota *, Kiyoshi Shibuya, Yoichi Tanaka, Manahito Aoki, Megumi Shiomi, Wataru Ando, Katsuya Otori and Takako Komiyama

Research and Education Center for Clinical Pharmacy, School of Pharmacy,
Kitasato University 5-9-1 Shirokane, Minato-ku, Tokyo 108-8641, Japan
* Correspondence: kubotar@pharm.kitasato-u.ac.jp

Abstract: The Japanese pharmaceutical curriculum was extended from four to six years in 2006. Students now receive practical communication-skills training in their fourth year, before progressing to train in hospital and community pharmacies in their fifth year. Kitasato University School of Pharmacy, Tokyo, had established a program to meet these aims before the 2006 guidance. In the present study, we discuss and evaluate the features of this communication-skills training program. This study enrolled 242 fourth-year pharmacy students at Kitasato University. Students filled out a questionnaire survey after completing the laboratory element of their undergraduate education. As part of training, students were asked to obtain patient data from a model medical chart, before performing simulated patient interviews covering hospital admission and patient counseling. These simulations were repeated in a small group, and feedback was provided to students by both the simulated patient and the faculty after each presentation. It was found that students were able to develop their communication skills through this approach. Thus, an effective system of gradual and continuous training has been developed, which allows students to acquire clinical and practical communication skills.

Keywords: pharmacy education; simulated patient; preliminary education; communication skill

---

1. Introduction

In 2006, the Japanese pharmaceutical curriculum was extended from four to six years [1], with each pharmacy college required to implement a new core curriculum [2,3]. Since then, students have received preliminary education and practical training in laboratory settings during their fourth year of study. Following this, students are assessed for knowledge, skill and attitude through common achievement tests, computer-based testing, and objective-structured clinical ability examinations (OSCEs) [4]. If successful, a student progresses to the fifth year when they engage in training at hospital and community pharmacies for eleven weeks each.

Kitasato University School of Pharmacy, a private school in Japan, has established fundamental and clinical education early. Currently, a six-year course is available through the Pharmaceutical Department and a four-year course is available through the Life Sciences and Drug Development Department. However, both the courses are undergoing constant evolution to address the changing needs of clinical pharmacy. An example of this is the drive to provide a more advanced pharmacist education to solve medical problems using basic research. To complement this, we have introduced several clinical programs to provide early exposure and preliminary practical education in the six-year pharmaceutical course. The required practical hospital training is provided at four hospitals affiliated to Kitasato University, but fourth-year students receive preliminary education in a laboratory setting over a four-month period. During this preliminary period, they learn about drug information evaluation, physical assessment, dispensing, intravenous preparation and patient counseling.

In laboratory practice, that is, one component of didactic curriculum, hands-on skill-based labs, simulated inpatient interviews and counseling were used to conduct training and develop an understanding of the patients' background and feelings. Many authors have demonstrated that the simulation of clinical teaching was effective [5–7]. Simulation is described as substitution of a real patient for trained–simulated patients enacting a patient experience [5–7]. Medicine and nursing schools use patient simulation to teach a broad range of clinically related skills [8,9]. Additionally, patient simulation (role play) is one of the teaching methods in pharmacy education. Moreover, pharmacy practice-related skills including communication have been recently expanded and incorporated in such training. Rickles reported that the use of simulated patients in teaching communication skills to pharmacy students was effective [7].

The aims of this study were as follows: (1) to introduce the advanced features of an element of this education program that seeks to develop communication and problem-solving skills; (2) to evaluate the perceived effectiveness of this education among students.

2. Materials and Methods

2.1. Objectives and Study Design

This study was conducted among 242 fourth-year pharmacy students at Kitasato University. The survey focused on the effects of the simulated patient, and requested that students evaluated the teaching method and gave reasons for their responses. The students filled out the questionnaires after their classes. The questions included were as follows: (1) was it effective that simulated patient played a role in simulation? (Multiple responses were chosen from five listed reasons.); (2) was the teaching method wherein the faculty added step-by-step comments within a group effective? (Multiple responses were chosen from four listed reasons.)

2.2. Overview of the Preliminary Education: Patient Interview and Counseling

This laboratory work was delivered to students over three days. For each session, 30 students were categorized into four groups, and one faculty member and one simulated patient were included per group, covering a different case each (see Table 1). On day one, the students were asked to obtain patient data from a model medical chart, confirm the patient's background, and list the patient's problems in an appropriate format. On day two, they simulated a patient interview covering hospital admission. For this, we used a classroom and set up four beds in it. Simulated patients sat on the beds and one student interviewed them. The other students, who were observers, surrounded the bed. During these, each student engaged in a simulated interview in their small group, before the other students who had observed them gave their feedback. Also, the simulated patient provided feedback about behaviors after each presentation, and the faculty staff provided feedback about additional points (see Figure 1 for an example). In this way, communication in the simulated interviews was improved in a step-by-step manner within each group. One representative from each group then simulated the patient interview in front of the whole class. On day three, the students simulated patient counseling regarding medicines for internal use, including intravenous therapy, using the same method that was followed on day two. Table 1 summarizes the details of the simulated patients and Figure 1 outlines the feedback process and concrete comments from the faculty. The simulated patients belong to the Institute of My Informed Consent (association for dispatching simulated patients), and have been trained to portray a character or a patient problem as described in a scripted case scenario.

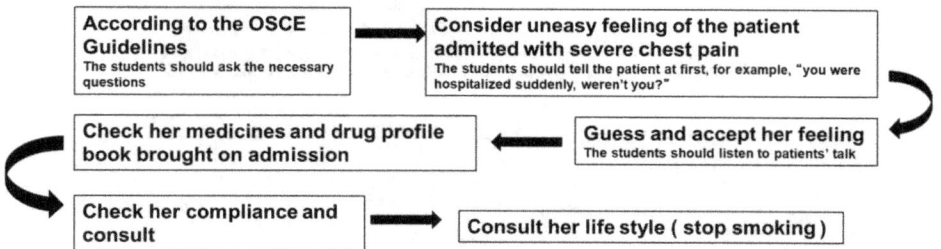

Case (1) 57y.o. Female, Angina, Patient interview on hospital admission

```
┌─────────────────────────────┐      ┌──────────────────────────────────┐
│ According to the OSCE       │ ───► │ Consider uneasy feeling of the     │
│ Guidelines                  │      │ patient admitted with severe chest │
│ The students should ask the │      │ pain                               │
│ necessary questions         │      │ The students should tell the patient│
│                             │      │ at first, for example, "you were    │
│                             │      │ hospitalized suddenly, weren't you?"│
└─────────────────────────────┘      └──────────────────────────────────┘

┌─────────────────────────────┐      ┌──────────────────────────────────┐
│ Check her medicines and     │ ◄─── │ Guess and accept her feeling       │
│ drug profile book brought   │      │ The students should listen to       │
│ on admission                │      │ patients' talk                      │
└─────────────────────────────┘      └──────────────────────────────────┘

┌─────────────────────────────┐      ┌──────────────────────────────────┐
│ Check her compliance and    │ ───► │ Consult her life style ( stop      │
│ consult                     │      │ smoking )                          │
└─────────────────────────────┘      └──────────────────────────────────┘
```

Figure 1. A representative feedback process followed by the faculty for patient simulations.

Table 1. Details of simulated patients.

Case	Patient's Background	Points of Interview	Points of Counseling
57-year-old female with angina	Patient admitted with severe chest pain Non-adherence	Patient's adherence Consider patient's feelings	Using nitroglycerin and isosorbide dinitrate tape Coping with non-adherence Advice to quit smoking
60-year-old female with diabetes	Patient had sudden episodes of increased blood sugar Patient took health food Patient was reluctant to undergo insulin therapy	Check the lifestyle and health food intake Consider patient's feelings	Explaining insulin and oral hypoglycemic drug Counseling to adopt healthy lifestyle
65-year-old male with ureteral stone	Severe pain Anxiety for drug intake due to adverse effect	Consider patient's feelings	Explain about the change of drug
68-year-old male with gallstone	Surgery for gallstone Discontinued anticoagulant agent before surgery Anxiety for surgery	Check discontinued drug Consider patient's feeling before surgery	Consider patient's condition after surgery

3. Results

Questionnaires were completed by all 242 students (response rate, 100%). Regarding whether it was considered effective to use a simulated patient, 99% responded positively. Frequent explanations for the high effectiveness (Figure 2) were that "they could simulate the experience just like with a real patient" (79.3%), "they could raise the presence" (77.3%), and "they could get the feedback from the perspective of patient" (66.5%). In response to whether teaching by faculty staff was effective when adding comments in the step-by-step group discussion, 98% of students answered positively. Among the most frequent reasons for this (Figure 3) were that "feedback from the faculty and simulated patient to peers was useful" (74.4%), "simulations performed by peers were helpful" (71.1%), and "communication points could be understood through the step-by-step analysis" (59.4%).

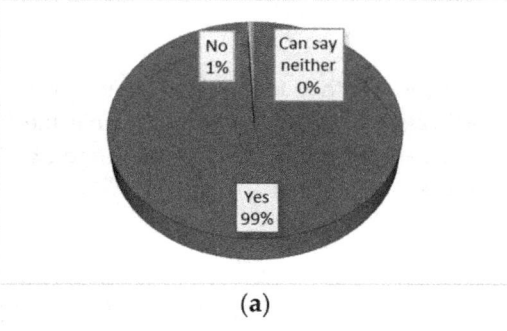

(a)

Figure 2. *Cont.*

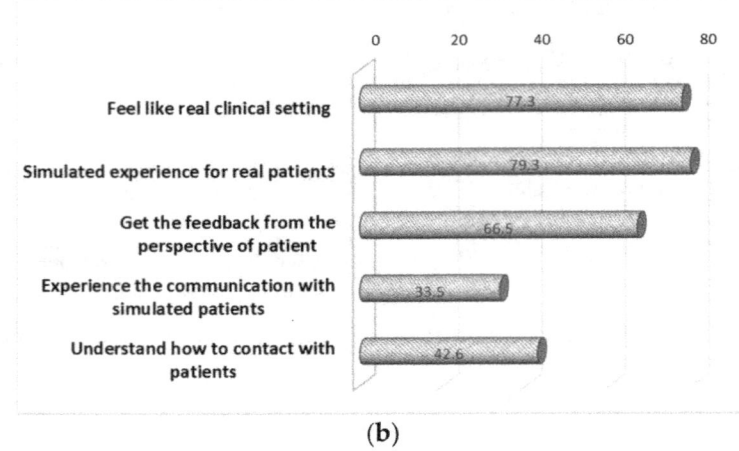

(b)

Figure 2. The effectiveness of using a simulated patient for interview and counseling. (**a**) Response to the question "was it effective that simulated patient played a role in simulation?" (**b**) The reasons for the response given to the question in (**a**); multiple responses were permitted.

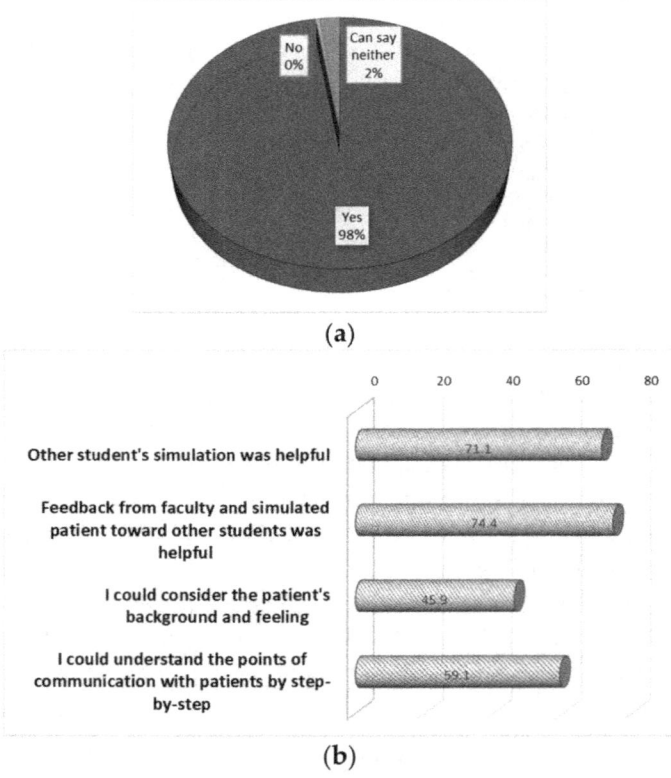

(a)

(b)

Figure 3. Evaluation of the simulation method for teaching about patient interviews and counseling. (**a**) Response to the question "was the teaching method wherein the faculty added step-by-step comments within a group effective?" (**b**) The reasons for the response given to the question in (**a**); multiple responses were permitted.

4. Discussion

The six-year education that was introduced in 2006 aimed to train pharmacists to have not only fundamental scientific knowledge but also a humanistic approach, medical ethics, refinement as a medical specialist, and problem-solving and practical skills.

Practical clinical training is required for at least six months in both hospital and community pharmacies before taking the national examination. This is in line with the 2010 recommendation by the Ministry of Health, Labor and Welfare in Japan, which stated that interprofessional collaboration with other healthcare professionals should be promoted [10]. Indeed, it is considered that the pharmacist should be an expert and authority in medications, being best-placed in medical teams to ensure patient safety and improve medical therapy. The six-year core curriculum therefore aims to improve medical knowledge, skills and attitudes, including key attributes like problem-solving and communication skills [3]. At Kitasato University School of Pharmacy, such programs had already been introduced before 2006, using simulated patients to improve communication skills. This was used as a preliminary education program before students entered clinical training at hospital and community pharmacies. Based on our experience and the results presented, the described training for inpatient interview and counseling is effective.

Hospital pharmacists should be skilled in interviewing patients on hospital admission, for medication counseling, and before discharge. When patients are admitted to hospital, pharmacists should ask about symptoms, disease progression, medication history, and experience of adverse events or allergy. However, as with any other healthcare professional, pharmacists should also consider the patient's background and feelings. To meet this requirement, each student must now have their skills and attitudes evaluated in OSCEs before they can continue training at hospital and community pharmacies [4]. Fifth-year students can then practice medication monitoring, interviews and counseling with the support of a trainer during their clinical experience at a hospital pharmacy [11].

In laboratory practice, simulated inpatient interviews and counseling were used to provide training and develop an understanding of the patients' backgrounds and feelings, paying attention to the requirements of OSCEs [4]. Simulation is an adaptable teaching method and can be used to incorporate a range of skills and knowledge in students pursuing pharmacy [12]. Barrow defined the term simulated patient in 1964, and reported that using a simulated patient instead of actual patients was useful as a teaching and assessment tool in the classroom [13]. Today, several pharmacy schools in Japan use simulated patients to deliver communication-skills education [14]. In the present cases, the simulated patients had received specialized training for each scenario. Most of the students (99%) reported that simulated patients were effective. The students felt like they communicated with real patients, and the simulation created an authentic environment. Moreover, simulated patients can repeat the clinical scenarios and cases can be offered to them on demand [15]. Perhaps most importantly, the students indicated that using these simulated patients was an effective method of role play and that they felt like they were communicating with real patients. Additionally, simulated patients can enhance patient safety because students practice clinical skills without involving actual patients, thereby reducing risk to actual patients [16]. Feedback from the simulated patients was also highly valued and was considered to help the students acknowledge the patient's perspective.

The communication-skills training in this study was delivered in large groups of 40 students per class because of staffing limitations. To deliver an effective teaching method, the simulations were then repeated in small groups of seven or eight students, in which students received feedback from their peers, the simulated patient and the faculty. Most students (98%) reported that this method was effective. Although students did not repeat simulations, they did feel that it was useful to observe their peers and to share in the feedback process. They also felt that the feedback from patients helped them to better understand communication dynamics. Simulated patients were closely matched to the patient scenario to enhance the clinical situation simulation. Additional feedback from the faculty staff supported learning from peers and patients, allowing them to improve in a step-by-step manner within a group. This step-by-step approach is important for students to improve their knowledge and communication skills.

All of the students could pass the part of OSCEs related to simulated inpatient interviews and counseling, and continue the clinical training at the hospitals after this experience. The teaching method advocated in this study, based on small-group discussion of simulated patient interviews, has several key requirements. Before training in the communication-skills laboratory, the details of interviews must be arranged and agreed with the simulated patient to ensure consistency and that learning objectives are met. During this, there is a need to ensure that the scenario includes relevant aspects of how the patient feels and his or her background, ensuring that questions are asked to obtain the patient's viewpoint during feedback. Faculty members must also work in collaboration with the simulated patient and share in the standardization of the teaching method and its goals.

5. Conclusions

The change in curriculum in 2006 requires that students engage in a gradual and continuous program to acquire clinical and practical skills. Overall, the available evidence suggests that simulated patients are suitable for use in communication-skills training. This study was limited to evaluate the efficacy of this training. We would further like to evaluate whether this clinical pharmacy training contributes to clinical practice in a hospital setting.

Author Contributions: R.K. provided all the data and information the revised the manuscript for important intellectual content. T.K. was responsible for the study practice. All other authors contributed to the data collection and interpretation, and critically reviewed the manuscript.

Acknowledgments: I am deeply grateful to Haruko Saeki, Institute of My Informed Consent, who coordinated the simulated patients.

References

1. Ministry of Education, Cultures, Sports, Science and Technology. Improving and Expanding Pharmaceutical Education. Available online: http://www.mext.go.jp/b_menu/shingi/chukyo/chukyo0/toushin/04021801.htm (accessed on 1 March 2018).
2. The Pharmaceutical Society of Japan. Model Core Curriculum for Pharmacy Education. Available online: http://www.pharm.or.jp/kyoiku/pdf/mdl_1408.pdf (accessed on 1 March 2018).
3. The Pharmaceutical Society of Japan. Model Core Curriculum for Pharmacy Practice. Available online: http://www.pharm.or.jp/kyoiku/pdf/mdl_1512.pdf (accessed on 1 March 2018).
4. Pharmaceutical Common Achievement Tests Organization. Available online: http://www.phcat.or.jp/en/ (accessed on 1 March 2018).
5. Lin, K.P.; Travlos, D.V.P.; Wadelin, J.W.P.; Vlasses, P.H.P. Simulation and introductory pharmacy practice experiences. *Am. J. Pharm. Educ.* **2011**, *75*, 209. [CrossRef] [PubMed]
6. Seybert, A.L. Patient simulation in pharmacy education. *Am. J. Pharm. Educ.* **2011**, *75*, 187. [CrossRef] [PubMed]
7. Rickles, N.M.; Tieu, P.; Myers, L.; Galal, S.; Chung, V. The impact of a standardized patient program on student learning of communication skills. *Am. J. Pharm. Educ.* **2009**, *73*, 4. [CrossRef] [PubMed]
8. Cant, R.P.; Cooper, S.J. Simulation-based learning in nurse education: Systematic review. *J. Adv. Nurs.* **2010**, *66*, 3–15. [CrossRef] [PubMed]
9. Norcini, J.; Boulet, J. Methodological issues in the use of standardized patients for assessment. *Teach. Learn. Med.* **2003**, *15*, 293–297. [CrossRef] [PubMed]
10. Ministry of Health, Labor and Welfare. To Promote Interprofessional Collaboration of the Healthcare Professions. Available online: http://www.mhlw.go.jp/shingi/2010/05/dl/s0512-6h.pdf (accessed on 1 March 2018).
11. Utsumi, M.; Hirano, S.; Fujii, Y.; Yamamoto, H. Evaluation of pharmacy practice program in the 6-year pharmaceutical education curriculum in Japan: Hospital pharmacy practice program. *J. Pharm. Health Care Sci.* **2015**, *1*, 18. [CrossRef] [PubMed]
12. Smithson, J.; Bellingan, M.; Glass, B.; Mills, J. Standardized patients in pharmacy education: An integrative literature review. *Curr. Pharm. Teach. Learn.* **2015**, *7*, 851–863. [CrossRef]
13. Barrows, H.S. An overview of the uses of standardized patients for teaching and evaluating clinical skills. *Acad. Med.* **1993**, *68*, 443–451. [CrossRef] [PubMed]

14. Egawa, T.; Shibata, T.; Taniguchi, R.; Ishimoto, A.; Okamatsu, S.; Matsuda, R. Development of systematic communication training program for preclinical training using dialog simulator1. *Jpn. J. Pharm. Health Care Sci.* **2010**, *36*, 476–485. [CrossRef]

15. Bradley, P. The history of simulation in medical education and possible future directions. *Med. Educ.* **2006**, *40*, 254–262. [CrossRef] [PubMed]

16. Kane-Gill, S.L.; Smithburger, P.L. Transitioning knowledge gained from simulation to pharmacy practice. *Am. J. Pharm. Educ.* **2011**, *75*, 210. [CrossRef] [PubMed]

13

Integrating Medication Therapy Management (MTM) Services Provided by Community Pharmacists into a Community-Based Accountable Care Organization (ACO)

Brian Isetts [iD]

Department of Pharmaceutical Care & Health Systems, University of Minnesota College of Pharmacy, 308 Harvard St., SE Minneapolis, MN 55455, USA; isett001@umn.edu

Academic Editors: Anandi Law and Micah Hata

Abstract: (1) Background: As the U.S. healthcare system evolves from fee-for-service financing to global population-based payments designed to be accountable for both quality and total cost of care, the effective and safe use of medications is gaining increased importance. The purpose of this project was to determine the feasibility of integrating medication therapy management (MTM) services provided by community pharmacists into the clinical care teams and the health information technology (HIT) infrastructure for Minnesota Medicaid recipients of a 12-county community-based accountable care organization (ACO). (2) Methods: The continuous quality improvement evaluation methodology employed in this project was the context + mechanism = outcome (CMO) model to account for the fact that programs only work insofar as they introduce promising ideas, solutions and opportunities in the appropriate social and cultural contexts. Collaborations between a 12-county ACO and 15 community pharmacies in Southwest Minnesota served as the social context for this feasibility study of MTM referrals to community pharmacists. (3) Results: All 15 community pharmacy sites were integrated into the HIT infrastructure through Direct Secure Messaging, and there were 32 recipients who received MTM services subsequent to referrals from the ACO at 5 of the 15 community pharmacies over a 1-year implementation phase. (4) Conclusion: At the conclusion of this project, an effective electronic communication and MTM referral system was activated, and consideration was given to community pharmacists providing MTM in future ACO shared savings agreements.

Keywords: community pharmacist interventions; value-based care models; medication therapy management

1. Introduction

The aim of this project was to integrate medication therapy management (MTM) services provided by community pharmacists into the clinical care teams and the health information technology (HIT) infrastructure for Medicaid recipients of a 12-county community-based accountable care organization (ACO). Southern Prairie Community Care (SPCC) of Southwest Minnesota invited colleagues from the University of Minnesota College of Pharmacy to collaborate on integrating medication management services into the redesigned care delivery and financing system of the 12-county SPCC Accountable Care Organization. This was a novel opportunity to engage community pharmacists in a feasibility test of change related to value-based care model integration and financing. Funding for this feasibility study was obtained from the Community Pharmacy Foundation.

The U.S. healthcare system is evolving from fee-for-service reimbursement to an outcomes-based payment system based on reductions in total cost of care and improvements in quality of care performance measures of the Centers for Medicare & Medicaid Services (CMS) Quality Payment Program (QPP) [1].

In this feasibility study, there was an existing reimbursement system in place for the provision of MTM services by pharmacists through the Minnesota Medicaid Program. This existing reimbursement mechanism helped to address a common challenge of providing MTM services. Other common challenges to the provision of MTM services include collaborative relationships with prescribers, billing difficulties, inadequate management support for MTM, and technology barriers such as access to patients' medical records and bi-directional exchange of health information [2].

The SPCC community-based care system has engaged multiple providers, payers and stakeholders since 2006 in building capacity to increase local control around service decisions made for vulnerable people living in the 12-county region. Local pharmacists contributing to SPCC work groups and planning committees during the stakeholder engagement process provided outcomes research data on the impact of MTMS provided by pharmacists, convincing SPCC decision-makers of the need to help patients confidently manage their medications. Pharmacist engagement in the SPCC stakeholder planning process focused attention on the need for building systems to improve the effective and safe use of medications and to reduce drug-related morbidity and mortality.

SPCC is accountable for the medical, facilities, and pharmacy costs of over 20,000 attributable Minnesota Medicaid recipients living in the 12-county region, and there are approximately 36,000 Medicaid recipients in the 12-county SPCC area. Attribution is a method for assigning patients to an ACO based on the utilization history of a patient. Medicaid recipients who are not attributable to the SPCC network typically receive care outside the 12-county area or outside of the SPCC network. It is noted that pharmacy costs constituted nearly one-fourth of total expenditures for SPCC Medicaid recipients, which is well above national averages for pharmaceutical expenditures reported by the Commonwealth Fund based on Organization for Economic Cooperation and Development (OECD) Health Data [3].

The objectives of this project were to: (1) ensure service level expectations of MTM services provided by community pharmacists; (2) equip pharmacists to function effectively in the SPCC healthcare teams; and (3) integrate the electronic documentation of community pharmacists providing MTMS into the SPCC HIT infrastructure. The significance of this initiative relates to community pharmacist integration in new care delivery models supporting the Medicare Access and Chip (Children's Health Insurance Program) Reauthorization Act (MACRA) reimbursement programs.

2. Materials and Methods

The methodological approach used in this project combined evidence-based medicine with the science of continuous quality improvement. The relationship of evidence-based medicine to the science of quality improvement can be described as consistently doing the right thing right. Pawson and Tilley pointeyearbookd out that evidence-based medicine is deeply vested in experimental design using an OXO evaluation approach of: observe a system (O), introduce a perturbation/intervention (X) to some participants but not others, and then observe again (O) [4]. Dr. Don Berwick, former CMS Administrator and champion of the Science of Quality Improvement, has noted that the OXO paradigm most commonly applied in the traditional toolkit of evidence-based medicine is, "a powerful, perhaps unequaled, research design to explore the efficacy of conceptually neat components of clinical practice—tests, drugs, and procedures. For other crucially important learning purposes, however, it serves less well" [5].

Previous research projects have replicated favorable clinical and economic outcomes of pharmacist integration in comprehensive, team-based medication management [6–11]. The evaluation question is no longer *if* pharmacist integration in care model innovation works, but *how* do we make it work more effectively and efficiently? The introduction of interprofessional and interdisciplinary systems for establishing a rational medication use system in which patients routinely achieve their goals of therapy with zero tolerance for preventable medication harms is a complex, multicomponent intervention—essentially a process of social change.

An alternative evaluation approach applied in this project was the context + mechanism = outcome (CMO) model. This evaluation approach accounts for the fact that programs only work insofar as they introduce promising ideas, solutions and opportunities in the appropriate social and cultural contexts [4,5]. One example of the CMO model in use on a large national scale involved concerted rapid cycle quality improvement to reduce medical harms and to decrease readmissions. Results from collaborations among federal partners and external stakeholders indicate that there were 2.1 million fewer patient harms and 87,000 deaths prevented, saving $19.8 billion in costs in the CMS Innovation Center—Partnership for Patients initiative. These improvements included an 8% reduction in Medicare 30-day fee-for-service readmissions and a 15% decrease in hospital acquired adverse drug events [12,13].

2.1. Study Design

This was a 24-month feasibility study that included an 8-month community outreach phase, a 12-month implementation phase and a 4-month evaluation phase, spanning from October 2014–September 2016. The study design focused on three major objectives. The first objective relates to understanding the care capacity of pharmacists working in the 12-county region, and coordinating service level expectations of MTMS provided by pharmacists. The second objective was preparing pharmacists to function effectively in high performing teams. The third objective was integrating the electronic documentation of community pharmacists providing MTMS into the SPCC HIT infrastructure.

2.1.1. Objective 1

Ensuring service level expectations of pharmacists providing MTMS was the responsibility of the Principal Investigator working in collaboration with colleagues from the MedEdge Rx (formerly UPlan) MTM Network. The MedEdge Rx Network coordinated communications among credentialed providers. Prior to project inception, it is noted that pharmacists throughout the 12-county region were formally introduced to the SPCC Accountable Care Organization initiative in December 2013 at a local Minnesota Pharmacists Association Pharmacy Night in which the SPCC CEO served as the keynote presenter.

This project represented an opportunity to build a rational medication use system within redesigned care delivery intended to integrate the resources of pharmacists living and working in the SPCC communities. The pharmacy workforce profile of the 12-county SPCC area includes approximately 80 pharmacists working in 34 community pharmacies, 15 critical access hospitals, three regional hospitals, and 25 area clinics. The 12 Minnesota counties in the SPCC area include (from North to South), Swift, Kandiyohi, Chippewa, Yellow Medicine, Lincoln, Lyon, Redwood Falls, Murray, Cottonwood, Rock, Nobles, and Jackson County. Pharmacists working in 15 community pharmacies and in 2 clinic pharmacies were credentialed providers of the MedEdge Rx MTM Network providing MTMS consistent with State of Minnesota MTM requirements at project inception [14]. All other pharmacists in the SPCC area were contacted in-person and/or by telephone encouraging them to complete MTMS training to become recognized providers by the State of Minnesota Department of Human Services (Minnesota DHS) and enrolled in the MedEdge Rx MTM Network.

Pharmacists in the 12-county region were provided with the opportunity to take Minnesota DHS-approved MTM training programs, if they had not already completed training. The MedEdge Rx MTM Network coordinated oversight for credentialing pharmacists in the SPCC region, providing access to peer mentors, and assessing and monitoring quality of care delivered by pharmacists. An Exempt Category 4 Institutional Review Board (IRB) application was reviewed by the University of Minnesota Human Research Protection Program [15].

2.1.2. Objective 2

This project was designed to equip MTM pharmacists to function effectively in high performing teams for making valuable contributions toward helping patients achieve their drug therapy treatment goals and resolve drug therapy problems. Pharmacists, healthcare teams, and patient advisors across the SPCC area were brought together to build relationships and capacity utilizing portions of the primary care version of Team Strategies and Tools to Enhance Performance and Patient Safety (TeamSTEPPS) [16]. Modified TeamSTEPPS training programs were offered on multiple times/dates so that pharmacists and SPCC providers could have flexibility in attending training programs. A TeamSTEPPS Master Trainer was utilized to lead this program with support from the Principal Investigator.

In addition, a series of periodic half-day workshops were produced to bring community care team members together for the purpose of accelerating progress toward community-based medication management collaborations. Each workshop program included an overview of comprehensive medication management generally and the SPCC MTM Network specifically, as well as small workgroup sessions focusing on areas of care coordination. Topics of focus throughout the SPCC MTM Workshop series included, conducting co-visits, promoting the MTM service to SPCC recipients, and clinical topics such as building community-based systems to assist patients with cardiovascular and mental health needs.

2.1.3. Objective 3

Pharmacist integration into health information technology (HIT) systems and infrastructure is vitally important to effective and efficient team-based care, although access to critical medical information has been historically challenging to obtain for community pharmacists. The third objective of this project was integrating the electronic documentation of community pharmacists providing MTMS into the SPCC HIT infrastructure. Important steps in addressing this objective included:

- Creating the legal and regulatory scaffolding supporting community pharmacist integration in the SPCC HIT system,
- Providing community pharmacists with access to the recently-released national encryption standard for securely exchanging clinical healthcare data and Protected Health Information (PHI) known as Direct Secure Messaging, and,
- Developing processes to help pharmacists more effectively identify SPCC attributable Medicaid recipients for MTM services.

The legal and regulatory infrastructure for pharmacist participation in the SPCC HIT system relates to meeting standard health provider conditions of participation including HIPAA-compliant Provider Participation and Business Associate Agreements. Access to Direct Secure Messaging ensures community pharmacist compliance with the electronic health record technical specifications of the Medicare Access and CHIP Reauthorization Act (MACRA). In addition, pharmacist access to accurate lists of recipients that are both eligible for reimbursement through the Minnesota Medicaid MTM Program, and attributable to the SPCC network would be beneficial in prioritizing SPCC recipients for MTM services.

Southern Prairie Community Care is officially recognized by the State of Minnesota as a Health Information Organization (HIO) under Minnesota Statutes § 2015 62J.4981 [17]. At the time of project inception, SPCC employed the use of a company by the name of Sandlot Solutions, Inc., to serve as its HIT integration vendor, consistent with State of Minnesota technical HIT specifications. The University of Minnesota executed a subcontractor agreement with Santa Rosa Consulting, Inc., the parent company of Sandlot Solutions Inc., to conduct a technology survey of SPCC MTM network pharmacies and to guide the pharmacy HIT integration process.

Integrating pharmacists into the SPCC HIT infrastructure began with a technology survey to assess interoperability and compliance with meaningful use standards. Results of the technology survey were then used to structure technology site visits to each of the SPCC MTM network pharmacies. Once interoperability capabilities were established, original project plans called for the health integration vendor to assist in delivering a Webex training session on procedures and protocols for exchanging electronic health information. The intent of this project was to provide pharmacies with read-only access to medical records of SPCC attributable Medicaid recipients, and if feasible, select one pharmacy to test the bi-direction transfer of medical records and MTM documentation.

3. Results

Final project results were significantly influenced by major SPCC events and challenges. These challenges were related to the SPCC HIT master integration plan and recurring key personnel transitions. These challenges are briefly discussed below as a pretext to presenting project results.

The most significant challenge occurred within the SPCC HIT integration process. As SPCC embarked upon an ambitious goal of creating a common medical records platform across providers, health systems and electronic medical record systems, a number of technical problems were encountered. The goal of creating a common medical record platform for physicians, clinics and MTM pharmacies remained elusive. Early during this project, it became evident that the SPCC timeline for HIT integration was fraught with challenges. The original plan called for HIT integration of physician practices and clinics, followed by SPCC MTM pharmacists and pharmacies. Then, early in 2016, the SPCC HIT Integration Vendor, Sandlot Solutions, abruptly announced it was going out of business [18]. The other significant challenge relates to recurring key personnel losses. Over the course of this project, numerous Care Coordination Integrators were employed and then moved on to other opportunities, and the SPCC Executive Director also departed.

3.1. Feasibility Evaluation

As described in the Methods section, the program evaluation question applied to this feasibility study is not *if* pharmacist integration in care model innovation works, but *how* it works more effectively and efficiently. Pharmacist integration in health system settings of hospitals, clinics, and nursing homes has been in progress for many years. However, community pharmacist integration in emerging community-based care delivery systems is a relatively recent innovation. Therefore, this program evaluation assessed feasibility from both a near-term and a long-term perspective.

The near-term feasibility evaluation utilized the three study objectives of; ensuring service level expectations for MTMS, pharmacist engagement in community-based healthcare teams, and integration into the SPCC Health Information Exchange (HIE). Peer review of MTMS documentation for the 32 SPCC recipient referrals revealed that Minnesota Department of Human Services documentation standards were met for these recipients [14]. Interviews conducted with MTM pharmacists and SPCC personnel at the conclusion of the study indicated that pharmacists at seven of the 17 SPCC MTM sites collaborated with community-based healthcare providers to provide MTM services. In addition, the feasibility of integration in the SPCC HIE system was, at least partially achieved, through pharmacist access to the SPCC Direct Secure Messaging System designed for secure communications among community-based providers.

Long-term feasibility was made possible by determining the number of SPCC MTM pharmacists continuing to care for SPCC recipients one year after study conclusion. This study was conducted from October 2014–September 2016. Post-study interviews were conducted with MTM pharmacists and SPCC personnel in September 2017 indicating that five of the 15 SPCC community pharmacy MTM sites, and both of the clinic-based MTM sites, were continuing to collaborate with health team members in their communities to provide MTM services. Additional results are presented below within each of the three study objectives.

Objective 1: Ensuring Service Level Expectations of Pharmacists Providing MTMS

3.2. Pharmacist Credentialing and Collaboration with MN Department of Human Services (DHS)

The University of Minnesota Human Research Protection Program served as the Institutional Review Board (IRB) for this project, and an Exempt Category 4 IRB application was submitted and reviewed in September of 2014. The goal for this project at inception was to have pharmacists at 12 sites approved by MN DHS as MTM providers. There were 24 pharmacists at 17 sites recognized by the Minnesota Department of Human Services and credentialed by the MedEdge Rx Network as MTM providers. The distribution of 17 sites includes 15 community pharmacies, one clinic pharmacy owned by a community pharmacy, and one pharmacy in a family practice clinic. And the distribution of community pharmacies includes 12 sites owned by regional chain pharmacies, and 4 independent pharmacy sites.

3.3. MTM Billing

The Minnesota Medicaid—Resource-based Relative Value Scale reimbursement system was applied to the care delivered by pharmacists in this project. Of the 20,000 attributable SPCC recipients, the approximate distribution of recipients across health plans included, Blue Cross/Blue Shield (BCBS) managed care Medicaid (~50%), other managed care Medicaid plans (~30%), and MN Department of Human Services (DHS) fee-for-service Medicaid (~20%). MTM claims were submitted as a medical care benefit on an electronic CMS Form 1500 platform, which is the same claims format used for all other health care services. Procedures for submitting MTM claims for MN DHS fee-for-service recipients through the MN-eCONNECT system have been used for the past 10 years. It is noted that SPCC, Blue Cross/Blue Shield and University of Minnesota researchers collaborated to facilitate MTM contracting, and to provide three WebEx training programs for BCBS on-line MTM billing. Reimbursement levels and other economic and clinical data for the 32 SPCC referred recipients receiving MTM services was not an objective of this feasibility project.

Objective 2: Equipping Pharmacists to Function Effectively in SPCC Healthcare Teams

3.4. Interprofessional Team Training and Integration

The effective delivery of MTM provided by pharmacists is dependent on collaborations with a patient's health care team. Interprofessional collaboration represents the "high-touch" element of high-touch/high-tech integration. A series of interprofessional training programs were conducted throughout the course of this project. As part of the community outreach phase, a general MTM Informational Webinar was provided to SPCC community care teams. Then, an interprofessional training program was held that brought pharmacists and SPCC healthcare providers together to start the process of MTM collaboration. During the implementation phase, an SPCC Care Coordinator/MTM Pharmacist workgroup meeting was held to plan the MTM referral process for SPCC recipients, followed by a Care Coordinator workshop and then an SPCC Behavioral Health MTM workgroup meeting.

3.5. Recipient Identification Including MTM Data Driven Intervention Strategy for High Priority Recipient Enrollment

The SPCC ACO presented their proposed Access Design Requirements to the Minnesota Department of Human Services (MN DHS) in February 2016. Pursuant to this formal review and approval, SPCC began preparing the attribution file, or list of eligible recipients, for all healthcare providers across the SPCC network. SPCC ACO leaders then developed a Data Driven Intervention Strategy (DDIS) using recipient's prior medical, hospital and pharmacy claims in the previous year to help them prioritize recipients for MTM referrals. The claims-based data elements for DDIS referrals included recipients in the top 20% of total cost of care or total pharmacy expenditures, or recipients with three or more hospital or emergency department visits over a six-month period.

The original plan to distribute each pharmacy's list of attributable MTM recipients was delayed on several occasions pending DDIS access design reviews by MN DHS. SPCC prioritized MTM recipient referrals based on total health expenditures, medication expenditures and previous hospitalization and emergency room visits. A total of 32 SPCC recipients received MTM services pursuant to referrals at five community pharmacy sites.

Objective 3: Integrating Electronic Documentation in the SPCC HIT Infrastructure

3.6. Health Information Technology (HIT) Integration

Integrating community pharmacists into the HIT infrastructure of the 12-county Southern Prairie Community Care (SPCC) Accountable Care Organization was a key objective of this project. One of the first HIT integration tasks completed early in the project was to have each MTM pharmacy execute HIPAA-compliant Business Associate Agreements and Health Information Exchange Agreements with SPCC. The University of Minnesota then contracted with Santa Rosa Consulting (the parent company of Sandlot Solutions) to assist in the HIT integration process. Santa Rosa Consulting was the same HIT consulting firm hired by SPCC to facilitate exchange of HIT in clinics and health systems across the 12-county ACO.

At the outset of the project there was an ambitious HIE integration plan for community pharmacists that included the following steps:

1   Design of a technology survey for SPCC pharmacies providing MTM services,
2   Technology site visits to SPCC pharmacies with the Health Information Exchange (HIE) Integration Vendor,
3   WebEx training to prepare pharmacies for receiving read-only access to the SPCC HIE infrastructure via a web based portal,
4   Development of technical design specifications for bi-directional data interchange between a pilot MTM pharmacy site and a central SPCC medical exchange platform.

Santa Rosa Consulting met their Step 1 and 2 statements of work. Results of the technology survey revealed that there would need to be a substantial investment to integrate the patient care documentation systems of SPCC MTM pharmacies to facilitate bi-directional data exchange. The primary challenge to bi-directional data exchange of SPCC MTM documentation was because pharmacist care plan HIE standards were not yet established at the time of this study. It is noted that the Pharmacist eCare Plan public/private initiative was recently launched to develop a standardized, interoperable document for exchange of medication management care plans and goals of therapy for pharmacists working in multiple environments [19].

However, the Step 3 and 4 objectives were not met due to insolvency of the HIE Vendor, and funds were reallocated for two alternative HIE integration approaches. A new health care communications portal advocated by the U.S. Department of Health & Human Services, Office of the National Coordinator for Health Information Technology (ONC), known as Direct Secure Messaging, was deployed throughout the SPCC region [20]. Direct Secure Messaging facilitates communications directly between health care providers, rather than relying on facsimile transmission via telephone lines. Each MTM pharmacy's startup costs for Direct Secure Messaging was paid by reallocating funds originally intended for the HIT Integration Vendor. A second approach was for SPCC MTM pharmacies to utilize Business Associate Agreements to gain direct access to their local health systems electronic medical record (EMR) system. At the conclusion of the project, one SPCC MTM community pharmacy was successful in securing read-only access to their local health system's EMR system.

3.7. Qualitative Indicators of Care Model Integration

There were a number of new collaborations and serendipitous events that occurred during this project serving as qualitative indicators of care model integration. As community pharmacists, social service providers, mental health professionals, and community health workers began collaborating around a new community-based model of care; there was evidence of team-based medication management similar to characteristics of integrated health systems employing pharmacists on health teams. Some of these indicators included:

- Pharmacist/Integration Coordinator MTM co-visits including one with a recipient utilizing 44 Emergency Department (E.D.) visits over a 6-month period. The result was that this recipient had no further E.D. visits over the implementation and evaluation phases of this project. There were two direct quotations from SPCC stakeholders related to the care of this recipient that are noteworthy. The Integration Coordinator performing the MTM co-visit noted that, 'I didn't know that pharmacists had this type of training to help patients with their medication problems." The other quote came from the Emergency Department Coordinator at a meeting six months after the MTM co-visit lamenting, 'We haven't seen (this recipient) in six months and we thought that (this person) had passed away.'

- MTM pharmacists at a community pharmacy site located inside a medical clinic were invited to join the clinic's Primary Care Provider Department with dedicated office space to provide MTM services. In addition, this invitation created the opportunity to create a post-graduate pharmacy residency experience at this site. During a Principal Investigator site visit shortly after the MTM pharmacist joined this practice, a primary care provider described elation in this newfound collaboration noting that, 'We always had pharmacists on our teams during my residency training in large health systems, and I never thought this was possible in a small rural setting.'

- Collaborations with the local Health Department to execute a Centers for Disease Control and Prevention (CDC) cardiovascular health outreach grant in which the Community Health Worker was co-located at the MTM Community Pharmacy.

- Placement of an SPCC Integration Coordinator inside one of the community pharmacy MTM sites.

- Placement of an SPCC Somali Cultural Liaison at one of the MTM community pharmacy sites located in a grocery store.

- The appointment of an SPCC MTM Pharmacist to serve on the Southern Prairie Center for Community Health Improvement Board of Directors.

4. Discussion and Future Implications

Although extenuating circumstances that occurred when the SPCC HIT Integration Vendor went out of business coupled with turnover of key SPCC personnel were disappointing, there are a number of highlights and lessons learned that are expected to be helpful in the future. Qualitative indicators and anecdotal reports from the SPCC MTM referrals were encouraging. As community pharmacists in the 12-county SPCC region strive to provide MTM services, discussions have progressed on including SPCC MTM pharmacies in shared savings agreements in the future. Minnesota was one of the first six CMS State Innovation Model (SIM) sites selected to accelerate progress towards value-based reimbursements. And shared savings agreements represent a bridge to global payment systems for achieving better care and better health at lower cost.

This feasibility study was designed to address multiple barriers to pharmacist integration in community-based care teams. As noted previously, common challenges to the provision of MTM services include reimbursement, collaborative relationships with prescribers, billing difficulties, inadequate management support for MTM, and technology barriers such as access to patients' medical records and bi-directional exchange of health information [2]. This study helped community pharmacies by incorporating reasonable reimbursement rates for MTM services, building collaborative relationships with prescribers, streamlining MTM billing and contracting, and addressing technological barriers to a limited extent.

It became apparent that inadequate management support was the common factor among the 10 community pharmacies that were unsuccessful in this project. The context + mechanism = outcome

(CMO) model applied in this study suggests that programs only work insofar as they introduce promising ideas, solutions and opportunities in the appropriate social and cultural contexts [4,5]. The five successful sites provided adequate management support by changing the cultural context of their community pharmacy business model so that the business of patient care could coexist and complement the business of prescription dispensing. This management support included reorienting all community pharmacy personnel to the business of patient care, allocating pharmacist time to caring for patients, and expanding pharmacy technician responsibilities to assist with patient recruitment, scheduling, billing and documentation. This means that future efforts to assist community pharmacies in building patient care practices will need to guide the implementation of effective change management. In other words, removing all other barriers to pharmacist integration in community-based care teams is insufficient without guiding management support for effective change management.

It is important to highlight the relationship of this project to the new physician-focused reimbursement system of the Medicare Access and CHIP Reauthorization Act (MACRA). The two MACRA reimbursement tracks of the Merit-based Incentive Payment System (MIPS) and the Advanced Alternative Payment Models (APM) are founded on achieving Quality Payment Program benchmark measures in the four broad categories of Quality, Improvement Activities, Advancing Care Information, and Cost. The Physician Quality Reporting System served as a backbone of MACRA, and over one-half of the nearly 300 MIPs and APM Program measures are dependent on the effective or safe use of appropriately indicated medications. The profession of Pharmacy has established an extensive research portfolio demonstrating the impact of medication therapy management services on economic, clinical, and humanistic outcomes. And steps taken in this project to integrate community pharmacists in a community-based ACO are expected to help accelerate collaborations with physicians to achieve MACRA benchmarks.

The elusive goal of Health Information Integration (HIE) was prominent in this feasibility study. Although the ambitious objective of bi-directional HIE was not achieved, the integration of MTM pharmacists into the SPCC Direct Secure Messaging infrastructure has the potential to accelerate use of the Pharmacist eCare Plan standards, when fully developed [19]. The Pharmacy HIT Collaborative has championed a national focus on ensuring the meaningful use of standardized electronic health records (EHR) that supports safe, efficient, and effective medication use, continuity of care, and providing access to the patient-care services of pharmacists with other members of the interprofessional patient care team [21]. The experiences and results of this project can help other health systems and community pharmacies understand the steps and challenges that will need to be addressed to achieve this Pharmacy HIT Collaborative vision.

Assessing the need for community pharmacist engagement in value-based healthcare delivery and financing is summarized in a White Paper produced under contract from the Pharmacy Quality Alliance. *Applying Value-based Incentive Models within Community Pharmacy Practice* presents the landscape for engaging community pharmacists in improving health care quality through innovative care delivery and payment models. Key concepts applied in this PQA White Paper included arrangements for pharmacists/pharmacies to share savings with ACO providers, and implementing value-based insurance programs in community pharmacies [22].

Limitations

One potential limitation of this feasibility study is that it was not designed to evaluate clinical or economic outcomes of MTM services. As noted in the Methods section, previous results of research projects demonstrating favorable clinical and economic outcomes of pharmacist integration in comprehensive, team-based medication management has shifted the evaluation question to *how* we can make this integration more effective and efficient. The fact that an existing reimbursement system was in place for the provision of MTM services by pharmacists through the Minnesota Medicaid Program facilitated the design of this feasibility study.

It is noted that the provision of MTMS for children was not a component of this feasibility study. Although pharmacists may provide MTMS for Minnesota Medicaid recipients under the age of 18, this patient population was not a focus of the SPCC attributable ACO population. Future feasibility studies related to the provision of MTMS for children in evolving MACRA care delivery and financing systems is warranted.

Although reducing the burden of ineffective medication use and drug-related morbidity and mortality may seem like a daunting task, there is a solution. Outcomes studies of MTMS provided by pharmacists working in interprofessional care teams have consistently demonstrated improved clinical outcomes, reduced healthcare expenditures, and favorable return on investment [6–11]. The fact that the U.S. healthcare system is leaving an antiquated fee-for-service reimbursement system behind in favor of value-based healthcare delivery and financing is good news for individuals who take medications. This project was designed to address community-based care system needs by ensuring service level expectations of MTM services provided by community pharmacists, equipping pharmacists to function effectively in SPCC community-based healthcare teams, and integrating the electronic documentation of community pharmacists providing MTMS into the SPCC HIT infrastructure.

Future research and pharmacy/pharmacist opportunities will be created by understanding the MTMS service level expectations of community-based care teams, establishing tools and resources for community pharmacists to function effectively in high-performing health teams, and by integrating the electronic documentation of community pharmacists providing MTMS into HIT infrastructure.

The health care industry is implementing a range of approaches for succeeding in risk-bearing and outcomes-based financing to shift payments from volume to value [23]. Competencies for effective and efficient team-based medication management in which pharmacists are integrated into community-based health teams is essential to achieving this value-based care model objective. The experiences and results of this study are expected to make an important contribution to building community-based medication management toolkits of the future.

5. Conclusions

Pharmacist integration in healthcare teams in hospitals, skilled nursing facilities, and clinics has grown steadily over the past 30 years. Community pharmacist integration in healthcare teams has unique challenges owing largely to distance, information access, and reimbursement. As healthcare delivery and financing transitions from expensive volume-based services and procedures in hospitals, emergency departments and large facilities, to community-based care delivery and value-based financing, there is a new opportunity for community pharmacists to develop patient care practices. This feasibility study of community pharmacist integration was enabled by a community-based ACO with strong support for community pharmacist integration in new care delivery and information exchange models, as well as the presence of a pharmacist reimbursement system for MTM services.

Although the daunting task of bi-directional exchange of health information between health systems and community pharmacists persist, there were small steps forward in terms of using Direct Secure Messaging to communicate with other community health team members, as well as the emergence of new Pharmacy eCare Plan standards for integrating pharmacists' MTM documentation into electronic health records. A significant lesson learned in this feasibility study is the importance of understanding the skills and abilities of all other care providers in a community and then working together in coordinated action similar to high performing health teams in large medical centers. Equally important are lessons learned from unsuccessful sites in that removing barriers of reimbursement, billing, collaborative prescriber relationships, and technology access are insufficient to advance community pharmacy practice without also guiding management support for social and cultural transformation so that the business of patient care can coexist and complement the prescription dispensing business.

Acknowledgments: Gary Schneider and colleagues of the MedEdge Rx MTM Network were instrumental in supporting the SPCC MTM Network and communicating with pharmacists throughout this study. Amy Pittenger, Associate Professor at the University of Minnesota College of Pharmacy and a TeamSTEPPS Master Trainer, assisted in designing the SPCC community-based interprofessional training programs for this study. Shelly Spiro, Executive Director of the Pharmacy HIT Collaborative, provided guidance related to the health information exchange components of this study. Norris Anderson, Chief Medical Officer, and colleagues of Southern Prairie Community Care devoted considerable time and resources to promoting and supporting MTM services provided by pharmacists in this study.

Author Contributions: Brian Isetts is the sole investigator and author of this manuscript, and has been responsible for all phases of this study.

Funding: This feasibility study was funded by the Community Pharmacy Foundation.

References

1. U.S. Department of Health & Human Services. Quality Payment Program. Available online: https://qpp.cms.gov/ (accessed on 25 August 2017).

2. American Pharmacists Association. *Medication Therapy Management Digest*; American Pharmacists Association: Washington, DC, USA, 2013.

3. The Commonwealth Fund. U.S. Health Care from a Global Perspective: Spending, Use of Services, Prices, and Health in 13 Countries. Available online: http://www.commonwealthfund.org/publications/issue-briefs/2015/oct/us-health-care-from-a-global-perspective (accessed on 8 October 2017).

4. Pawson, R.; Tilley, N. *Realistic Evaluation*; Sage Publications Ltd.: London, UK, 1997.

5. Berwick, D.M. The Science of Improvement. *JAMA* **2008**, *299*, 1182–1184. [CrossRef] [PubMed]

6. Chisholm-Burns, M.A.; Graff Zivin, J.S.; Lee, J.K.; Spivey, C.A.; Slack, M.; Herrier, R.N.; Hall-Lipsy, E.; Abraham, I.; Palmer, J. Economic effects of pharmacists on health outcomes in the United States: A systematic review. *Am. J. Health-Syst. Pharm.* **2010**, *67*, 1624–1634. [CrossRef] [PubMed]

7. Isetts, B.J.; Brown, L.M.; Schondelmeyer, S.W.; Lenarz, L.A. Quality assessment of a collaborative approach for decreasing drug-related morbidity and achieving therapeutic goals. *Arch. Intern. Med.* **2003**, *163*, 1813–1820. [CrossRef] [PubMed]

8. Isetts, B.J.; Brummel, A.R.; Ramalho de Oliveira, D.; Moen, D.W. Managing drug-related morbidity and mortality in a patient-centered medical home. *Med. Care* **2012**, *50*, 997–1001. [CrossRef] [PubMed]

9. Isetts, B.J.; Schondelmeyer, S.W.; Artz, M.B.; Lenarz, L.A.; Heaton, A.H.; Wadd, W.B.; Brown, L.B.; Cipolle, R.J. Clinical and economic outcomes of medication therapy management services: The Minnesota experience. *J. Am. Pharm. Assoc.* **2008**, *48*, 203–211. [CrossRef] [PubMed]

10. Gattis, W.A.; Hasselblad, V.; Whellan, D.J.; O'Connor, C.M. Reduction in heart failure events by the addition of a clinical pharmacist to the heart failure management team: Results of the pharmacist in heart failure assessment recommendation and monitoring (PHARM) study. *Arch. Intern. Med.* **1999**, *159*, 1939–1945. [CrossRef] [PubMed]

11. Cranor, C.W.; Christensen, D.B. The Asheville Project: Long-Term Clinical and Economic Outcomes of a Community Pharmacy Diabetes Care Program. *J. Am. Pharm. Assoc.* **2003**, *43*, 173–184. [CrossRef]

12. U.S. Department of Health & Human Services, Agency for Healthcare Research and Quality. Saving Lives and Saving Money: Hospital-Acquired Conditions Update. 1 December 2015. Available online: https://www.ahrq.gov/professionals/quality-patient-safety/pfp/interimhacrate2014.html?utm_source=HHSPressRelease65&utm_medium=HHSPressRelease&utm_term=HAC&utm_content=65&utm_campaign=CUSP4CAUTI2015 (accessed on 8 October 2017).

13. Centers for Medicare & Medicaid Services, Center for Medicare and Medicaid Innovation. Project Evaluation Activity in Support of Partnership for Patients: Task 2 Evaluation Progress Report. 10 July 2014. Available online: https://partnershipforpatients.cms.gov/about-the-partnership/what-is-the-partnership-about/lpwhat-the-partnership-is-about.html (accessed on 23 July 2017).

14. Minnesota Department of Human Services. Medication Therapy Management Services (MTMS). Available online: http://www.dhs.state.mn.us/main/idcplg?IdcService=GET_DYNAMIC_CONVERSION& RevisionSelectionMethod=LatestReleased&dDocName=dhs16_136889 (accessed on 8 October 2017).

15. University of Minnesota—Human Research Protection Program. Available online: http://www.irb.umn. edu/ (accessed on 8 October 2017).

16. Agency for Healthcare Research and Quality (AHRQ). TeamSTEPPS Primary Care Version. Available online: http://www.ahrq.gov/professionals/education/curriculum-tools/teamstepps/primarycare/ (accessed on 8 October 2017).

17. State of Minnesota. Office of the Revisor of Statutes. 2015 Minnesota Statutes, 62J.4981 Certificate of Authority to Provide Health Information Exchange Services. Available online: https://www.revisor.mn. gov/statutes/?id=62J.4981&year=2015 (accessed on 8 October 2017).

18. Modern Healthcare. Chicago-Area HIE Sues IT Vendor over Shutdown Plans. 20 April 2016. Available online: http://www.modernhealthcare.com/article/20160420/NEWS/160429995 (accessed on 8 October 2017).

19. HealthIT.gov Interoperability Proving Ground. Pharmacist eCare Plan. Available online: https://www. healthit.gov/techlab/ipg/node/4/submission/1376 (accessed on 8 October 2017).

20. HealthIT.gov Interoperability Portfolio. Direct Project. Available online: https://www.healthit.gov/policy-researchers-implementers/direct-project (accessed on 8 October 2017).

21. Pharmacy Health Information Technology Collaborative. Pharmacist's Role in HIT. Available online: http://www.pharmacyhit.org/ (accessed on 8 October 2017).

22. Pringle, J.A. Perspectives: Applying Value-Based Incentive Models within Community Pharmacy Practice. Available online: http://pqaalliance.org/images/uploads/files/VBI_Paper_FINAL_20140522_v3--0.pdf27 (accessed on 8 October 2017).

23. McClellan, M.B.; Leavitt, M.O. Vital directions from the National Academy of Medicine: Competencies and tools to shift payments from volume to value. *JAMA* **2016**, *316*, 1655–1656. [CrossRef] [PubMed]

14

Competence-Based Pharmacy Education in the University of Helsinki

Nina Katajavuori, Outi Salminen, Katariina Vuorensola, Helena Huhtala, Pia Vuorela and Jouni Hirvonen *

Faculty of Pharmacy, University of Helsinki, P.O. Box 56, 00014 Helsinki, Finland;
nina.katajavuori@helsinki.fi (K.N.); outi.salminen@helsinki.fi (S.O.); katariina.vuorensola@helsinki.fi (V.K.);
helena.huhtala@helsinki.fi (H.H.); pia.vuorela@helsinki.fi (V.P.)
* Correspondence: jouni.hirvonen@helsinki.fi

Academic Editor: Jeffrey Atkinson

Abstract: In order to meet the expectations to act as an expert in the health care profession, it is of utmost importance that pharmacy education creates knowledge and skills needed in today's working life. Thus, the planning of the curriculum should be based on relevant and up-to-date learning outcomes. In the University of Helsinki, a university wide curriculum reform called 'the Big Wheel' was launched in 2015. After the reform, the basic degrees of the university are two-cycle (Bachelor–Master) and competence-based, where the learning outcomes form a solid basis for the curriculum goals and implementation. In the Faculty of Pharmacy, this curriculum reform was conducted in two phases during 2012–2016. The construction of the curriculum was based on the most relevant learning outcomes concerning working life via high quality first (Bachelor of Science in Pharmacy) and second (Master of Science in Pharmacy) cycle degree programs. The reform was kicked off by interviewing all the relevant stakeholders: students, teachers, and pharmacists/experts in all the working life sectors of pharmacy. Based on these interviews, the intended learning outcomes of the Pharmacy degree programs were defined including both subject/contents-related and generic skills. The curriculum design was based on the principles of constructive alignment and new structures and methods were applied in order to foster the implementation of the learning outcomes. During the process, it became evident that a competence-based curriculum can be created only in close co-operation with the stakeholders, including teachers and students. Well-structured and facilitated co-operation amongst the teachers enabled the development of many new and innovative teaching practices. The European Union funded PHAR-QA project provided, at the same time, a highly relevant framework to compare the curriculum development in Helsinki against Europe-wide definitions of competences and learning outcomes in pharmacy education.

Keywords: curriculum; learning outcomes; competency; stakeholders; generic skills

---

1. Introduction

In order to meet the expectations of an expert in the health care profession, it is of utmost importance that pharmacy education also creates the knowledge and skills needed in working life and to serve society. Pharmacists are in responsible positions within the health care system and therefore high quality, competence-based pharmacy education is needed [1–5].

Competence can be defined as a specialized system of abilities, proficiencies, or skills that are necessary to reach a specific goal. The term also refers to special functional competencies which are needed in a particular area of expertise [6]. In competence-based curriculum, four features are emphasized: focus on outcomes, emphasis on abilities, a reduced emphasis on time-based training and learner centeredness [7]. Thus, a competence-based curriculum in higher education aims at responding to the needs of the working life. In a competence-based curriculum the defined learning outcomes describe what the students are expected to know, understand and/or be able to do after completing a degree or in order to attain a passing grade in a course [8]. The definition of the learning outcomes take into account not only the expertise in the field, but also the knowledge and skills required for employment [9]. Furthermore, the discipline's latest developments and trends, as well as the changing learning needs and requirements of employers, need to be taken account [10].

The defined learning outcomes describe the knowledge, skills, and attitudes thought to be essential for a professional individual in their working life [11]. It is possible to divide the competencies into three categories: (1) Discipline-specific knowledge and skills; (2) Generic knowledge and skills for knowledge work; and (3) Knowledge and skills related to the expert identity (e.g., [10,12]). Carefully defined learning outcomes should aid the students to better understand what kind of knowledge and skills are needed in their profession after graduation and to direct their learning during (and after) their studies, and thus, aid the students to study more effectively and in a deep-level manner [8].

Learning outcomes should be defined for the whole study programs in the University, but also for each study-module and individual course within the program. Thus, the defined learning outcomes are more general at the program level, and more specified in the module and course levels ([8] Biggs & Tang 2011). The defined learning outcomes for the program affect both the curriculum design and teaching. The curriculum structure, as well as the teaching methods, should be derived from and linked to the specified learning objectives [2,8,13]. Furthermore, the assessment should be criterion-based and should validly be related to learning outcomes. John Biggs [2,13] coined the term "constructive alignment" to describe this kind of high quality curriculum design. In a constructively aligned curriculum the learning outcomes, course contents, teaching methods, and assessment are aligned and foster students' deep-level learning. In other words, constructive alignment highlights the importance of applying the defined competencies and learning outcomes to real-life teaching practices throughout the curriculum.

An extensive education reform, called 'the Big Wheel', was launched at the University of Helsinki in 2015. The aim of this reform is to create competence-based curricula with defined learning outcomes for all the study programs in the University in order to equip the students with the most relevant knowledge and skills needed in today's working life. In addition, the reform aims at producing the most qualified programs, education, and teaching practices throughout the University in order to foster the students' deep-level learning via the constructive alignment. Each study program (Bachelor and Master) has a degree program director and a steering group to ensure the quality of the programs. The competence-based teaching in the multidisciplinary programs makes it possible for a student to reach the ability to "think big", to perceive the whole picture and to assess connections in different contexts. There is also an increasing need to develop broadly such skills as critical thinking, information analysis, and communication (see [5,9,10]).

Faculty of Pharmacy, University of Helsinki, offers Bachelor's, Master's, and Doctoral Degree programs in pharmacy education. Students complete the Bachelor's Degree (180 credits) in three years and Master's Degree (additional 120 credits) in five years. The studies include a compulsory 3 + 3 month work practice in a community and/or hospital pharmacy during their second and third study-years. The majority of the graduating students find a job in community pharmacies, followed by hospital pharmacies, drug industry and research, education, and administration.

In the Faculty of Pharmacy, the curriculum reform was launched already in 2012, before the Big Wheel reform of the entire University of Helsinki commenced. There was a true need to define the competencies and to create learning outcomes for the Bachelor's and Master's programs in Pharmacy. The teachers, students, and employers all pointed out the need to update teaching contents and practices according to the rapidly developing knowledge and practices in various fields of pharmacy profession. These renewals in Helsinki can be directly related to and compared with the process and outcomes of the PHAR-QA project. This article summarizes these developmental activities and is focused on the processes of the reforms as well as on the outcomes.

2. Process of the Curriculum Reform

The learning outcomes for both the Bachelor's and Master's degree programs were created during 2012–2016. In addition, contents and practices of teaching were reformed to meet the intended learning outcomes in order to follow the principles of constructive alignment [3,8,13]. The curriculum reform took place in two phases: the first (2012–2014) focused on the Bachelor's program and the second (2015–2017) on the Master's program. Both the renewals were conducted by a named team, which consisted of senior lecturers in pharmacy education, a senior lecturer in higher education, and a member of administrative staff. The teams cooperated closely with the Educational Committee of the Faculty and organized several hearings and interviews for all the professors, teachers, and students in the Faculty.

In the beginning of the reform, the team carefully studied all the relevant information about the recent evaluations and research reports of pharmacy education and study subjects together with feedback from curriculum and course evaluations. In addition, the team benchmarked exemplary educational units on health care and management in order to find out the best practices for conducting the educational reform. Based on this familiarization, specific aims for the curriculum reform were formed: (1) to create the learning outcomes for the Bachelor's and Master's programs which would meet the needs of working life; (2) to create a more challenging curriculum and to develop teaching and assessing methods which would foster students' deep level learning and active work by students; and (3) to increase the flexibility of the curriculum and the amount of optional studies and thereby strengthen the professional orientation and identity of the students.

In order to define the learning outcomes, the team arranged hearings for all the relevant parties in autumn 2012. The needs of the working life representatives were found out by interviewing a broad sample of stakeholders in the field of pharmacy. For example, community and hospital pharmacies, the pharmaceutical industry, and authorities in the pharmacy sector were interviewed. The team interviewed also faculty teachers in each discipline, pharmacy students, and international staff of the faculty. The interviews were conducted as focus group discussions. In each interview, there were three to nine participants and they lasted for 60–120 min. Furthermore, all the professors of the faculty were interviewed individually in order to hear their visions in more detail and to engage them to the reform. More than 30 interviews were performed with 83 interviewees altogether.

The interviews explored the competencies, knowledge, and skills a pharmacy student should gain by graduation in order to excel in working life in the field of pharmacy. Detailed notes were written during every interview and the notes written were visible to all the participants in the discussions. The notes were commented on and corrected during the discussion if needed. The data of the interviews was analyzed by content analysis method by grouping and categorizing similar themes. In spring 2013, based on the analyses, the team formulated a draft of the learning outcomes including both subject/contents knowledge and generic skills for the Bachelor's and Master's programs (see [9,10]). The learning outcomes were further developed, defined, and finalized in several workshops during the spring and autumn 2013. All the interviewed stakeholders, teachers, and students of the faculty were invited to these workshops. The aims of the workshops were to inform about the process and also to discuss important and current themes which rose up from the interviews or from the process. In this respect, the process resembled the iterative character of the Delphi methodology in the PHAR-QA project. Also, the next steps in the reform were decided upon together in the workshops (Figure 1).

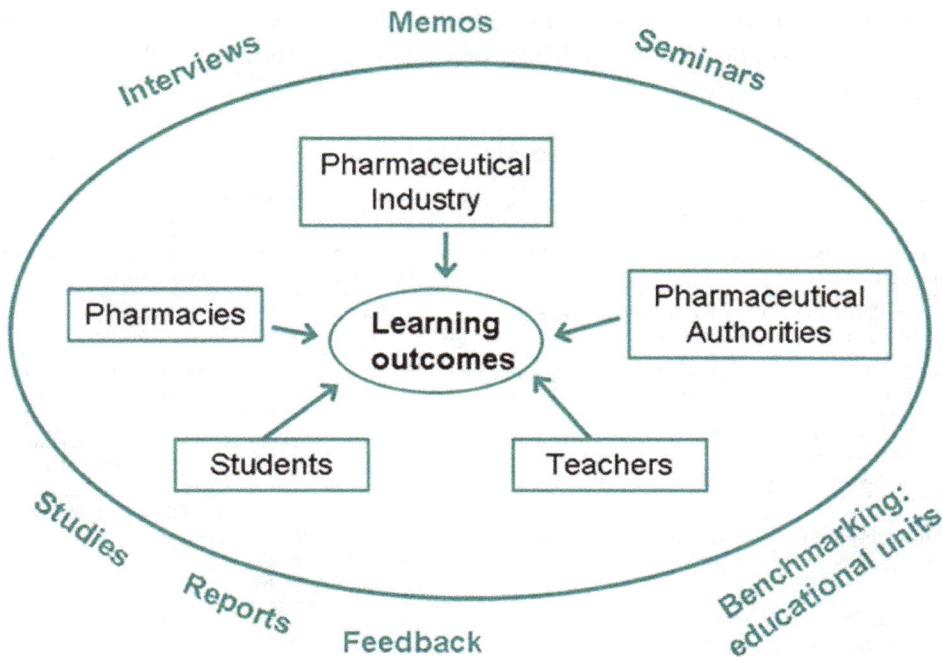

Figure 1. Defining the learning outcomes for Bachelor's and Master's programs in pharmacy.

3. The Outcomes of the Curriculum Reform

Formation of the new curriculum was a communal process between the University and working life. The curriculum, its contents, and the learning outcomes for the degree programs were discussed and processed together with teachers, stakeholders, and students (see [3,8]). The atmosphere during the process was enthusiastic and allowed everyone to participate in the process. An increased and systematic co-operation between the university teachers was grounded during the curriculum reform process in order to foster communal learning (e.g., [14,15]). As a result, many of the new practices developed during the curriculum reform were created in longitudinal processes in close co-operation with teachers. In addition, closer co-operation between the university teachers and the stakeholders was established.

3.1. The Learning Outcomes

The learning outcomes for the programs were defined and, for the first time, the learning outcomes for the programs in pharmacy education in Helsinki also included generic skills (Table 1). When the learning outcomes are defined for the program-level, they are at a more general level. More detailed learning outcomes should be defined at module and course levels of the program [8]. Importance of generic skills in working life were highly emphasized in the interviews. Although the backgrounds of the interviewees were quite different, the learning outcomes proposed by different stakeholders were surprisingly uniform. In addition to critical thinking and problem solving skills, the importance of professionalism rose up in the interviews. Pharmacy students should develop their professional identity during the studies. That includes the importance of realizing one's role in a health care system and understanding the significance and versatility of the pharmacy field. The core of the pharmaceutical knowledge was, however, to be focused on drug(s) and medication and the education should give a strong basis for this pharmaceutical knowledge and expertise. Defined generic learning outcomes seem to be uniform also at an international level, as shown by Bzowyckyj and Janke [5].

The objectives of education leading to the degrees of Bachelor's and Master's of Science (Pharmacy) are: (1) To produce experts for pharmaceutical work in all branches of healthcare and provide the knowledge and skills needed to maintain and improve their expertise; (2) To ensure pharmaceutical expertise, the degrees aim to provide students with the general knowledge and skills described below. Directive 2005/36/EC outlines the knowledge to be acquired through the education leading to the Master's of Science (Pharmacy) degree.

Table 1. Learning outcomes for the degrees of Bachelor's and Master's of Science (Pharmacy).

Bachelor's of Science (Pharmacy)	
Learning outcomes concerning knowledge of students who have completed the degree:	**Learning outcomes concerning generic skills of students who have completed the degree:**
Can apply basic knowledge of the natural sciences and biomedicine in pharmaceutical work	Have developed a professional identity and understand their expert role and duties in healthcare
Have a comprehensive command of pharmacotherapy, from the manufacture of medications to their safe and appropriate use	Are capable of critical thinking, that is, can assess information and apply the results of research in their work
Understand the field of pharmacy as a whole, including employment prospects as well as the role and significance of pharmacy in Finnish and other societies and healthcare systems	Have good problem-solving skills, can tolerate uncertainty, and can acquire information independently
Have the language and communication skills required for expert pharmaceutical work	Understand the necessity of lifelong learning, are motivated to enhance their expertise and can act in a self-directed, creative, ethical, and responsible manner in compliance with the principles of sustainable development
Understand the basic economic principles of business operations and the social functions of healthcare	Can communicate and interact both with customers and in multi-professional groups
Master's of Science (Pharmacy)	
Learning outcomes concerning knowledge	**Learning outcomes concerning generic skills**
Students who have completed the degree have expanded the knowledge and skills acquired through their Bachelor's of Science (Pharmacy) degree, in addition to which they:	
Profoundly understand the broad scope of the discipline of pharmacy and have a command of its key phenomena, theories, and concepts	Can work as experts, trainers, and developers in multiprofessional groups in both the pharmaceutical industry and the healthcare sector in Finland and abroad
Have a command of the basics of pharmaceutical development, understand the process of pharmaceutical development, and can apply their knowledge as experts in pharmaceutical development and pharmacotherapy	Have a command of key research methods as well as the research-based work method, can draw scientific conclusions and can produce scientific texts
Have acquired good theoretical competence and methodological knowledge in their specialist area	Have acquired the competences needed for research work in their specialist area as well as the competences for independent work in an international multi-professional research community
Can work in an expert environment in compliance with the principles of expert leadership and have the competence to develop in supervisory positions	Can think critically and analytically and apply research-based knowledge in their work, and have acquired good argumentation and problem-solving skills
Have a command of the basic concepts of business administration and understand the realities of business, particularly from the perspective of pharmaceutical medicine	Understand the potential provided by their expertise in various international environments

3.2. Curriculum Structures

In order to meet the defined learning outcomes and to foster the constructive alignment in teaching, the curriculum structure was modified first. For the Bachelor's program (the first three study years), a strand model was created by grouping the courses with similar contents to the same strand, to diminish the overlapping of the courses and to promote the smooth continuum of the studies (Figure 2). Coordinators for the four strands in the curriculum, the strand leaders, were nominated in 2014 to lead this process and to develop the constructive alignment and collaboration in the curriculum development and practices. To increase the professional identity of the pharmacy students, the amount of optional studies was increased in the new curriculum. In addition, the optional studies were grouped into three study paths, namely (1) community and hospital pharmacy; (2) industrial pharmacy and pharmaceutical authorities; and (3) research and scientific thinking.

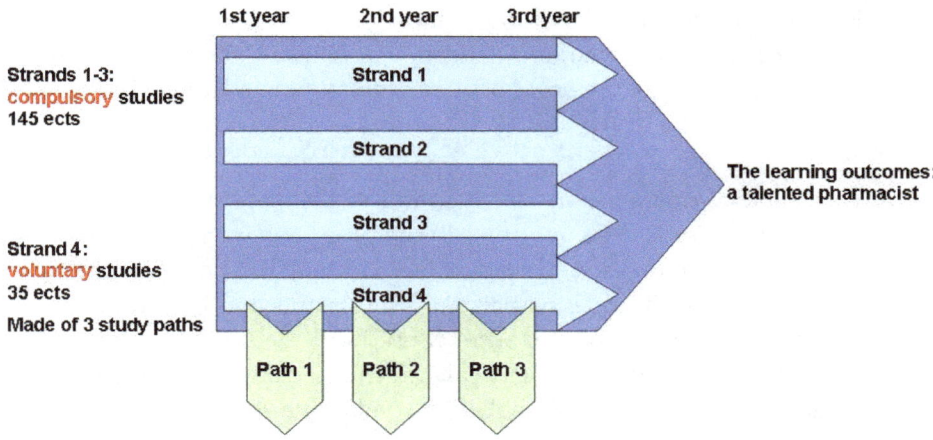

Figure 2. The strand model in Bachelor's program in the University of Helsinki.

During the Master's program (fourth and fifth study years) the first autumn includes compulsory studies incorporated to one large module, called "Drug Development and Use" (Figure 3). Parallel to this module, there are other compulsory modules including business, economics, analytics and statistics, and also preparation of a personal learning portfolio. The whole term is implemented in close collaboration of all the responsible teachers lead by a named coordinator. In the beginning of the spring term, the students select one specializing study line from seven different disciplines within the field of pharmacy. During these advanced major subject studies the students prepare their Master's Thesis. The program also contains advanced level optional studies.

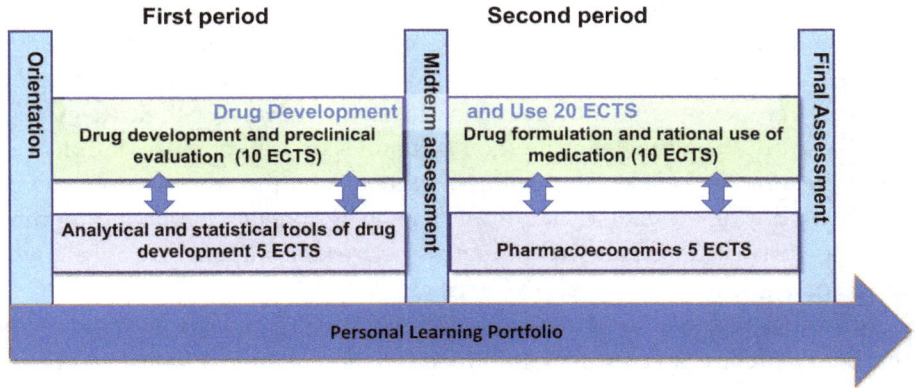

Figure 3. The compulsory studies during the fourth year of Master's Program in Pharmacy in the University of Helsinki.

As a result of the Big Wheel reform, steering groups with degree program directors were nominated for the Bachelor's and Master's programs in the end of the year 2016. These groups co-operate with each other and lead all the teaching and education development practices from now on, while different working groups, like strand leaders, fall within the guidance of these steering groups.

3.3. Projects Based on the Defined Learning Outcomes during the Pharmacy Education

A few projects extending over the whole curriculum were established to respond to the requested theoretical and generic learning outcomes, and further, to foster students' deep-level learning:

(1) teachers' workshops within and between the strands in Bachelor's program and during the first term of the Master's program; (2) student group work emphasizing the generic skills; (3) portfolio working; (4) progress testing; and (5) the proof demonstration of knowledge/skills.

3.3.1. Engagement of the Teachers to Constructive Alignment in Curriculum Design

In order to foster the co-operation in teaching and to develop the teaching and assessment methods, the new strand model and the modules in the programs were discussed and developed in workshops lead by the nominated strand leaders (see [14,16,17]). The new learning outcomes of the programs were implemented and defined also for the strands and individual courses. Several workshops within the strands and modules were carried out including discussions between the teachers about the learning outcomes, constructive alignment, teaching, and assessing methods which would foster students' deep level learning, challenge-level of the studies and the work-load of the learning tasks.

These workshops created an enthusiastic atmosphere between the teachers. Co-operation and alignment between courses were achieved and teaching and assessment methods were developed. The amount of the lectures was reduced, and new teaching methods like flipped classroom, different assignments, and projects, were introduced to the courses. Assessment methods were also diversified to include also self and peer evaluation, oral assessment, and evaluation of the project works. In addition, the timing of the teaching and assessments were coordinated (see [8]).

From now on, the nominated steering groups of the programs followed the work of the teachers in the strand groups as well as in the module groups and make sure that the teaching and evaluation of the programs were based on the learning outcomes and followed the principles of constructive alignment.

3.3.2. Fostering the Learning of Generic Skills

In order to help students to achieve the defined learning outcomes, to encourage their deep-level learning, and to achieve generic skills (Table 1), a systematic and explicit approach was integrated to the theoretical studies facilitating students' active learning process (see [8–10]).

In the very beginning of their studies, students are divided into small groups. Within these groups, they study together the whole academic year practicing generic skills and solving complicated theoretical problems related to theoretical courses. Four challenging theoretical courses throughout the first study year were selected for this purpose. Each course has a specific theme for the generic skills exercises like group forming, learning methods and scheduling, presentation of results of the assignments, and preparation for an examination. Instructions for the groups are given via the Moodle learning environment during the courses and the groups work independently on assignments without teachers. With proper instructions and well-thought exercises the students are able to work in groups without tutoring and solve the theoretical problems given in the courses.

Student groups produce materials and memorandums to the Moodle. In these memos, students reflect on their study process and present solutions for the theoretical assignments. The students' outputs are addressed during the lectures afterwards and the teachers also give feedback of the tasks collectively via the Moodle.

The group meetings succeeded well and the students felt that the groups are effective in helping to understand the theory and to learn generic skills. On the other hand, some students have had problems in understanding the significance of the group work and allocating time for the meetings. Teachers' experiences have been positive: students' study success and group working skills have been significantly improved compared to previous years, and less individual tutoring is needed. In the future, the group assignments will be developed further by selecting the most relevant and closely connected assignments to the theoretical courses. The solid basis for group working is established during the first study year. Different kinds of group assignments continue throughout the study program. In the second study year, learning of the generic skills is highlighted by different kinds of self-evaluations related to the theoretical courses.

3.3.3. The Learning Portfolio in the Study Programs

A portfolio is a tool to plan and document ones' education, work demonstrations and skills. A portfolio can include in-depth reflection of ones' development and transferable skills. In higher education, portfolios can be used as a tool to evaluate how well the theoretical and generic skills are achieved during the curriculum [18,19].

In order to visualize the learning and development of the students, a portfolio for the pharmacy programs was introduced (Table 2). In the portfolio, the student reflects on his/her learning with respect to the learning outcomes twice during the academic year. In addition, the student makes personal plans for studies, reflects on learning skills, completes the progress test (Section 3.3.4.) once a year, and summarizes the overall development during the studies via the demonstration of proof (Section 3.3.5). Also, the student reflects his/her knowledge and skills with regards to future employment. In the Master's program, the student also writes an application with a motivation letter for the main discipline for their advanced studies. All these assignments and instructions are given via Moodle.

Table 2. The contents of the student portfolio of the pharmacy programs.

Portfolio of the Pharmacy Programs
Reflection of learning in respect to the learning outcomes
Student's personal study plans
Reflection of the student's learning skills
Progress testing
Summarization of the development (years 1–3)
Demonstration of proof
Application for the main discipline with a motivation letter
Summarization of the development (years 4–5)

3.3.4. Progress Testing throughout the Curriculum

A progress test is a longitudinal educational assessment tool which gives feedback to both the student and the teacher about the development of knowledge during the learning process. The progress test is comprised of multiple choice questions, which assess the substance-specific knowledge, and is administered to all students at the same time at regular intervals throughout the program studies. The differences between students' knowledge level is shown in the test scores: the further a student has progressed in the curriculum, the higher the score. The results of the progress test provide a longitudinal, repeated assessment of the success on theoretical learning outcomes of the entire curriculum [20–22].

In the Faculty of Pharmacy, the strand leaders evaluate the results of the progress test. The idea is based on multidisciplinary questions, which measure a deeper understanding of substance concepts and foster the multidisciplinary nature of the questions. The progress test was launched in spring 2015 and it has now been implemented during the first three years of studies. The test acts as an evaluation tool for the degree program, and the students are actively using the progress test to evaluate their own development. The teachers have already began to see which areas of theoretical studies are well learned and which need brushing up. The degree program directors have gained evidence for the development and improvement of the curriculum. Thus, the progress test works nicely in two ways, reciprocally, to aid both the students and teachers alike. Most importantly, by using the progress test, the degree program directors and the steering groups are able to monitor how well theoretical learning outcomes have been reached during the studies. Preliminary findings suggest that the student learning curve is improving steadily as the studies progress, and it seems that the predetermined learning outcomes can indeed be reached by the end of the studies.

3.3.5. The Demonstration of Proof

During the reform process, a practical test called the 'demonstration of proof' was created to evaluate both the theoretical and generic skills developed throughout the curriculum, and will be launched for the very first time in spring 2017. The practical test is a two-phase two-day event based on group work. The first phase will include group discussions about the development and strengths of students during their studies and with regards to their employment in the future. In the second phase, the students are given an inspirational stimulus describing a real-life challenge in the field of pharmacy. The students need to create a solution to the challenge, which could be an innovation, a product, a practice, or a procedure, which could be implemented further. The students need to use the theoretical knowledge and generic skills they have learned during their studies and work as a team, just like in real working life. The students will present their solutions to a panel, which consists of teachers and stakeholders. The panel evaluates the students' presentations and rewards the most innovative and creative solutions.

The aim of this practical is to summarize the theoretical and generic learning outcomes of the study program. Never before have the learning outcomes been assessed at the end of the studies as a whole. The constructive alignment of the teaching and assessment methods should be implemented not only at the course level, but also in the program level. A final book exam, or even a practical exam, which only measures learning-by-heart type learning, does not answer properly to the question of how learning outcomes have been reached. It is more likely that this type of group activity will demonstrate better the constructive alignment and the achievement of the learning outcomes. The intention is to develop a similar kind of practice for the Master's program as well. [3,8,13,23].

4. Conclusions

During the reform process, it became clear that it is absolutely necessary to involve all the stakeholders including teachers and students when reforming the curriculum. Although the reform process was demanding and time-consuming, it was inspiring at the same time. Even though the process was unforeseeable, the teams could hold the processes together by carefully managing, planning, and changing them in the case of altering circumstances.

The reform process was able to produce the intended learning outcomes. For the first time in Helsinki, the learning outcomes for the programs in pharmacy included also the generic skills, in addition to the theoretical skills. The learning outcomes enable the curriculum to be built based on constructive alignment and to create the knowledge and skills needed in working life. Increased co-operation with the stakeholders will aid in reaching the intended learning outcomes.

In the Faculty of Pharmacy, many processes—such as workshops for teachers, organized group work for students, learning portfolios, progress tests, and demonstration of proof—were developed in order to foster student's deep-level learning, to visualize the development of the students, to evaluate and reach the learning outcomes, to ensure the implementation of the constructive alignment and high quality of the study programs. In order to secure the quality of the programs and to create a sense of community and co-operation between the teachers, it is important to nominate committed responsible persons for the sub-structures of the curriculum. In the Faculty of Pharmacy, the nominated program directors with steering groups and strand leaders follow up and make sure that the programs fulfill the criteria of high quality education.

The University of Helsinki has participated and kept a keen eye on European level educational development, especially the Pharmine and PHAR-QA projects. Health and patient care orientations and development of generic skills, in addition to subject specific knowledge of drugs, are megatrends that request active follow-up, pedagogic capacity, and active measures to keep pharmacy education as one of the front-runners in University education.

Author Contributions: Nina Katajavuori made a first version of the manuscript which was written together with Outi Salminen and Katariina Vuorensola. Jouni Hirvonen commented and finalized the manuscript and Helena Huhtala and Pia Vuorela commented the manuscript.

References

1. International Pharmaceutical Federation. Fip Statement of Policy on Good Pharmacy Education Practice. 2000. Available online: http://www.fip.org/www/uploads/database_file.php?id=188&table_id= (accessed on 25 March 2017).
2. Fallows, S.; Steven, C. Building employability skills into the higher education curriculum: A university-wide initiative. *Educ. Train.* **2000**, *42*, 75–83. [CrossRef]
3. Biggs, J.; Tang, C. *Teaching for Quality Learning at University: What the Student Does*, 2nd ed.; Society for Research into Higher Education & Open University Press: Buckingham, UK, 2003.
4. Tynjälä, P.; Slotte, V.; Nieminen, J.; Lonka, K.; Olkinuora, E. From University to working life: Graduates' workplace skills in practice. In *Higher Education and Working life—Collaborations, Confrontations and Challenges*; Tynjälä, P., Välimaa, J., Boulton-Lewis, G., Eds.; Elsevier: Amsterdam, The Netherlands, 2006; pp. 77–88.
5. Bzowyckyj, A.S.; Janke, K.K. A Consensus Definition and Core Competencies for Being an Advocate for Pharmacy. *Am. J. Pharm. Educ.* **2013**, *77*, 24. [CrossRef] [PubMed]
6. Weinert, F.E. Concept of Competence: A Conceptual clarification. In *Defining and Selecting Key Competencies*; Rychen, D.S., Sagalnik, L.H., Eds.; Hogrefe & Huber: Seattle, WA, USA, 2001.
7. Frank, J.R.; Snell, L.S.; Cate, O.T.; Holmboe, E.S.; Carraccio, C.; Swing, S.R.; Harris, P.; Glasgow, N.J.; Campbell, C.; Dath, D.; et al. Competency-based medical education: Theory to practice. *Med. Teach.* **2010**, *32*, 638–645. [CrossRef] [PubMed]
8. Biggs, J.; Tang, C. *Teaching for Quality Learning at University*, 4th ed.; Society for Research into Higher Education & Open University Press: Buckingham, UK, 2011.
9. Jones, A. Generic attributes as espoused theory: The importance of context. *High. Educ.* **2009**, *58*, 175–191. [CrossRef]
10. Badcock, P.B.T.; Philippa, E.P.; Harris, K.-L. Developing generic skills through university study: A study of arts, science and engineering in Australia. *High. Educ.* **2010**, *60*, 441–458. [CrossRef]
11. Tuxworth, E. Competence based education and training: Backgroung and origins. In *Competence Based Education and Training*; Burke, J.W., Ed.; Falmer Press: Sussex, UK, 1989.
12. Kemper, D. Nurturing generic capabilities through a teaching and learning environment which provides practise in their use. *High. Educ.* **2009**, *57*, 37–55. [CrossRef]
13. Biggs, J. Enhancing teaching through constructive alignment. *High. Educ.* **1996**, *32*, 1–18. [CrossRef]
14. Shulman, L. Teaching as community property. *Change* **1993**, *25*, 6–7. [CrossRef]
15. Kahn, P.; Goodhew, P.; Murphy, M.; Walsh, L. The Scholarship of Teaching and Learning as collaborative working: A case study in shared practice and collective purpose. *High. Educ. Res. Dev.* **2013**, *32*, 901–914. [CrossRef]
16. Davis, B. A conceptual model to Support Curriculum Review, Revision, and Design in an Associate Degree Nursing Program. *Nurs. Educ. Perspect. (Natl. Leag. Nurs.)* **2011**, *32*, 389–394. [CrossRef]
17. Lakkala, M.; Toom, A.; Ilomäki, L.; Muukkonen, H. Re-designing university courses to support collaborative knowledge creation practices. *Australas. J. Educ. Tech.* **2015**, *31*, 521–536. [CrossRef]
18. Tillema, H.H. Portfolios as Developmental Assessment Tools. *Int. J. Train. Dev.* **2001**, *5*, 126–135. [CrossRef]
19. Gadbury-Amyot, C.C.; Bray, K.K.; Austin, K.J. Fifteen years of portfolio assessment of dental hygiene student competency: Lessons learned. *J. Dent. Hyg.* **2014**, *88*, 267–274. [PubMed]
20. Van Diest, R.; Dalen, J.V.; Bak, M.; Schruers, K.; Vleuten, C.V.D.; Muijtjens, A.; Scherpbier, A. Growth of knowledge in psychiatry and behavioural sciences in a problem-based learning curriculum. *Med. Educ.* **2004**, *38*, 1295–1301. [CrossRef] [PubMed]
21. Verhoeven, B.H.; Snellen-Balendong, H.A.; Hay, I.T.; Boon, J.M.; van der Linde, M.J.; Blitz-Lindeque, J.J.; Hoogenboom, R.J.I.; Verwijnen, G.M.; Wijnen, W.H.F.W.; Scherpbier, A.J.J.A.; et al. The versatility of progress testing assessed in an international context: A start for benchmarking global standardization? *Med. Teach.* **2005**, *27*, 514–520. [CrossRef] [PubMed]
22. Freeman, A.; van der Vleuten, C.; Nouns, Z.; Ricketts, C. Progress testing internationally. *Med. Teach.* **2010**, *32*, 451–455. [CrossRef] [PubMed]

15

Assessing the Perceptions and Practice of Self-Medication among Bangladeshi Undergraduate Pharmacy Students

Md. Omar Reza Seam [1], **Rita Bhatta** [1], **Bijoy Laxmi Saha** [1], **Abhijit Das** [1] ⓘ, **Md. Monir Hossain** [1], **S. M. Naim Uddin** [2], **Palash Karmakar** [1,*], **M. Shahabuddin Kabir Choudhuri** [3] **and Mohammad Mafruhi Sattar** [3]

[1] Department of Pharmacy, Noakhali Science and Technology University, Sonapur, Noakhali 3814, Bangladesh; omarrezaseam@gmail.com (M.O.R.S.); phar_rita@yahoo.com (R.B.); bijoylaxmi.saha@yahoo.com (B.L.S.); abhijitdas@nstu.edu.bd (A.D.); monirjupharmacy@gmail.com (M.M.H.)

[2] Department of Pharmacy, University of Chittagong, Chittagong 4331, Bangladesh; pharma.naim@yahoo.com

[3] Department of Pharmacy, Jahangirnagar University, Savar, Dhaka 1342, Bangladesh; mskchoudhuri@juniv.edu (M.S.K.C.); mafruhi1968@yahoo.com (M.M.S.)

* Correspondence: pk@nstu.edu.bd

Abstract: Objectives: To evaluate the perceptions and extent of practicing self-medication among undergraduate pharmacy students. **Methods:** This cross-sectional, questionnaire-based study was conducted over a six month period (January to June 2016) among undergraduate pharmacy students in five reputable public universities of Bangladesh. It involved face-to-face interviews regarding self-medication of 250 respondents selected by simple random sampling. **Results:** Self-medication was reported by 88.0% of students. Antipyretics (58.40%) were mostly preferred for the treatment of fever and headaches. The major cause for self-medication was minor illness (59.60%, $p = 0.73$) while previous prescriptions were the main source of knowledge as well as the major factor (52.80%, $p = 0.94$) dominating the self-medication practice. The results also demonstrated 88.80% of students had previous knowledge on self-medication and 83.60% of students always checked the information on the label; mainly the expiry date before use (85.60%). A significant ($p < 0.05$) portion of the students (51% male and 43% female) perceived it was an acceptable practice as they considered self-medication to be a segment of self-care. Furthermore, students demonstrated differences in their response level towards the adverse effect of drugs, the health hazard by a higher dose of drug, a physician's help in case of side effects, taking medicine without proper knowledge, and stopping selling medicine without prescription. **Conclusions:** Self-medication was commonly used among pharmacy students primarily for minor illnesses using over-the-counter medications. Although it is an inevitable practice for them it should be considered an important public health problem as this practice may increase the misuse or irrational use of medicines.

Keywords: self-medication; pharmacy students; awareness; perception; Bangladesh

---

1. Introduction

Self-medication is a human trait in which an individual (or a member of the individuals' family) selects and uses medicines or any other substances for the treatment of self-recognized or self-diagnosed physical or psychological ailments [1]. Conventionally it has been described as the intake of drugs, herbs or other home remedies on an individual's own persuasion or taking the advice of another person without consulting a physician [2,3]. Thus it forms an integral part of patients' self-care which in fact is the first choice and is one of the most crucial tools when an individual encounters common health problems that do not require a doctor's visit [4,5]. Due to insufficient medical facilities, the free accessibility of over-the-counter (OTC) drugs in the local market and the impoverished national drug regulatory policy, it is now becoming a very common occurrence in numerous countries of the world. Other reasons for self-medication are the shortage of time to visit a physician, inability to get a quick appointment, mild illness, long distance of hospitals and clinics from home, and finally unaffordable doctor's fees. Moreover, extraction of much information from online sources, magazines or periodicals makes people courageous about treating their own illness [6]. However, people are endangering their lives by practicing self-medication as it can lead to habituation, lethal allergic reactions, under dosage of medication which may not alleviate the symptom, and also over dosage that can cause collateral injury to different organs [7].

The substances which are most extensively self-medicated are OTC drugs and dietary supplements. Besides analgesics, antimalarials, antibiotics, and cold syrups are intermittently used for self-administration [8]. Sometimes some psychoactive drugs like recreational drugs, alcohol, and comfort foods are self-medicated to alleviate the symptoms of mental distress, stress, and anxiety [9]. The practice of self-medication has become very familiar throughout the world [10–13] with a high prevalence rate in developing countries [14,15]. Some studies have found that the amplitude of self-prescribing rate with antibiotics in Asia is 4–7.5% which is higher that of 3% in northern Europe [16]. Although self-medication, when practiced precisely can save time and is also cost effective to the patients where professional care is relatively expensive and not readily available, there are several critical health hazard issues that should be considered before endorsing the potential benefits of self-medication [7,17,18]. Sometimes it may lead to wastage of resources, boost up resistance to pathogens, and cause severe health problems, including adverse drug reaction, addiction, and ultimately death [7].

There are no examples of data relating health hazards and health care utilization including the practice of self-medication among young adults, but it is expected that they are highly motivated towards self-administration of drugs by the internet and media [19]. A study carried out by the university students of Karachi, Pakistan demonstrated that the propensity of self-prescribing of medications among medical students was 77.7%, and was 83.3% for non-medical students [20]. So the study on self-practice of medications among university pharmacy undergraduates is imperative as they are that segment of the population who are well educated and have access to all the information regarding their health. Moreover study on the tendency of self-medication practice among pharmacy undergraduates is essential as they are the oncoming drug prescribers and health educationalist [5].

Over-the-counter (OTC) drugs are the only drugs which can be self-prescribed and sold in convenience stores, grocery stores, and health shops without prescription as they are less hazardous [21]. In Bangladesh paracetamol, ORS saline, metronidazole, ranitidine, omeprazole, aspirin, and diaclofenac sodium etc. are accepted to be sold as OTC drugs. However, due to immoral drug sellers and improper regulation, 90% of stocked drugs are sold without any prescription and therefore the phenomenon of self-medication is a common topic in our country [21]. Besides there have been very confined researches conducted regarding the impact of self-medication practice among university pharmacy undergraduates [15].

Considering all this evidence, this research work focuses on assessing the perceptions about self-medication practice among the pharmacy students of Bangladesh. The study also compares the attitudes toward and the extent of practicing self-care between male and female students, as well as the year in pharmacy school.

2. Methods

2.1. Study Design

This population-based cross-sectional study was carried out to investigate the knowledge, attitudes and practice of self-medication among the undergraduate pharmacy students of Bangladesh from January to June, 2016. The study was conducted by using both qualitative and quantitative data.

2.2. Study Area

To conduct the study, the pharmacy department of five public universities of Bangladesh namely Dhaka University, Jahangirnagar University, Chittagong University, Comilla University, and Noakhali Science and Technology University were chosen as the study area. The above mentioned universities were chosen by the field investigators based on the availability and accessibility of the participants. Time and distance were also the key factors for the selection of the study areas.

2.3. Study Participants

The study included 250 undergraduate students (131 male and 119 female) enrolled in a Bachelor of Pharmacy program who understood English, aged between 18–25 years and were permanent residents of Bangladesh, with different socioeconomic backgrounds from five different public universities. Both residential and nonresidential students were selected randomly, i.e., we did not consider whether the students were resident or non-resident in different halls of the university. Before data collection each and every participant was clearly informed about the purpose of the study and a written consent was taken from each of the respondents.

2.4. Participants and Eligibility Criteria

This study included only those respondents who were easily available for data collection and interested to provide information willingly. Those who did not feel comfortable to give information were excluded from the study.

2.5. Sampling and Sample Size

A simple random sampling technique was used for the selection of study participants. The sample size was calculated assuming that 50% of the undergraduate pharmacy students had a tendency of self-medication practice with 5% margin of error and 95% confidence interval. The sample size was calculated to be 232. However, to ensure more representative data, we selected a larger sample size of 250 for this study.

2.6. Data Collection

The procedure of data collection was segmented into three steps. The first step was to fill out the questionnaire including socio-demographic information by the study subjects. The second step was to discuss the study protocol, and the final step was to cross-check the questionnaires filled by the respondents. The questionnaire was adopted from a formerly published study which was developed, standardized, and previously used by Kumar et al. [4] for undergraduate pharmacy students. The questionnaire was divided into four segments and consisted of 16 close-ended and 11 open-ended questions. Section 1 contained questions related to socio-demographic information of the respondents. Section 2 included questions about the practice of self-medication by the respondents. Section 3 was concerned with the knowledge and awareness related questions of the respondents while Section 4 was on questions related to the perception of the respondents regarding self-medication practice.

The questionnaire was distributed to the selected student together with a written consent form that explained the purpose of the research and assured them of their confidentiality. The interviews lasted for 15 min and included a range of questions about self-medication along with an explanation about self-medication, its main principles, as well as evidence based and practical demonstration. The questionnaire was constructed in English and translated to Bengali by the interviewers to make the questions easily understandable to the participants during the interview. They were asked to complete the questionnaire immediately. The authors were present on hand to answer questions or clarify any doubts that they might have.

2.7. Statistical Analysis

Data analyses were conducted using SPSS software version 20.0 (SPSS Inc., Chicago, IL, USA). Descriptive statistics was used for the calculation of proportions. The Chi-square test was performed to measure the association between the demographic characteristics and responses to understanding, perceptions and self-use of medication. The p values were calculated by the Chi-square test. An alpha level of 0.05 or less was considered significant. The Microsoft excel program was used for data analysis and for chart, graph, and diagram preparation.

3. Results

3.1. Demographic Characteristics

Table 1 shows that 52.40% of the students were male while female students comprised 47.60%. Among all the pharmacy students 26% was from the 1st year, 26.00% from the 2nd year, 26.00% from the 3rd year, and 22.00% from the 4th year. The lowest number of students was in the age group <18 years with a percentage of 5.20% while the highest number of students was in the 21–25 years age group with a percentage of 63.60%. Another 31.20% of students was in the age group 18–20 years. Among the respondents 80.40% of respondents was from an urban area and 19.60% was from a rural area.

Table 1. Demographic characteristics of respondents.

Item	Sub Group	Number (n)	Percentage (%)
Sex	Male	131	52
	Female	119	48
Year of study	1st year	65	26
	2nd year	65	26
	3rd year	65	26
	4th year	55	22
Age group	<18 year	13	5
	18–20 year	78	31
	21–25 year	159	64
Area of residence	Urban	201	80
	Rural	49	20

3.2. Practice of Self-Medication

Table 2 describes the practice of self-medication by pharmacy students (from 1st year to 4th year) from five reputable public universities of Bangladesh. From the table we get a clear scenario that the majority of students reported practicing self-medication (88.0%). The practice of self-medication among both male and female students (45.20% and 42.80% respectively) was almost similar with no significant difference ($p > 0.05$).

Table 2. Practice of self-medication of the respondents.

Item	Response	Male		Female		Total (%)	p-Value
		n	%	n	%		
Practice of self-medication	Yes	113	45.20	107	42.80	220 (88.0)	0.44
	No	18	7.20	12	4.80	30 (12.0)	

n indicates the number of respondents. p value was determined using Chi-square Test. $p < 0.05$ was considered significant when compared between male and female groups.

3.3. Purpose of Self-Medication Practice

Table 3 demonstrates that the use of self-medication practice for different complications differed insignificantly ($p > 0.05$) between male and female students. It can also be seen from the table that students used self-medication for headache (71.20%); cough, cold/flu (61.20%); diarrhea (47.60%); pain (42.80%); stomach ache (32.80%); vomiting (32.00%); rash/allergies (23.60%), and skin problems (16.40%) respectively. Here the percentage of using self-medication for fever was highest and the value was least for ear problems.

Table 3. Purpose of practicing self-medication of the respondents.

Items	Male		Female		Total (%)	x^2 Value	p Value
	n	%	n	%			
Indications for Using Self-Medication							
Headache	89	35.60	89	35.60	178 (71.20)	1.59	0.66
Cough, Cold/Flu	75	30.00	78	31.20	153 (61.20)	1.41	0.72
Fever	98	39.20	93	37.20	191 (76.40)	1.62	0.67
Stomach ache	34	13.60	48	19.20	82 (32.80)	1.88	0.62
Diarrhea	66	26.40	53	21.20	119 (47.60)	2.76	0.43
Menstrual Symptoms	0	0	12	4.80	12 (4.80)	-	-
Rash/Allergies	26	10.40	33	13.20	59 (23.60)	2.46	0.49
Anxiety/Depression	7	2.80	10	4.00	17 (6.80)	3.29	0.45
Ear Problems	3	1.20	2	0.80	5 (2.00)	2.10	1.00
Vomiting	37	14.80	43	17.20	80 (32.00)	4.54	0.21
Eye infections	7	2.80	9	3.60	16 (6.40)	3.81	0.13
Skin problems	27	10.80	14	5.60	41 (16.40)	1.02	0.83
Tooth ache	17	6.80	11	4.40	28 (11.20)	0.41	1.00
Insomnia	3	1.20	3	1.20	6 (2.40)	3.13	1.00
Pain	51	20.40	56	22.40	107 (42.80)	5.20	0.15
Reason for Self-Medication							
Minor illness	72	28.80	77	30.80	149 (59.60)	1.35	0.73
Sufficient pharmacological knowledge	27	10.80	21	8.40	48 (19.20)	1.56	0.74
Quick relief	40	16.00	37	14.80	77 (30.80)	2.17	0.56
Lack of time to consult doctor	35	14.00	29	11.60	64 (25.60)	3.99	0.26
Cost effectiveness	22	8.80	10	4.00	32 (12.80)	1.28	0.86
Easy availability of medicine	52	20.80	36	14.40	88 (35.20)	3.02	0.39
Emergency use	34	13.60	46	18.40	80 (32.00)	2.19	0.53
Type of Self-Prescribed Medicine							
Analgesics	63	25.20	60	24.00	123 (49.20)	0.60	0.93
Antipyretics	44	17.60	53	21.20	146 (58.40)	2.44	0.48
Antidiarrheals	48	19.20	50	20.00	98 (39.20)	2.64	0.44
Antiemetics	13	5.20	20	8.00	33 (13.20)	4.30	0.22
Antibiotics	27	10.80	12	4.80	39 (15.60)	1.73	0.66
Antacids	71	28.40	75	30.00	97 (38.80)	3.58	0.31
Sedatives	11	4.40	12	4.80	23 (9.20)	4.38	0.20
Anti-allergic	36	14.40	37	14.80	73 (29.20)	3.15	0.38
Vitamins	40	16.00	39	15.60	79 (31.60)	7.62	0.05
Ophthalmic preparations	1	0.40	3	1.20	4 (1.60)	-	1.00
Cosmetic products	21	8.40	34	13.60	55 (22.00)	1.72	0.64

Data is represented both as number and percentage (%). n indicates the number of respondents. p values from Chi-square or Fisher Exact tests for comparisons between male and female groups.

The purpose of self-practicing of medications by the students was categorized into seven broad categories (Table 3). The majority of the students (59.60%) used self-medication because they thought that they did not need to see a doctor for a minor illness. Easy availability of medicines (32.20%) and emergency use (32.00%) were the secondary reasons for practicing self-medication. Meanwhile quick relief (30.80%), lack of time to consult doctor (25.60%), sufficient pharmacological knowledge (19.20%), and cost effectiveness (12.80%) were other reasons behind self-medication of drugs. The table shows some high values on the purpose of using self-medication, but none of the values was significant ($p > 0.05$).

Different categories of medicine which were self-medicated by the students for the treatment of ailments are listed in Table 3. From the table it is clear that the use of different classes of drugs showed no difference in use between males and females. Among the drugs the rate of antipyretic consumption was highest (58.40%) by the students whereas analgesics (49.20%); anti-diarrheal (39.20%);

antacid (38.80%); vitamins (31.60%); anti-allergic (29.20%); cosmetics (22.00%), and anti-diabetics (15.60%) were also used by them. It was found that among different types of drugs students used ophthalmic preparations the least with a percentage of 1.60%.

3.4. Sources of Information on Self-Medication Practice

Figure 1 represents the pharmacy students' (1st to 4th year) source of information on the medications self-prescribed by them. From the diagram we get a clear picture that the majority of the male and female students considered an old prescription for common illness (56% and 58% respectively) and academic knowledge (62% and 55% respectively) as their primary sources of information on self-medicated drugs. It was an interesting finding that male students gathered information about medicines from friends (32%), internet (35%), and advertisement (30%) and this rate was higher in comparison to female students.

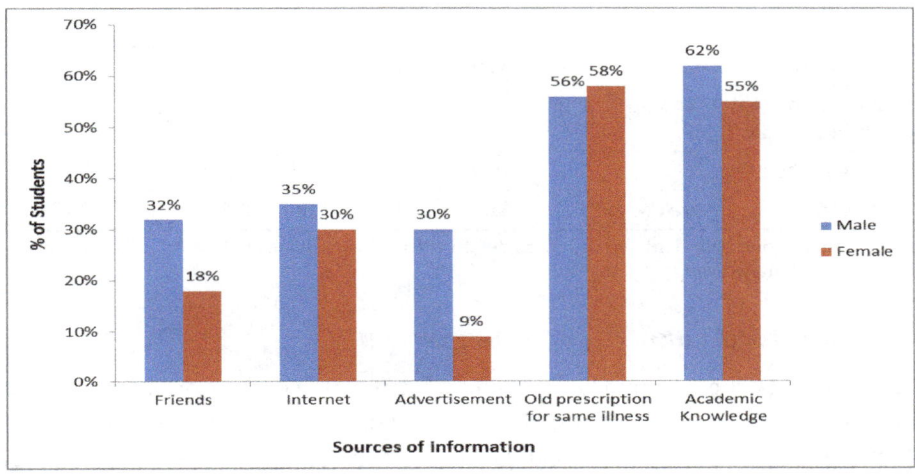

Figure 1. Sources of information on self-medicated drugs. Data is represented as percentage (%) for the two groups.

3.5. Factors Influencing Self-Medication Practice

Table 4 represents a pharmacy student's opinion on the factors (predefined categories from the survey) which influence the practice of self-medication. A major portion of the students (52.80%) said that they had self-prescribed a drug based on the previous doctor's prescription for the same disease. Another 50.80% students had previous experience of practicing self-medication while the opinions of family members (45.20%) and of friends (15.20%) were also influential factors for self-medication practice by the students. Advertisement (6.00%) and recommendation by local people (5.60%) were the least influential factors for self-prescription of medications.

Table 4. Influencing factors for the selection of medications for self-practice by the respondents.

Factors	Male		Female		Total (%)	x^2 Value	p Value
	n	%	n	%			
Opinion of family members	52	20.80	61	24.40	113 (45.20)	1.74	0.63
Opinion of friends	27	10.80	11	4.40	38 (15.20)	1.62	0.65
Recommendation by local people	10	4.00	4	1.60	14 (5.60)	1.14	0.57
Previous doctor's prescription	58	23.20	74	29.60	132 (52.80)	0.40	0.94
Own experience	75	30.00	52	20.80	127 (50.80)	9.08	0.03 *
Advertisement	12	4.80	3	1.20	15 (6.00)	1.63	0.44

n indicates the number of respondents. p value was determined using Chi-square Test.* $p < 0.05$ was considered significant when compared between male and female groups.

3.6. Knowledge on Self-Medication Practice

Table 5 is concerned with the information relating to pharmacy students' perceived knowledge on self-medication practice. The table illustrates that most of the students who had self-prescribed medication for different diseases knew about self-medication (88.80%) previously. Among the students 83.6% had a tendency to check the package insert while 85.6% students had a sound attitude towards checking the expiry date of the drug before using it. Furthermore 67.6% students had concerns about the importance of completing the course of the drug. All the results differed significantly ($p < 0.05$) when compared between male and female students.

Table 5. Knowledge of the students on self-medication.

Modality	Male		Female		Total (%)	x^2 Value	p Value
	n	%	n	%			
Idea about self-medication	130	52.00	92	36.80	222 (88.80)	8.84	0.03 *
Knowledge about dose completion of self-prescribed medications	90	36.00	79	31.60	169 (67.60)	14.16	0.00 *
Checking of the insert	120	48.00	89	35.60	209 (83.60)	7.54	0.03 *
Checking of the expiry date before use	110	44.00	104	41.60	214 (85.60)	8.17	0.04 *

n indicates the number of respondents. p value was determined using Chi-square Test. * $p < 0.05$ was considered as significant male and female groups.

3.7. Attitude towards Self-Medication

Figure 2 represents the pharmacy students' (1st to 4th year) approach on self-prescription of medication for self-healthcare. From the figure it is clear that the students' concept about self-medication was classified into three categories namely good practice, acceptable practice, and not acceptable practice. Both male (51%) and female (43%) considered self-medication an acceptable practice while another 17% male and 13% female students considered self-practice of medication was good. Moreover the diagram also shows that 32% male and 44% female students thought self-medication was not an acceptable practice.

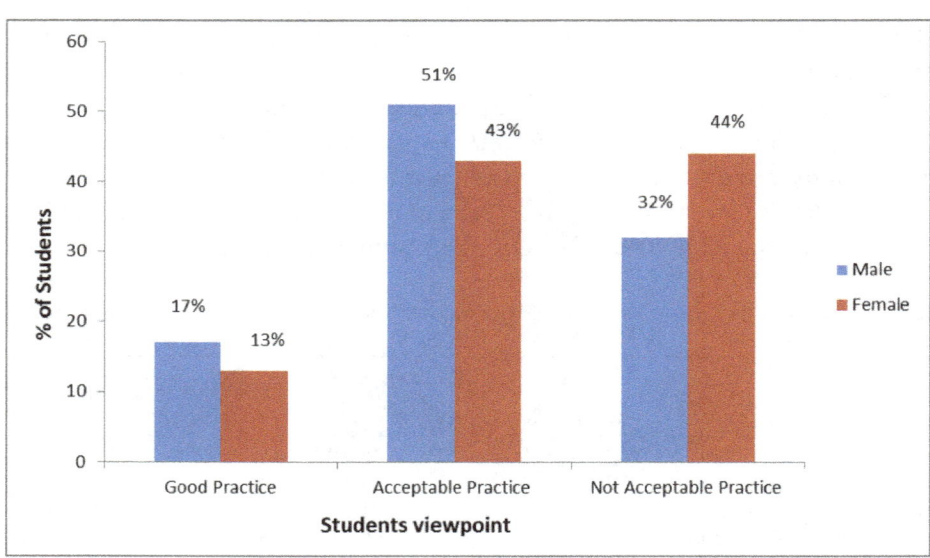

Figure 2. Attitude of the students towards self-medication. Data is represented as percentage (%) for the two groups.

Table 6 represents the students' attitudes on self-medication among 1st to 4th year pharmacy students of five reputed public universities. The answer level is given as "yes" and "no". The majority of students had a positive attitude on self-medication. A very negligible number of students had a negative attitude.

Table 6. Attitude of the students towards Self-medication.

Modality	Year of Study	Yes/No (n)	x^2 Value	p Value
Part of self-care	1st	44/21	3.27	0.12
	2nd	47/19		
	3rd	47/19		
	4th	45/10		
Advice of self-medication to your family and friends	1st	29/36	0.50	0.98
	2nd	27/38		
	3rd	26/39		
	4th	25/30		
Idea about which drugs have side effects	1st	37/28	6.35	0.22
	2nd	49/16		
	3rd	48/17		
	4th	37/18		
Concern that increasing drug dose can be health hazardous	1st	45/20	12.80	0.00 *
	2nd	56/9		
	3rd	59/6		
	4th	48/7		
In the case of side effects a physicians help must be needed	1st	59/6	3.29	0.66
	2nd	63/2		
	3rd	61/4		
	4th	49/6		
Mild medical problems do not need drug treatment	1st	21/44	9.25	0.02 *
	2nd	29/36		
	3rd	24/41		
	4th	32/23		
Physicians can be overlooked	1st	43/22	11.26	0.00 *
	2nd	40/25		
	3rd	40/25		
	4th	21/34		
Taking without proper knowledge is harmful	1st	54/11	4.09	0.16
	2nd	60/5		
	3rd	60/5		
	4th	50/5		
Stopping selling medicine without prescription	1st	56/9	6.01	0.03 *
	2nd	56/9		
	3rd	58/7		
	4th	54/1		

n indicates the number of respondents. p value was determined using Chi-square Test. * $p < 0.05$ was considered significant for male and female groups.

The tabulated results show differences in response level of the students to some survey items such as self-medication is a part of self-care; the idea about drugs side effects; health hazard on increased dose of a drug; physician's help in case of side effects; taking medicine without proper knowledge, and stopping selling medicine without prescription. The observed answers were significant ($p < 0.05$) in the case of concern about the impact of increased dose of drug, for no need of drug treatment in mild medical cases, for overlooking physicians and not selling drugs without prescription, while for other modalities the results were not significant ($p > 0.05$).

4. Discussion

People have always been very cautious about their personal health status and for this they have used self-medication, a feature of healthcare, from ancient times. Although self-medication has many pros and cons it depends on who uses it and how it is used for self-treatment [4]. We focused on pharmacy students because they have adequate knowledge of medicine in theory and are more cautious about the safety of drugs which is lacking in other student groups or in the general population. Thus a pharmacy student's view on the self-medication practice can be considered as a major factor to judge the characteristics of their future prescription pattern.

Students of Bangladesh frequently use self-medication and gender difference has not been shown to have any influence on the practice of self-medication. The reason behind insignificant gender differences in the overall exercise of self-medication may be the study format that allowed the respondents to select drugs by themselves [5]. In our study we found that about 88.0% of the students self-practice different types of medication. A similar type of study was conducted by Kumar et al. [4] in coastal south India and signified that the amplitude of self-medication practice was 78.90% among medical students. Other similar studies also demonstrated the prevalence rate of self-medication ranged between 57.1% and 92% among the medicals students in India [22]. Several research works carried out in other developing countries revealed that the prevalence of self-medication was 38.5% and 43.2% among medical, pharmacy, and health science students in Ethiopia [22,23], 51% among citizens in Slovenia [24], 55.3% and 55% among medical students in Pakistan [25] and Egypt [26] respectively, 56.9% among medical undergraduate students in Nigeria [27], and 80.9% among female university students in Malaysia [28]. The major influential reason behind the higher propensity of self-medication might be the unregulated easy availability of all categories of medicine without prescription.

Similar to some previously published articles [22,29–31], headache, common cold, fever, pain, and vomiting were the most common symptoms for self-administration of medications mentioned by the respondents. It was quoted in our research report that the most common cause for self-treatment with drugs was the insignificance of the illness which did not require a doctor's visit. Similar outcomes were reported by the study conducted in India [7,32]. This type of attitude of the respondents may be attributed to a disregard and absence of consciousness about the advancement of diseases. Sometimes the people who practice medication for self-treatment may suffer from a serious illness as the symptoms of many diseases are primarily mild but wrong diagnosis and treatment may promote serious health hazards. However, in agreement with other studies, easy availability of medicines [4,6], quick relief [16], and time saving [33] were found to be the other causatives for preferring self-medication practice.

As stated earlier, antipyretics, analgesics, antacids, and antidiarrheal drugs were the most common classes of drugs self-prescribed for treatment by almost all of the respondents in our study. Almost identical observations were found in the studies conducted in India [4,34], Pakistan [32], Iran [35], and Ethiopia [8] where these common classes of drugs were frequently used by medical students. Meanwhile, the use of antibiotics was different to that of analgesics and antipyretics. This tendency is because of the knowledge of pharmacy graduates on the resistance and side effects of antibiotics. It is well known that proper medicinal knowledge can promote a good prescribing pattern of pharmacists. However, at the same time inappropriate or irrational use of these drugs can lead to various hazardous effects including the reduction in the capability of microbial flora to resist detrimental microorganisms, the development of multidrug resistance, addiction, toxicity, and other related syndromes [32]. Therefore, such kind of practice should be discouraged.

Our study found that the key factor for self-medication practice by the participants was their adequate pharmacological knowledge which they had gathered from their academic courses. These findings are similar to those from studies conducted in Nepal [7], India [4,33], Malaysia [36], Ethiopia [8], and Pakistan [32]. The second major source of information on self-prescribed drugs was from previous prescriptions for the same illness and this result was analogous to the findings of the study conducted in India [4,33]. Further, other researches conveyed in India [34] and Ethiopia [8] reported the internet as another common source of knowledge on self-prescribed medicines which was the third common source of information in our study results.

The fact that majority (52.80%) of the respondents gathered information about self-medication from the previously prescribed medicines of physicians was consistent with the research work conducted earlier [37]. However as the respondents were younger, they were also influenced by other sources like previous illness experiences, opinions of family members, friends and local people, and advertisement. This result resembles formerly conducted research findings [23,37]. All the students irrespective of the year of the study reported that they were completely aware of the treatment procedure using self-medication. They were also cautious about completing the dose of the medicine, checking the instructions given on the insert before using and also looking for the expiry date of the drug before using it. Less awareness was noted among 1st year students which was similar to the findings of Kalyan et al. [38] and Sontakke et al. [34] Non-inclusion of pharmacology as a subject in the 1st year curriculum could be the reason.

In this research work, about 73.2% of the respondents believed the practice of self-medication to be part of their own health-care and the proportion was higher than the reports from India [34], Ethiopia [22], and Pakistan [25]. Self-medication can only be considered a part of self-care if legitimate use of medicaments can be ensured. It may lead to accidental drug toxicity as there is always a risk of using expired drugs and also sharing with friends or taking medicines that have been actually prescribed for other problems [4,29,32,39].

5. Limitations

The study had some limitations as we faced some complications during the survey. First, we covered only five universities due to shortage of time for the research work. If we had conducted the study in more universities we would have got a more extensive scenario on the self-medication practice among the university students of Bangladesh. Second, many students were busy with their examinations, and lab work for training purposes; so collecting data from them was slightly difficult. Third, students of 1st year and 2nd year were less familiar with some terminologies and complication were created during the understanding of the questionnaire. They had to be given extra explanation. Finally, social desirability bias may have impacted the responses since the interviews were done in person Also the survey did not distinguish between the uses of OTC drugs in self-medication vs. prescription drugs such as antibiotics and may have resulted in confusion among respondents. The survey was not revalidated after translation and may have resulted in some changes in the survey items.

6. Conclusions

This descriptive study has demonstrated that self-practice of medication is very common among undergraduate pharmacy students of five renowned universities which was facilitated by the easy availability of drugs and information from previous prescriptions. The use of antibiotics, antidepressants, and sedative among a small segment of students without proper follow up or lab tests by healthcare providers may lead to serious health hazards, not only to the students themselves but also to those to whom they suggest the medication. Therefore, it is the sole responsibility of the health care professionals and drug regulatory authorities to ensure the safe use of drugs and control the exercise of self-administration of medications by describing the total impact of the drugs on the body to the students. As the study was confined to the pharmacy student population, further research is needed to test the prevalence of self-medication practices among the general population and how these differ by type of medication. Furthermore steps should be taken to monitor the drug selling system by stake holders especially of those drugs with potentially harmful effects.

Acknowledgments: The authors are thankful to the management and students of participated institutions for their cordial help. Authors also would like to thank all the volunteer students of the Department of Pharmacy of Noakhali Science and Technology University for their warm support for this research work.

Author Contributions: Md. Omar Reza Seam and Bijoy Laxmi Saha carried out the data collection process and conducted the research work. Bijoy Laxmi Saha wrote the manuscript. Palash Karmakar, M. Shahabuddin Kabir Choudhuri, Mohammad Mafruhi Sattar, and Abhijit Das carried out conception and design of the study, statistical analysis, and interpretation of data. Rita Bhatta, Md. Monir Hossain and S. M. Naim Uddin helped in the data collection procedure, revised the manuscript, and gave guidance to improve the quality of the final manuscript. All authors read and approved the final manuscript.

References

1. Ruiz, M.E. Risks of self-medication practices. *Curr. Drug Saf.* **2010**, *5*, 315–323. [CrossRef] [PubMed]
2. Bennadi, D. Self-medication: A current challenge. *J. Basic Clin. Pharm.* **2013**, *5*, 19–23. [CrossRef] [PubMed]
3. Hernandez-Juyol, M.; Job-Quesada, J.R. Dentistry and self-medication: A current challenge. *Med. Oral* **2002**, *7*, 344–347. [PubMed]
4. Kumar, N.; Kanchan, T.; Unnikrishnan, B.; Rekha, T.; Mithra, P.; Kulkarni, V.; Papanna, M.K.; Holla, R.; Uppal, S. Perceptions and practices of self-medication among medical students in coastal South India. *PLoS ONE* **2013**, *8*, e72247. [CrossRef] [PubMed]
5. Klemenc-Ketis, Z.; Hladnik, Z.; Kersnik, J. A cross sectional study of sex differences in self-medication practices among university students in Slovenia. *Coll. Antropol.* **2011**, *35*, 329–334. [PubMed]
6. Kumari, R.; Kiran, K.D.; Bahl, R.; Gupta, R. Study of knowledge and practices of self-medication among medical students at Jammu. *J. Med. Sci.* **2012**, *15*, 141–144.
7. Mehta, R.K.; Sharma, S. Knowledge, attitude and perception of self-medication among medical students. *IOSR J. Nurs. Health Sci.* **2015**, *4*, 89–96.
8. Afolabi, A.O. Factors influencing the pattern of self-medication in an adult Nigerian population. *Ann. Afr. Med.* **2008**, *7*, 120–127. [CrossRef] [PubMed]
9. Harris, K.M.; Edlund, M.J. Self-medication of mental health problems: New evidence from a national survey. *Health Serv. Res.* **2005**, *40*, 117–134. [CrossRef] [PubMed]
10. Angeles-Chimal, P.; Medina-Flores, M.L.; Molina-Rodriguez, J.F. Self-medication in a urban population of Cuernavaca, Morelos. *Salud Publ. Mex.* **1992**, *34*, 554–561.
11. Figueiras, A.; Caamano, F.; Gestal-Otero, J.J. Sociodemographic factors related to self-medication in Spain. *Eur. J. Epidemiol.* **2000**, *16*, 19–26. [CrossRef] [PubMed]
12. Hayran, O.; Karavus, M.; Aksayan, S. Help-seeking behavior and self-medication of a population in an urban area in Turkey: Cross sectional study. *Croat. Med. J.* **2000**, *41*, 327–332. [PubMed]
13. Martins, A.P.; Miranda, A.C.; Mendes, Z.; Soares, M.A.; Ferreira, P.; Nogueira, A. Self-medication in a Portuguese urban population: A prevalence study. *Pharmacoepidemiol. Drug Saf.* **2002**, *11*, 409–414. [CrossRef] [PubMed]
14. Chang, F.R.; Trivedi, P.K. Economics of self-medication: Theory and evidence. *Health Econ.* **2003**, *12*, 721–739. [CrossRef] [PubMed]
15. Alam, N.; Saffoon, N.; Uddin, R. Self-medication among medical and pharmacy students in Bangladesh. *BMC Res. Notes* **2015**, *8*, 763. [CrossRef] [PubMed]
16. Sawalha, A.F. Assessment of self-medication practice among university students in Palestine: Therapeutic and toxicity implications. *IUG J. Nat. Stud.* **2015**, *15*, 267–282.
17. Kiyingi, K.; Lauwo, J. Drugs in the home: Danger and waste. *World Health Forum* **1992**, *14*, 381–384.
18. Loyola Filho, A.I.; Lima-Costa, M.F.; Uchoa, E. Bambui project: A qualitative approach to self-medication. *Cad. Saude Publ.* **2004**, *20*, 1661–1669. [CrossRef]
19. Mumtaz, Y.; Jahangeer, S.; Mujtaba, T.; Zafar, S.; Adnan, S. Self-medication among university students of Karachi. *J. Liaquat Univ. Med. Health Sci.* **2011**, *10*, 102–105.
20. Castel, J.M.; Laporte, J.R.; Reggi, V.; Aguirre, J.; Buschiazzo, P.M.; Coelho, H.L.; Batista, M.D.C.D.; Carvalho, M.L.; Righi, R.E.; Prieto, J.C.; et al. Multicenter study on self-medication and self-prescription in six Latin American countries. *Clin. Pharmacol. Ther.* **1997**, *61*, 488–493. [CrossRef]
21. Babu, M.M. Factors contributing to the purchase of over the counter (OTC) drugs in Bangladesh: An empirical study. *Int. J. Third World Med.* **2008**, *6*, 9–24.
22. Abay, S.M.; Amelo, W. Assessment of self-medication practices among medical, pharmacy, and health science students in Gondar university, Ethiopia. *J. Young Pharm.* **2010**, *2*, 306–310. [CrossRef] [PubMed]
23. Gutema, G.B.; Gadisa, D.A.; Kidanemariam, Z.A.; Berhe, D.F.; Berhe, A.H.; Hadera, M.G.; Hailu, G.S.; Abrha, N.G.; Yarlagadda, R.; Dagne, A.W. Self-medication practices among health sciences students: The case of Mekelle university. *J. Appl. Pharm. Sci.* **2011**, *1*, 183–189.

24. Smogavec, M.; Softic, N.; Kersnik, J.; Klemenc-Ketis, Z. An overview of self-treatment and selfmedication practices among Slovenian citizens. *Zdr. Vestnik* **2010**, *79*, 757–763.

25. Zafar, S.N.; Syed, R.; Waqar, S.; Irani, F.A.; Saleem, S. Prescription of medicines by medical students of Karachi, Pakistan: A cross-sectional study. *BMC Public Health* **2008**, *8*, 162. [CrossRef] [PubMed]

26. El Ezz, N.; Ez-Elarab, H. Knowledge, attitude and practice of medical students towards self-medication at Ain Shams university, Egypt. *J. Prev. Med. Hyg.* **2011**, *52*. [CrossRef]

27. Fadare, J.O.; Tamuno, I. Antibiotic self-medication among university medical undergraduates in northern Nigeria. *J. Public Health Epidemiol.* **2011**, *3*, 217–220.

28. Ali, S.E.; Ibrahim, M.I.; Palaian, S. Medication storage and self-medication behaviour amongst female students in Malaysia. *Pharm. Pract.* **2010**, *8*, 226–232. [CrossRef]

29. Hughes, C.M. Monitoring self-medication. *Expert Opin. Drug Saf.* **2003**, *2*, 1–5. [CrossRef] [PubMed]

30. Nandha, R.; Chhabra, M.K. Prevalence and clinical characteristics of headache in dental students of a tertiary care teaching dental hospital in northern India. *Int. J. Basic Clin. Pharmacol.* **2013**, *2*, 51–55. [CrossRef]

31. Sarahroodi, S.; Maleki-Jamshid, A.; Sawalha, A.F.; Mikaili, P.; Safaeian, L. Pattern of self-medication with analgesics among Iranian university students in central Iran. *J. Family. Community Med.* **2012**, *19*, 125–129. [CrossRef] [PubMed]

32. Hughes, C.M.; McElnay, J.C.; Fleming, G.F. Benefits and risks of self medication. *Drug Saf.* **2001**, *24*, 1027–1037. [CrossRef] [PubMed]

33. Souza, L.A.; da Silva, C.D.; Ferraz, G.C.; Sousa, F.A.; Pereira, L.V. The prevalence and characterization of self-medication for obtaining pain relief among undergraduate nursing students. *Rev. Lat. Am. Enfermagem.* **2011**, *19*, 245–251. [CrossRef] [PubMed]

34. Sontakke, S.D.; Bajait, C.S.; Pimpalkhute, S.A.; Jaiswal, K.M.; Jaiswal, S.R. Comparative study of evaluation of self-medication practices in first and third year medical students. *Int. J. Biol. Med. Res.* **2011**, *2*, 561–564.

35. Lukovic, J.A.; Miletic, V.; Pekmezovic, T.; Trajkovic, G.; Ratkovic, N.; Aleksic, D.; Grgurevic, A. Self-medication practices and risk factors for self-medication among medical students in Belgrade, Serbia. *PLoS ONE* **2014**, *9*, e114644. [CrossRef] [PubMed]

36. Kayalvizhi, S.; Senapathi, R. Evaluation of the perception, attitude and practice of self medication among business students in 3 select cities, south India. *IJEIMS* **2010**, *1*, 40–44.

37. Pereira, C.M.; Farias Alves, V.; Freire Gasparetto, P.; Carneiro, D.S.; de Carvalho, D.D.G.R.; Ferreira Valoz, F.E. Self-medication in health students from two Brazilian universities. *Rev. Sul-Bras. Odontol.* **2012**, *9*, 361–367.

38. Kalyan, V.S.; Sudhakar, K.; Srinivas, P.; Sudhakar, G.; Pratap, K.; Padma, T.M. Evaluation of self-medication practices among undergraduate dental students of tertiary care teaching dental hospital in south India. *J. Educ. Ethics Dent.* **2013**, *3*, 21–25. [CrossRef]

39. Sharif, S.I.; Ibrahim, O.H.M.; Mouslli, L.; Waisi, R. Evaluation of self-medication among pharmacy students. *Am. J. Pharmacol. Toxicol.* **2012**, *7*, 135–140. [CrossRef]

16

Community Pharmacists' Knowledge Regarding Donepezil Averse Effects and Self-Care Recommendations for Insomnia for Persons with AD

Marketa Marvanova [1],*,† (iD) **and Paul Jacob Henkel** [2],†

[1] Department of Pharmacy Practice, School of Pharmacy/College of Health Professions, North Dakota State University, Department 2650, P.O. Box 6050, Fargo, ND 58108-6050, USA

[2] Department of Geographical and Historical Studies, University of Eastern Finland, FI-80101 Joensuu, Finland; suomenpoika@yahoo.com

* Correspondence: marketa.marvanova@ndsu.edu

† These authors contributed equally to this study.

Abstract: Alzheimer's disease (AD) impacts millions of individuals worldwide. Since no cure is currently available, acetylcholinesterase inhibitors are symptomatic therapy. This study assessed community pharmacists' knowledge regarding donepezil adverse effects (AEs) and self-care recommendations for insomnia management for persons with AD treated with rivastigmine. This is a cross-sectional, standardized telephone survey of community pharmacists ($n = 862$) in three study areas: West Virginia, North Dakota/South Dakota, and Southern Oregon/Northern California. Pharmacists' degree, sex, and pharmacists' AD-related knowledge were assessed. In-stock availability of donepezil and rivastigmine formulations was assessed. Analyses were performed using Stata 10.1. Only 31.4% pharmacists were able to name ≥ 2 donepezil AEs. Only four donepezil AEs were named by at least 13% of pharmacists: nausea (36.1%), dizziness (25.1%), diarrhea (15.0%), and vomiting (13.9%). All other AEs were named by fewer than 7% of respondents. Only 62.9% of pharmacists ($n = 542$) provided appropriate recommendations: melatonin (40.3%), referral to physician (22.0%), or sleep hygiene (0.6%). Over 12% of pharmacists ($n = 107$) provided inappropriate recommendations (anticholinergic agent or valerian root) and 21.5% of pharmacists were unable to provide any recommendation. We identified significant gaps in community pharmacists' knowledge regarding donepezil AEs and non-prescription insomnia recommendation needing significant improvement to ensure high-quality AD-related care.

Keywords: community pharmacist; pharmaceutical care; Alzheimer's disease; cognitive enhancer; acetylcholinesterase inhibitor; donepezil; rivastigmine; anticholinergic agent

1. Introduction

Alzheimer's disease (AD) is the most common type of irreversible dementia causing 70% of dementia cases among persons over the age of 70 [1,2]. About 50 million people worldwide are diagnosed with AD, 4.5 million residing in the United States (US); and this number is expected to rise in the coming decades [1–3]. Advanced age is the greatest risk factor for development of late-onset AD [2]. In the US, this will mean an estimated 7.1 million persons with AD in 2025 [1]. Currently, no disease-modifying therapy is available, so treatment is symptomatic utilizing cognitive enhancers from two pharmacologic classes: acetylcholinesterase inhibitors (AChEIs) (i.e., donepezil, galantamine, rivastigmine), and NMDA-receptor antagonist (memantine) [4–9]. Use of AChEIs in persons with AD can have modest beneficial effects on cognitive, global, daily functioning [10]. However, caring for a person with AD requires more than medications to achieve maximum therapeutic benefits.

Pharmacists are medication experts, responsible for ensuring safe and effective medication use in seeking positive treatment outcomes [11–13]. Pharmacists practicing in local community pharmacies are among the most accessible healthcare professionals and can play a significant role in provision of primary care for community-dwelling individuals. One-third of individuals with dementia are estimated to be living at home [1]; therefore, they, their family members, or caregivers are likely to be regular clients of local community pharmacies. In the US, states such as West Virginia (WV), North Dakota (ND), and South Dakota (SD), as well as large areas of California and Oregon, are predominantly rural with elderly populations above the national average. Given pharmacists' medication expertise and role in chronic disease management, and the growing population of older adults in the US [14], pharmacists should possess the requisite knowledge to provide high-quality, contemporary care for AD.

All community pharmacists should be able to counsel patients on common disease states and disease management, treatment expectations, drug adverse effects (AEs), and interactions. They also should provide safe and effective self-care recommendations alongside general medication dispensing. Currently, no matter where community pharmacists practice, they are likely to serve persons with AD and/or their caregivers. Therefore, it is necessary for pharmacists to have sufficient knowledge and appropriate skills for providing AD-related care [15–17]. Recent evidence suggests improvement in pharmacists' knowledge regarding AD and its pharmacological management is needed [18–20].

The study objectives were to understand the knowledge of community pharmacists regarding donepezil AEs and self-care recommendations for insomnia for persons with AD treated with rivastigmine. This knowledge is intended to serve as an indication of potential quality of actual AD-related services in the community that a community-dwelling person with AD, a family member, or a caregiver would receive.

2. Materials and Methods

Study Design

This is a cross-sectional study of community pharmacists and pharmacies utilizing a standardized telephone survey, revised from Marvanova and Henkel [18]. The study population consists of a 100% sample of pharmacies in three high-elderly study areas: WV ($n = 502$), ND ($n = 179$), and SD ($n = 180$), and select counties of Northern California (N.CA.) ($n = 212$), and Southern Oregon (S.OR.) ($n = 93$). A list of community pharmacies in surveyed areas was obtained from individual states' Boards of Pharmacy. One pharmacist was interviewed from each pharmacy. The research study was approved as exempt by the University Institutional Review Board.

Pharmacies were cold contacted by telephone during business hours between August and October 2014. Prospective participants were informed that information provided would be used for academic research purposes only, and that participation was voluntary and would remain anonymous. If the pharmacist was unavailable, contact was re-attempted on the same day or a later date. If the time was inconvenient, the pharmacist was provided the opportunity to select a time/day when they would be available. Pharmacists were not informed about the survey questions prior to actual administration as we wanted to assess knowledge without allowing for preparation. Knowledge data was gathered by speaking directly to a pharmacist, taking less than two minutes, but without restriction on interview length. In-stock availability of cognitive enhancers was then obtained from the pharmacist, but if the pharmacist was busy, pharmacy technicians were allowed to provide this information. Two trained, fourth-year pharmacy student assistants obtained pharmacist and pharmacy demographic information and then asked questions on pharmacists' knowledge regarding AChEI AE(s) and self-care recommendation for insomnia in individual with AD treated with an AChEI. These items were assessed using open-ended questions: "What are the most important AEs to counsel a new patient on regarding donepezil?" and "What non-prescription (non-Rx) recommendation would you provide for a dementia patient currently using rivastigmine patch, for his/her insomnia?"

respectively. We assessed in-stock availability of several donepezil formulations (10 mg tablet, 10 mg orally-disintegrating tablet, and donepezil 23 mg tablet), and rivastigmine formulations (9.5 mg/h patch, and 3 mg capsule) to ascertain practice-based medication familiarity. Information was entered in Microsoft Excel, coded, cleaned, and uploaded into Stata 10.1. where descriptive statistics and logistic regression analyses were performed.

3. Results

3.1. Characteristics of Respondents

A total of 862 responses (74%) were obtained from 1166 eligible community pharmacies and are summarized in Table 1. Respondents were balanced between male (50.3%) and female (49.7%). Just under half (43.5%) had terminal Bachelor of Science in Pharmacy (B.S.), while 56.5% had a Doctor of Pharmacy (Pharm.D.). One or more donepezil formulation(s) (donepezil 10 mg tablet, donepezil 23 mg tablet and/or donepezil 10 mg orally-disintegrating tablet) was in-stock in 88.6% of surveyed pharmacies. Rivastigmine formulations (rivastigmine 3 mg capsule and/or 9.5 mg/24 h patch) were in-stock in fewer pharmacies (28.6% and 47.1%, respectively).

Table 1. Pharmacists Characteristics.

Characteristic	n	%
Sex		
Male	434	50.3%
Female	428	47.7%
Pharmacy Terminal Degree		
Bachelor of Science in Pharmacy	375	43.5%
Doctor of Pharmacy	487	56.5%
Study Areas		
Northern California	119	13.8%
Southern Oregon	58	6.7%
North Dakota	109	12.7%
South Dakota	156	18.1%
West Virginia	420	48.7%

3.2. Pharmacists' Knowledge Regarding Donepezil AEs

While over half of surveyed pharmacists (61.7%, $n = 513$) were able to name ≥ 1 AE, less than one third (31.4%, percent ($n = 261$) were able to name ≥ 2 AEs, and only 15.7 percent ($n = 131$) were able to name ≥ 3 AEs. (Table 2) Respondents' ability to name individual, evidence-based AEs is shown in Table 3. Only four donepezil AEs were named in any significant numbers: nausea (36.1%); dizziness (25.1%); diarrhea (15.0%); and vomiting (13.9%). Other AEs were named by fewer than 7% of respondents (headache 3.8%, insomnia 6.4%, anorexia 6.6%, muscle cramps 1.4%, weight loss 1.6%, and fatigue 3.0%). Only 0.6% of all surveyed pharmacists named lower heart rate ($n = 5$), 0.2% lower blood pressure ($n = 3$), or 1.2% vivid dreams ($n = 10$). While the number of AEs named was low in all areas, logistic regression analyses identify that, compared to those in the ND/SD study area, respondents in the N.CA./S.OR. study area were more likely to name ≥ 2 AEs (OR = 1.70; 95% CI = 1.17–2.54) and ≥ 3 AEs (OR = 2.77; 95% CI = 1.62–4.74), and those in the West Virginia study area more likely to name ≥ 1 AEs (OR = 1.51; 95% CI = 1.07–2.14), ≥ 2 AEs (OR = 2.16; 95% CI = 1.57–2.98), and ≥ 3 AEs (OR = 2.86; 95% CI = 1.81–4.52). Overall, pharmacists with a Pharm.D. were more likely to name ≥ 1 AEs (OR = 1.65; 95% CI = 1.24–2.197), ≥ 2 AEs (OR = 1.86; 95% CI = 1.37–2.52), and ≥ 3 AEs (OR = 2.01; 95% CI = 1.34–3.01) compared to those with a B.S.

Table 2. Pharmacists' Knowledge of Donepezil Adverse Effects.

Knowledge of AEs	Mean	SD
Common AEs [a]	1.17	1.27
Number of AEs Named	N	%
$\geq$ 1 AEs	513	61.7%
$\geq$ 2 AEs	261	31.4%
$\geq$ 3 AEs	131	15.7%

Abbreviations: Adverse effects (AEs). [a] Donepezil adverse effects with incidence rates of $\geq$5%: nausea, diarrhea, headache, vomiting, insomnia, anorexia, dizziness, muscle cramps, weight loss, fatigue [4].

Table 3. Pharmacists' Knowledge of Individual Donepezil Adverse Effects.

Common Adverse Effects [a]	n	%
Nausea	311	36.1%
Diarrhea	129	15.0%
Headache	33	3.8%
Vomiting	120	13.9%
Insomnia	55	6.4%
Anorexia	57	6.6%
Dizziness	216	25.1%
Muscle Cramps	12	1.4%
Weight Loss	14	1.6%
Fatigue	26	3.0%
Other Adverse Effects [b]	**n**	**%**
Bradycardia [c]	5	0.6%
Vivid Dreams	10	1.2%

[a] Adverse effects with reported incidence rates of $\geq$5%: nausea, diarrhea, headache, vomiting, insomnia, anorexia, dizziness, muscle cramps, weight loss, fatigue [4]. These adverse effects are also listed in order from highest to lowest reported incidence rate; [b] Adverse effects with reported incidence rate <3% [4]; [c] Rare but severe adverse effect [4].

3.3. Pharmacists' Knowledge Regarding Self-Care Recommendations

When providing a non-Rx sleep-aid recommendation, 12.4% of pharmacists (n = 107) provided inappropriate recommendations: valerian root and doxylamine, diphenhydramine, or another first-generation antihistamine. More than 20 percent of pharmacists were unable to provide any recommendation. Only 62.9% of pharmacists (n = 542) provided appropriate recommendations: melatonin (40.3%) or referral to physician (22.0%), along with sleep hygiene (0.6%). A small number of pharmacists (3.3%) refused to answer (Table 4). There was no difference among study areas with regard to provision of an inappropriate recommendation. Pharmacists with a Pharm.D. were less likely to make an inappropriate recommendation (OR = 0.43; 95% CI = 0.28–0.66), more likely to recommend melatonin (OR = 2.08; 95% CI = 1.56–2.77), and less likely to say "don't know" (OR = 0.67; 95% CI = 0.48–0.93).

Table 4. Pharmacists' Non-Prescription Sleep-Aid Recommendations.

Recommendation	n	%
APPROPRIATE	542	62.9%
Melatonin	347	40.3%
Refer to Physician	190	22.0%
Sleep Hygiene	5	0.6%
INAPPROPRIATE	107	12.4%
Anticholinergic Agent [a]	104	12.1%
Valerian Root	3	0.4%
DON'T KNOW	185	21.5%
REFUSE	28	3.3%

[a] Anticholinergic agent: any over-the-counter product containing diphenhydramine, doxylamine, or first generation antihistamine

4. Discussion

Community pharmacists are highly accessible and, over the past few decades, their role has significantly expanded from traditional medication dispensing into provision of a variety of clinical services [11,12,17,21,22]. For community-dwelling persons with AD, there are potentially beneficial clinical services that community pharmacists/pharmacies can provide to ensure appropriate medication use and positive health outcomes [13,16,20]. Maintaining continuous pharmacological treatment of patients with Alzheimer's disease can be difficult because of low persistence of treatment with AChEIs due to perceived medication inefficacy, unrealistic treatment expectations, and/or GI AEs [23–26]. Medication education and pharmacist-counseling have been associated with improved adherence and treatment persistence with AChEIs [27–29]. Inappropriate medications among community-dwelling persons with AD are relatively common including over-the-counter first-generation antihistamines with central anticholinergic AEs that can negatively impact cognition [30,31]. High-quality patient education on AChEIs and appropriate self-care recommendations for non-cognitive problems associated with dementia are a good starting point.

Donepezil is a widely-prescribed cognitive enhancer because of its once daily dosing and FDA-approval for all AD stages [4]. Most surveyed pharmacies had donepezil in-stock. Donepezil, as well as other AChEIs, increase synaptic acetylcholine and postsynaptic cholinergic neurotransmission in the brain due to decreased breakdown of acetylcholine [4–7,32]. However, these medications also increase peripheral cholinergic activity that leads to GI AEs (i.e., nausea, vomiting, diarrhea, and/or anorexia) and bradycardia [4–7,33]. Additional AEs commonly reported with donepezil are dizziness, headache, weight loss, muscle cramps, and fatigue. These AEs are usually transient during dose initiation or increase [4–7]. A community pharmacist's role is to provide medication education to patients and caregivers. All pharmacists practicing in the US should be able to provide effective counseling on medication AEs, more so for commonly stocked medications (i.e., donepezil).

Despite donepezil being in-stock, knowledge regarding AEs among surveyed pharmacists was poor. While pharmacists with a Pharm.D. named more AEs than their B.S. peers, and pharmacists in the WV and N.CA./S.OR. study areas named more AEs than those in the ND/SD study area, neither degree nor area was associated with meaningfully improved knowledge regarding AEs. A patient or caregiver will typically see a community pharmacist after receiving a prescription for donepezil. Community pharmacists play a role in dispensing AChEIs but also providing medication-related information, especially important for those with filling a medication for the first time. Inadequate pharmacist knowledge regarding donepezil GI AEs can potentially result in patient distress or early discontinuation [27,29], or to lack of understanding on how to potentially decrease AEs (e.g., taking medication with food, dividing daily dose and taking separately). Patients or caregivers should be informed that these AEs are usually transient and improve with continuous medication use [4]. Lack of knowledge regarding donepezil AEs could reduce effectiveness of pharmacist counseling, negatively impacting adherence or treatment persistence [27–29].

Because of age-related physiologic changes, number of comorbidities, and/or co-administration of other medications, persons with AD might be at increased risk for donepezil interactions leading to potentially serious problems such as bradycardia, syncope and falls, bradyarrhythmia, and/or atrioventricular (AV) block [4]. Lower heart rate is rare; however, it can be a serious donepezil AE, especially for individuals with pre-existing bradycardia, AV heart block, or concomitant medications affecting heart rate (i.e., beta-blockers, non-dihydropyridine calcium channel blockers, or amiodarone) [4]. Only 5 (0.6%) surveyed pharmacists named this as an AE on which they would counsel a person with AD filling donepezil for the first time.

An inappropriate recommendation of a first-generation antihistamine for management of insomnia in a person with AD treated with rivastigmine was made by 12.4% of pharmacists. There was no difference in rates of inappropriate recommendations among study areas, but pharmacists with a Pharm.D. were 57 percent less likely to make an inappropriate recommendation compared to those with a B.S. Given the central anticholinergic properties of this class of medications as well as AEs profile, this recommendation can negatively impact a patient [31]. Addition of diphenhydramine to a treatment regimen with rivastigmine (or AChEIs) is associated with reduced clinical effect of the cognitive enhancer due to central anticholinergic effect [6,7,30,34]. Diphenhydramine administration can also be associated with increased risk for cognitive AEs (i.e., memory and learning impairment), especially in older adults and those with pre-existing cognitive problems/deficit [31,35,36] and can actually worsen cognitive status and perceived efficacy of AChEIs, increasing risk for medication discontinuation. We also considered valerian root an inappropriate recommendation ($n = 3$) due to its pharmacologic properties that can increase risk for drug interactions, lower tolerability for older adults, and minimal clinical data on its use in dementia [36,37].

Melatonin was recommended by two out of five of pharmacists. Given the pathophysiology of AD and possible association of disrupted circadian rhythm [38], melatonin can be an appropriate recommendation that would not interact with disease state or medications [36,39–41]. However, efficacy of melatonin in AD has mixed results [37,42]. Over 20% of pharmacists were unable to provide any recommendation. Given community pharmacists' role in self-care for community-dwelling individuals, this is substandard performance. While no harmful recommendation was made, neither was a helpful recommendation nor guidance offered. To provide an appropriate self-care recommendation for non-cognitive complications of AD, it is crucial for pharmacists to have knowledge regarding AD pathophysiology and treatment management so they can consider effectiveness, AEs, and interactions prior to providing a recommendation. Unfortunately, Rx and non-Rx medications with central anticholinergic effects are commonly used by community-dwelling older adults as well as persons with AD [30,31,43–45]. Pharmacists should play a role in decreasing anticholinergic drug prescribing for and utilization by vulnerable persons with AD. They should be proactive in increasing awareness regarding potential harm of these medications, recognizing and managing potentially inappropriate medications in persons with AD, and not contributing to this problem by making inappropriate recommendations.

This study did not comprehensively assess AD knowledge but rather assessed two specific roles of community pharmacists: medication counseling and self-care recommendations, both part of care for community-dwelling persons with AD. The study was cross-sectional, thus was unable to comprehensively assess provision of complex AD care. Knowledge was not assessed for all cognitive enhancers. But as donepezil is the most widely available, knowledge is highly likely to better than for other AChEIs.

5. Conclusions

Community pharmacists can play a beneficial role in AD-related pharmaceutical care, managing drug therapy through patient counseling and providing recommendations able to lead to optimal drug use and positive health outcomes. Knowledge of surveyed community pharmacists was grossly inadequate. Significant gaps in knowledge were identified regarding AChEIs. Given the large and still growing population with AD, the importance of medication counseling, and community pharmacists' role in ensuring medication efficacy, tolerability, and safety for individuals with AD, knowledge improvement is needed regarding AChEIs including AEs, interactions, and self-care recommendations for insomnia in persons with AD. The findings seem to indicate a potential need for continuing education for community pharmacists in Alzheimer's disease management. The authors are currently concluding a study on pharmacists' decision-making, community information-seeking, and continuing education utilization related to AD.

Acknowledgments: The authors thank Sarah Kim and Nazish Raja, for their assistance with data collection.

Author Contributions: Marketa Marvanova: conceived and co-designed the project; obtained IRB study approval, performed and supervised the study; provided scientific input for data analysis; co-designed assessment tools; co-wrote the manuscript. Paul Henkel: conceived and co-designed the project; performed and supervised the study; performed the statistical analysis; co-designed assessment tools; co-wrote the manuscript.

References

1.   Alzheimer's Association. 2017 Alzheimer's Disease Facts and Figures. Available online: http://preview.alz.org/ri/documents/facts2017_report(1).pdf (accessed on 2 June 2017).
2.   Swerdlow, R.H. Pathogenesis of Alzheimer's disease. *Clin. Interv. Aging* **2007**, *2*, 347–359. [PubMed]
3.   Alzheimer Disease International. *Policy Brief: The Global Impact of Dementia 2013–2050*; Alzheimer Disease International: London, UK, 2013. Available online: https://www.alz.co.uk/research/GlobalImpactDementia2013.pdf (accessed on 30 March 2017).
4.   Aricept (Donepezil Hydrochloride) Tablets Package Insert. Eisai Inc. (updated 2015). Available online: http://labeling.pfizer.com/ShowLabeling.aspx?id=510 (accessed on 18 May 2017).
5.   Razadyne (Galantamine Hydrobromide) Tablets Package Insert. Janssen Pharmaceuticals, Inc. (updated 2013). Available online: http://www.janssen.com/us/sites/www_janssen_com_usa/files/products-documents/razadyne_er_1.pdf (accessed on 18 May 2017).
6.   Exelon (Rivastigmine Tartrate) Capsules Package Insert. Novartis Pharmaceuticals Corporation (updated 2015). Available online: http://pharma.us.novartis.com/product/pi/pdf/exelon.pdf (accessed on 18 May 2017).
7.   Exelon (Rivastigmine Transdermal System) Patch Package Insert. Novartis Pharmaceuticals Corporation (updated February 2015). Available online: http://www.pharma.us.novartis.com/product/pi/pdf/exelonpatch.pdf (accessed on 18 May 2017).
8.   Namenda (Memantine HCl) Tablets for Oral Use, Package Insert. Forest Pharmaceuticals, Inc. (updated October 2013). Available online: https://www.allergan.com/assets/pdf/namenda_pi (accessed on 18 May 2017).
9.   Doody, R.S.; Stevens, J.C.; Beck, C.; Dubinsky, R.M.; Kaye, J.A.; Gwyther, L.; Mohs, R.C.; Thal, L.J.; Whitehouse, P.J.; DeKosky, S.T.; et al. Practice Parameter: Management of Dementia (an Evidence-Based Review). Report of the Quality Standards Subcommittee of the American Academy of Neurology. *Neurology* **2001**, *56*, 1154–1166. [CrossRef] [PubMed]
10. Tricco, A.C.; Vandervaart, S.; Soobiah, C.; Lillie, E.; Perrier, L.; Chen, M.H.; Hemmelgarn, B.; Majumdar, S.R.; Straus, S.E. Efficacy of cognitive enhancers for Alzheimer's disease: Protocol for a systemic review and network meta-analysis. *Syst. Rev.* **2012**, *1*, 31. [CrossRef] [PubMed]

11. Morrison, C.M.; Glover, D.; Gilchrist, S.M.; Casey, M.O.; Lanza, A.; Lane, R.I.; Patanian, M. A Program Guide for Public Health: Partnering with Pharmacists in the Prevention and Control of Chronic Diseases. National Center for Chronic Disease Prevention and Health Promotion, 2012. Available online: http://www.cdc.gov/dhdsp/programs/spha/docs/pharmacist_guide.pdf (accessed on 15 June 2017).

12. Giberson, S.; Yoder, S.; Lee, M.P. Improving Patient and Health System Outcomes through Advanced Pharmacy Practice: A Report to the U.S. Surgeon General. 2011. Available online: http://www.accp.com/docs/positions/misc/improving_patient_and_health_system_outcomes.pdf (accessed on 8 June 2017).

13. Skelton, J.B. White paper on expanding the role of pharmacists in caring for individuals with Alzheimer's disease: APhA Foundation Coordinating Council to Improve Collaboration in Supporting Patients with Alzheimer's Disease. *J. Am. Pharm. Assoc.* **2008**, *48*, 715–721. [CrossRef] [PubMed]

14. United States Census Bureau. Available online: https://www.census.gov/quickfacts/table/PST045216/38 (accessed on 10 May 2017).

15. Stafford, A. The pharmacist's role in supporting people living with dementia in the community. *Aust. Pharm.* **2015**, *34*. Available online: http://www.detectearly.org.au/wp-content/uploads/2015/02/The-pharmacists-role-in-supporting-people-living-with-dementia.pdf (accessed on 8 June 2017).

16. Rickles, N.M.; Skelton, J.B.; Davis, J.; Hopson, J. Cognitive memory screening and referral program in community pharmacies in the United States. *Int. J. Clin. Pharm.* **2014**, *36*, 360–367. [CrossRef] [PubMed]

17. Manolakis, P.G.; Skelton, J.B. Pharmacists' contributions to primary care in the United States collaborating to address unmet patient care needs: The emerging role for pharmacists to address the shortage of primary care providers. *Am. J. Pharm. Educ.* **2010**, *74*, S7. [CrossRef] [PubMed]

18. Marvanova, M.; Henkel, P. Community pharmacists' knowledge of Alzheimer's disease care in high- and low-income Chicago. *J. Am. Pharm. Assoc.* **2017**. [CrossRef] [PubMed]

19. Zerafa, N.; Scerri, C. Knowledge and pharmacological management of Alzheimer's disease by managing community pharmacists: A nationwide study. *Int. J. Clin. Pharm.* **2016**, *38*, 1416–1424. [CrossRef] [PubMed]

20. Barry, H.E.; Parsons, C.; Passmore, A.P.; Hughes, C.M. Community pharmacists and people with dementia: A cross-sectional survey exploring experiences, attitudes, and knowledge of pain and its management. *Int. J. Geriatr. Psychiatry* **2013**, *28*, 1077–1085. [CrossRef] [PubMed]

21. Hemberg, N.; Huggins, D.; Michaels, N.; Moose, J. Innovative Community Pharmacy Practice Models in North Carolina. *N. C. Med. J.* **2017**, *78*, 198–201. [CrossRef] [PubMed]

22. Kelling, S.E.; Rondon-Begazo, A.; DiPietro Mager, N.A.; Murphy, B.L.; Bright, D.R. Provision of Clinical Preventive Services by Community Pharmacists. *Prev. Chronic Dis.* **2016**, *13*, E149. [CrossRef] [PubMed]

23. Campbell, N.L.; Perkins, A.J.; Gao, S.; Skaar, T.C.; Li, L.; Hendrie, H.C.; Fowler, N.; Callahan, C.M.; Boustani, M.A. Adherence and Tolerability of Alzheimer's Disease Medications: A Pragmatic Randomized Trial. *J. Am. Geriatr. Soc.* **2017**, *65*, 1497–1504. [CrossRef] [PubMed]

24. Gardette, V.; Andrieu, S.; Lapeyre-Mestre, M.; Coley, N.; Cantet, C.; Ousset, P.J.; Grand, A.; Monstastruc, J.L.; Vellas, B. Predictive factors of discontinuation and switch of cholinesterase inhibitors in community-dwelling patients with Alzheimer's disease: A 2-year prospective, multicentre, cohort study. *CNS Drugs* **2010**, *24*, 431–442. [CrossRef] [PubMed]

25. Arlt, S.; Lindner, R.; Rösler, A.; von Renteln-Kruse, W. Adherence to medication in patients with dementia: Predictors and strategies for improvement. *Drugs Aging* **2008**, *25*, 1033–1047. [CrossRef] [PubMed]

26. Umegaki, H.; Itoh, A.; Suzuki, Y.; Nabeshima, T. Discontinuation of donepezil for the treatment of Alzheimer's disease in geriatric practice. *Int. Psychogeriatr.* **2008**, *20*, 800–806. [CrossRef] [PubMed]

27. Nanaumi, Y.; Onda, M.; Tsubota, K.; Tanaka, R.; Mukai, Y.; Matoba, S.; Tanaka, Y.; Arakawa, Y. Effectiveness of Pharmacists' Comprehensive Assessment of Medication Profiles in Dementia Patients. *Yakugaku Zasshi* **2015**, *135*, 1057–1067. [CrossRef] [PubMed]

28. Nanaumi, Y.; Matoba, S.; Onda, M.; Tanaka, R.; Tsubota, K.; Mukai, Y.; Sakurai, H.; Hayase, Y.; Arakawa, Y. Pilot study of dementia medication compliance conducted among pharmacists providing home visits which evaluates the degree of drug compliance, as defined by numerous attributes, between patients at home and patients in a medical facility. *Yakugaku Zasshi* **2012**, *132*, 387–393. [CrossRef] [PubMed]

29. Watanabe, N.; Yamamura, K.; Suzuki, Y.; Umegaki, H.; Shigeno, K.; Matsushita, R.; Sai, Y.; Miyamoto, K.; Yamada, K. Pharmacist-based Donepezil Outpatient Consultation Service to improve medication persistence. *Patient Prefer Adherence* **2012**, *6*, 605–611. [PubMed]

30. Sverdrup Efjestad, A.; Ihle-Hansen, H.; Hjellvik, V.; Blix, H.S. Comedication and Treatment Length in Users of Acetylcholinesterase Inhibitors. *Demen Geriatr. Cogn. Dis. Extra* **2017**, *7*, 30–40. [CrossRef] [PubMed]

31. American Geriatrics Society 2015 Beers Criteria Update Expert Panel. American Geriatrics Society 2015 Updated Beers Criteria for Potentially Inappropriate Medication Use in Older Adults. *J. Am. Geriatr. Soc.* **2015**, *63*, 2227–2246.

32. Ghezzi, L.; Scarpini, E.; Galimberti, D. Disease-modifying drugs in Alzheimer's disease. *Drug Des. Dev. Ther.* **2013**, *7*, 1471–1478.

33. Hogan, D.B.; Bailey, P.; Black, S.; Carswell, A.; Chertkow, H.; Clarke, B.; Cohen, C.; Fisk, J.D.; Forbes, D.; Man-Son-Hing, M.; et al. Diagnosis and treatment of dementia: 5. Nonpharmacologic and pharmacologic therapy for mild to moderate dementia. *CMAJ* **2008**, *179*, 1019–1026. [CrossRef] [PubMed]

34. Kogut, S.J.; El-Maouche, D.; Abughosh, S.M. Decreased persistence to cholinesterase inhibitor therapy with concomitant use of drugs that can impair cognition. *Pharmacotherapy* **2005**, *25*, 1729–1735. [CrossRef] [PubMed]

35. Blokland, A. Acetylcholine: A neurotransmitter for learning and memory? *Brain Res. Rev.* **1995**, *21*, 285–300. [CrossRef]

36. Schroeck, J.L.; Ford, J.; Conway, E.L.; Kurtzhalts, K.E.; Gee, M.E.; Vollmer, K.A.; Mergenhagen, K.A. Review of Safety and Efficacy of Sleep Medicines in Older Adults. *Clin. Ther.* **2016**, *38*, 2340–2372. [CrossRef] [PubMed]

37. Lefebvre, T.; Foster, B.C.; Drouin, C.E.; Krantis, A.; Livesey, J.F.; Jordan, S.A. In vitro activity of commercial valerian root extracts against human cytochrome P450 3A4. *J. Pharm. Pharm. Sci.* **2004**, *7*, 265–773. [PubMed]

38. Saeed, Y.; Abbott, S.M. Circadian Disruption Associated with Alzheimer's Disease. *Curr. Neurol. Neurosci. Rep.* **2017**, *17*, 29. [CrossRef] [PubMed]

39. Salami, O.; Lyketsos, C.; Rao, V. Treatment of sleep disturbance in Alzheimer's dementia. *Int. J. Geriatr. Psychiatry* **2011**, *26*, 771–782. [CrossRef] [PubMed]

40. Wu, Y.H.; Swaab, D.F. Disturbance and strategies for reactivation of the circadian rhythm system in aging and Alzheimer's disease. *Sleep Med.* **2007**, *8*, 623–636. [CrossRef] [PubMed]

41. Asayama, K.; Yamadera, H.; Ito, T.; Suzuki, H.; Kudo, Y.; Endo, S. Double blind study of melatonin effects on the sleep-wake rhythm, cognitive and non-cognitive functions in Alzheimer type dementia. *J. Nippon. Med. Sch.* **2003**, *70*, 334–341. [CrossRef] [PubMed]

42. McCleery, J.; Cohen, D.A.; Sharpley, A.L. Pharmacotherapies for sleep disturbances in dementia. *Cochrane Database Syst. Rev.* **2016**. [CrossRef]

43. Kachru, N.; Carnahan, R.M.; Johnson, M.L.; Aparasu, R.R. Potentially inappropriate anticholinergic medication use in older adults with dementia. *J. Am. Pharm. Assoc.* **2015**, *55*, 603–612. [CrossRef] [PubMed]

44. Bhattacharya, R.; Chatterjee, S.; Carnahan, R.M.; Aparasu, R.R. Prevalence and predictors of anticholinergic agents in elderly outpatients with dementia. *Am. J. Geriatr. Pharmacother.* **2011**, *9*, 434–441. [CrossRef] [PubMed]

45. Abraham, O.; Schleiden, L.; Albert, S.M. Over-the-counter medications containing diphenhydramine and doxylamine used by older adults to improve sleep. *Int. J. Clin. Pharm.* **2017**. [CrossRef] [PubMed]

17

Community Pharmacy Use by Children across Europe

Mitch Blair [1] and Arjun Menon [2],* 🆔

[1]   Department of Paediatrics, Imperial College London, London SW7 2AZ, UK; m.blair@imperial.ac.uk
[2]   Imperial College School of Medicine, Imperial College London, London SW7 2AZ, UK
*   Correspondence: arjun.menon13@imperial.ac.uk

Abstract: The use of community pharmacies across Europe has potential to alleviate the burden on overstretched healthcare providers. Children and young people (0–18 years) account for a large number of primary care attendances. This narrative literature review between January 2000 and December 2017 examines the use of community pharmacy by paediatric patients in Europe. The results report both positive and negative perceptions of community pharmacy by parents and children, opportunities for an extended role in Europe, as well as the need for further training. The main limitations were the inclusion of English language papers only and an initial review of the literature carried out by a single researcher. It remains to be seen whether a 'new-look' role of the community pharmacist is practical and in alignment with specific European Commission and national policies.

Keywords: community pharmacy; pharmacist; children; parent; Europe

---

1. Introduction

Community pharmacy is a field of primary care medicine, which serves a large proportion of the European population. As of 2016, there were an estimated 400,000 community pharmacists in Europe visited by 46 million citizens daily [1,2], representing almost 10% of the 508 million people living in the European Union (EU) [3]. In general, the core pharmacy services across the EU include dispensing medication, medication management, emergency care (e.g., emergency contraception), as well as minor ailment management [1,2]. An example of this is in Slovakia, where up to 74% of emergency room attendances were due to lack of available alternative primary care services [4]. Further to this, in the United Kingdom (UK), the National Health Service (NHS) reported that 18 million general practitioner (GP) appointments and 2.1 million emergency department (ED) visits could have been treated at a community pharmacist and would have saved the health service £850 million in 2017 alone [5]. The paediatric population in particular have contributed to the rise in ED attendances with the UK seeing an increase in attendances of 28% from 1999 to 2010 [6]. A large part of this was attributed to the failure of other primary care services in dealing with children that had minor illnesses [6]. There is an opportunity for community pharmacists to redefine their role in the management of childhood illness. They can be the first port of call for illnesses and alleviate the burden of treating non-severe pediatric presentations in other over-stretched primary care facilities [7].

A number of pharmacists in Europe provide services such as routine vaccinations, chronic disease management, smoking cessation, early screening, and testing of disease [1,2]. In Belgium for example, asthma patients prescribed inhaled corticosteroids were given two follow up appointments with a community pharmacist [8]. This pilot programme was shown to benefit up to 36,000 patients, with the service potentially expanding to other chronic conditions [8]. In the UK, 1.1 million children suffer from asthma, with the NHS spending over £1 billion on the disease annually [9]. With the condition being so manageable in the community setting, it is surprising that community pharmacists do not deal with a greater number of cases to prevent hospital admissions. Another example is in Ireland where over 50,000 patients (a tenth of people vaccinated) were given the flu vaccine by community pharmacists in 2014 [1,2]. In 2015, owing to the success of the scheme, the pharmacist remit was increased to include pneumococcal and shingles vaccines as well [10]. Children are the most common recipients of such vaccines and therefore, it is important to understand why a community pharmacist does not manage more of these vaccinations for children across Europe.

This literature review aims to understand how community pharmacy is currently being utilised by children, young people, and parents across Europe. Furthermore, it will possibly give insight into the current role of the community pharmacist in paediatric treatment, and how this role might change in the future.

2. Materials and Methods

The researchers, with the assistance of the librarian, developed appropriate search parameters and identified the most relevant databases for the review, to be conducted over two weeks in December 2017. The researchers looked for data published between January 2000 and December 2017. An extensive exploratory search was performed and the literature was thoroughly assessed and synthesised in order to generate conclusions and consider future steps.

Electronic databases were searched including PubMed, EMBASE, OVID, and HMIC (for grey literature), with each one being thoroughly searched using as many permutations of the following key words: "community pharmacy", "community pharmacist", "pharmacy", "pharmacist", "children", "paediatric", "parent", "carer", "over-the-counter", and "Europe". The databases were searched by combining Boolean logic with truncation marks to generate a comprehensive set of literature. The initial literature was then subject to the specific inclusion/exclusion criteria seen in Table 1 to identify results that were in line with the objectives of the study. Once articles were obtained through database searching, the references of these articles were then screened to ensure that no relevant literature was missed from the databases. A handful of relevant articles were identified through this method, in addition to the ones found via databases. Figure 1 provides an in-depth view of how the literature was screened and selected for synthesis in the form of a narrative review, through a PRISMA flowchart [11]. It should be noted that all the studies included in the synthesis were screened individually and collectively for publication bias and selective reporting and this is reported in the results section below.

Table 1. Inclusion and exclusion criteria for the literature at each stage of the research.

Inclusion Criteria	Exclusion Criteria	Justification
At search string level:		
Papers published between January 2000 and December 2017		The role of community pharmacists compared to present day use may be significantly different
Any article type		This allows for a comprehensive review
Full paper available		The full paper needs to be analysed in order for the review to be robust
At title/abstract level:		
	Paper does not specifically relate to use of community pharmacy by children	This literature review aimed to study the utilisation of community pharmacy by paediatric populations (0–18 years) in Europe
English language paper		The resources were not sufficient to fully translate papers
Europe		This literature review aimed to study the utilisation of community pharmacy by paediatric populations (0–18 years) in Europe

Table 1. *Cont.*

Inclusion Criteria	Exclusion Criteria	Justification
At full-text level:		
Paper analyses utilisation of community pharmacy by children		These articles are relevant to the study
	Paper only mentions community pharmacy as the location of a study	This study aims to explore the utilization of community pharmacies as a primary care service

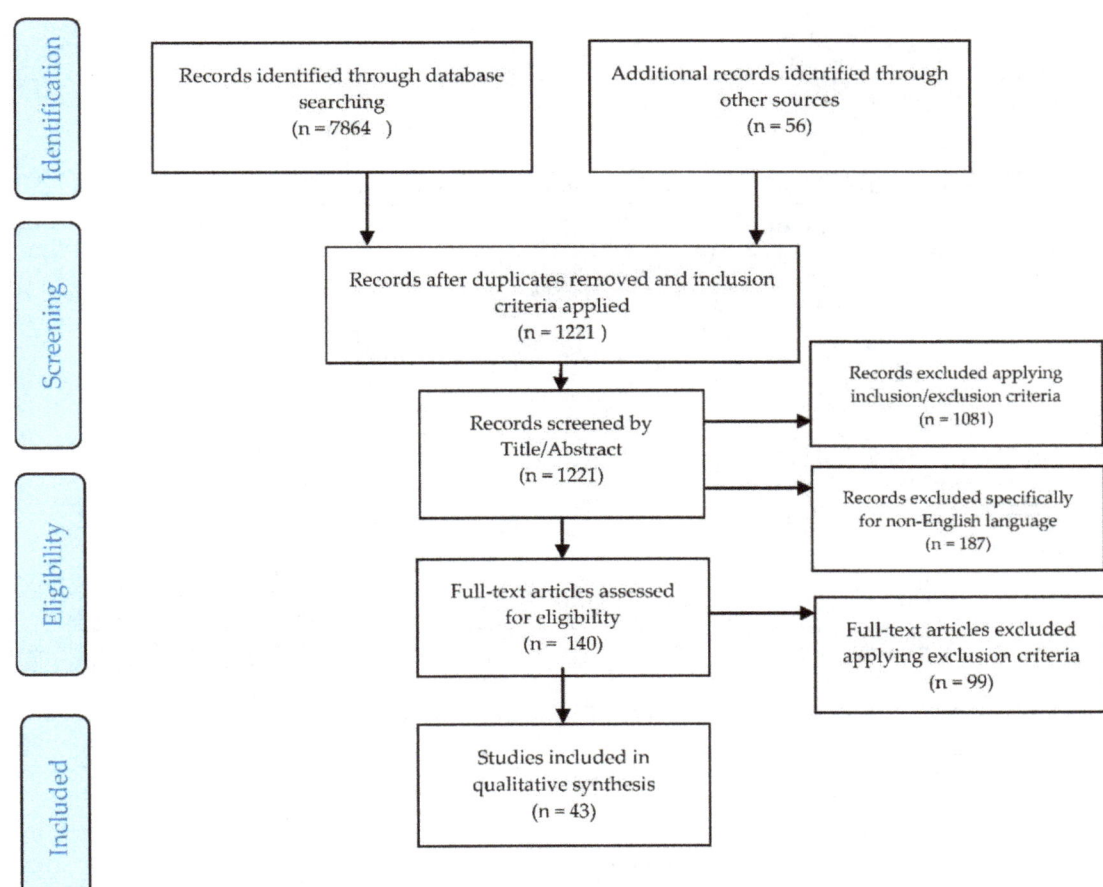

Figure 1. PRISMA flowchart [11] of how the literature was filtered to end up with the relevant articles for synthesis.

3. Results

Table 2 below demonstrates the number of studies from each country that were included in the synthesis.

In total, 43 studies were included in the synthesis as shown in the tables and PRISMA flowchart above. These studies demonstrated no clear publication bias or selective reporting. Non-English language studies ($n = 187$) were excluded due to translation resource restrictions. Table 3 gives an overview of all the results included, showing the type of study conducted as well as the key findings.

Table 2. Number of studies included in synthesis stratified by country.

Country	Number of Studies Included in Synthesis
United Kingdom (England, Scotland, Wales, Northern Ireland)	19
Sweden	5
Netherlands	4
France	4
Germany	3
Finland	2
Greece	1
Iceland	1
Belgium	1
Spain	1
Italy	1
Croatia	1

Table 3. Description of the synthesized studies.

Reference as in Text	AuthorNo (Year)	Type of Paper/Study	Population Size	Main Study Finding
[12]	Hammond (2004)	Cross-sectional questionnaire-based study	3984	Pharmacists are a good source of information for unwell children
[13]	Hodgson (2004)	Cross-sectional questionnaire-based study	85	87% of mothers find pharmacist advice for sick children helpful
[14]	Gray (2011)	Cross-sectional mixed methods study	134 questionnaires, 39 interviews	82% of parents find pharmacist advice somewhat helpful regarding medication
[15]	Bamford (2015)	Grey literature (Charity report)	Not applicable	Parents prioritise other information sources over pharmacists
[16]	Holappa (2012)	Cross-sectional questionnaire-based study	4020	44% of parents seek pharmacist advice for their sick children
[17]	Gray (2017)	Cross-sectional mixed methods study	Not provided	Most parents prefer receiving written (50%) or spoken (29%) advice from pharmacists
[18]	Plachouras (2010)	Cross-sectional questionnaire-based study	174	Inappropriate dispensing of antibiotics by pharmacists possibly led to widespread antibiotic resistance
[19]	Stakenborg (2016)	Cross-sectional focus group-based study	24	Parents trust their own knowledge more than advice from pharmacists
[20]	Gidman (2014)	Cross-sectional focus group-based study	26	Parents did not want to bring children to pharmacies due to presence of substance misuse patients in the clinic
[21]	Parsons (2013)	Cross-sectional questionnaire-based study	99	Parents found that pharmacies lack privacy compared to other primary care services
[22]	Guegan (2010)	Literature review	Not provided	Pharmacists have a trusted relationship with young patients formed over multiple encounters
[23]	Karamanidou (2016)	Cross-sectional interview-based study	15	Expanded role for pharmacists in oral contraceptive pill (OCP) provision and HPV vaccine
[24]	Terry (2016)	Cross-sectional observational study	1623	9% of ED attendances could have been dealt with in pharmacies
[25]	Carr (2007)	Pre-post interventional pilot study	50	Effective example of pharmacist led intervention in childhood eczema
[26]	Jacome (2003)	Pre-post interventional pilot study	164	Effective example of pharmacist-led intervention in childhood asthma
[27]	Gay (2006)	Randomised control trial	100	Ineffective example of pharmacist-led intervention for Type 1 Diabetes
[28]	Koster (2015)	Cross-sectional interview-based study	170	Regular attendance of children when collecting medication can improve medication adherence
[29]	Terry (2012)	Literature review	24 references	Increasing the communication between pharmacies and other primary care interfaces
[30]	de Jong-van den berg (2008)	Explorative comparative study	Not provided	Effective example of pharmacist-led intervention in the reduction of neural tube defects (NTDs)

Table 3. *Cont.*

Reference as in Text	AuthorNo (Year)	Type of Paper/Study	Population Size	Main Study Finding
[31]	Deacon (2011)	Statistics report (Epilepsy)	Not applicable	Incidence of epilepsy in children
[32]	Bilbow (2016)	Grey Literature (Charity report)	Not applicable	Incidence of attention deficit hyperactivity disorder (ADHD) in children
[33]	Perucca (2005)	Literature review	55 references	Medications for ADHD and epilepsy have a high rate of adverse events
[34]	Tobaiqy (2010)	Cross-sectional questionnaire-based pilot study	72	Exploring wider pharmacist involvement in the UK Yellow Card scheme
[35]	Stewart (2005)	Prospective questionnaire-based study	267	The pharmacist as a useful resource for therapeutic drug monitoring
[36]	Aston (2017)	Cross-sectional questionnaire-based study	76	23.7% of pharmacists performed medicine use reviews (MURs) for children's medication
[37]	Liley (2016)	Pre-post interventional pilot study	15	Increased use of MURs by pharmacists seems to improve children's asthma control
[38]	Ylinen (2010)	Cross-sectional questionnaire-based study	4032	50% of children use over-the-counter (OTC) medication
[39]	Clavenna (2009)	Retrospective cohort study	1,542,203	48% of children receive 1 drug prescription a month
[40]	Italia (2015)	Retrospective cohort study	3013	31.6% of children used an OTC drug in the last month
[41,42]	Koelch (2008)/ Du (2009)	Retrospective cohort study	17,450	30% of prescription medications for children were being used without proper prescription
[43,44]	Smith (2008)/ Smith (2008)	Systematic literature review (searching for randomised controlled trials)	3492	The various causes of mortality from children using cough medicines
[45]	Holmstrom (2014)	Cross-sectional questionnaire-based study	77	Careless and casual behavior of children towards OTC use
[46]	Stewart (2007)	Prospective questionnaire-based study	482	40% of pharmacists prescribed drugs off-label
[47]	Mukkatash (2011)	Cross-sectional questionnaire-based study	563	The need for clinical trials to change paediatric formulations, to reduce off-label prescribing
[48]	Hanna (2016)	Cross-sectional questionnaire-based study	90	Only 77% of pharmacists knew to use an adrenaline auto-injector for food anaphylaxis
[49]	Raffin (2016)	Cross-sectional questionnaire-based study	500	Pharmacist perpetuate a corticosteroid phobia in the population
[50]	Rees (2017)	Cross-sectional mixed methods study	2191	Medication errors occur at a much higher rate in community pharmacies than other primary care interfaces
[51]	Bardage (2013)	Cross-sectional questionnaire-based study	1098	6% of pharmacists provided inappropriate medication to febrile children
[52]	Lapeyre-Mestre (2004)	Cross-sectional questionnaire-based study	176	12.9% of pharmacists provided contra-indicated medication to children
[53]	Venables (2015)	Cross-sectional focus group-based study	4	60% of pharmacists were very dependent on product monographs
[54]	Driesen (2009)	Cross-sectional questionnaire-based study	101	Only 30% of pharmacists prescribed oral rehydration solution (ORS) to children with severe diarrhoea

The results are described by theme.

3.1. Perceptions

3.1.1. Parental Perception

Pharmacists are regularly compared by parents, to other sources of information about medication [12]. A UK study found that 87% of the time, mothers report such advice in dealing with minor illness in children, to be 'helpful' in managing the problem [13]. Another stated that 82% of parents reported that they have received 'very helpful' or 'helpful' advice from pharmacists regarding non-prescription medications, while 90% of the advice given had been fully understood by parents [14].

However, there are still variable levels of public trust in pharmacy services. Parents prioritise health information from the Internet and GPs over and above that given by pharmacists [15]. A study in Finland showed that only 44% of parents sought advice on treating their ill children from pharmacists compared to 70% who would seek a physician's advice [16]. If parents were to receive advice from health care professionals however, they preferred receiving written advice from a pharmacist or doctor (50%), or spoken advice from a pharmacist (29%) [17].

Parents identified various reasons for not trusting community pharmacist advice. In Greece, parents were hesitant to utilise pharmacists because of the lackadaisical attitude to antibiotic sale without prescription, possibly leading to wide scale resistance and adverse events [18]. A separate study in Netherlands indicated that parents did not trust explanations of doses and administration of drugs from a pharmacist, instead trusting their own limited knowledge more [19]. In addition to this, UK parents felt that pharmacists simply 'lacked adequate knowledge' specifically for their children [12].

Furthermore, the setting of the actual pharmacy may have an important effect on perception of the service. Parents felt that having substance users loitering in pharmacies, while awaiting harm reduction services and advice, was extremely intimidating to both their children and themselves [20]. This complemented the results of a study across the UK, which indicated that parents of young children found that pharmacies 'lacked privacy' that may otherwise be found at other primary care interfaces [21].

3.1.2. Young People

Children and young people across Europe have their own opinions on community pharmacists. A 2014 study of over 4000 adolescents across France, Germany, Portugal, and the UK demonstrated that pharmacists are more highly trusted by this age group than any other age group [15]. This notion was further confirmed by a UK trial of pharmacy-based OCP provision [21]. Following the trial, a staggering 97% of adolescent girls reporting being 'very comfortable' or 'comfortable' in discussing contraception with a pharmacist, while 87.5% were satisfied with the service they received [21]. In fact, owing to the trusted relationship that pharmacists are likely to share with patients from repeat encounters [22], they argue that they should have an expanded role in administering HPV vaccines and giving OCP to adolescent girls [23].

3.2. Potential Opportunities

The literature identified several opportunities for pharmacists to deal with paediatric patients in various capacities.

3.2.1. Acute Minor Illness

The literature identifies the possibility of an increased role for pharmacists in dealing with acutely unwell children. One UK study showed that 9% of ED attendees were appropriate for treatment by community pharmacists instead [24]. Similarly, 15% of consultations with children attending general practices in the UK were deemed unnecessary as opposed to just 6% in adults [12]. These studies demonstrate an opportunity for the diversion of children from other primary care services to the community pharmacy.

3.2.2. Chronic Disease

Several studies highlighted the important role pharmacists could play in the management of chronic paediatric disease. Pharmacist intervention in childhood eczema was trialled in a study, resulting in a statistically significant reduction in the severity of all symptoms. Furthermore, 78% of parents found the advice given to be 'very helpful' or 'helpful', with a marked increase in effective emollient use [25]. A similar pharmacist-led intervention was trialled in Spain, with the aim of improving childhood asthma control [26]. The intervention led to an increase in quality of life measures by 0.81 points, as well as a significant reduction in poorly controlled asthma by 1.15 points compared to the control group [26]. However, in the control of type 1 diabetes in children, patients in the pharmacist-led intervention group were shown to have no significant difference in their HbA1c compared to the control group [27]. Researchers suggested that this was due to poor follow-up attendance among the intervention group [27].

In order for pharmacists to have a truly meaningful impact on the management of chronic conditions, they need to foster stronger relationships with adolescents [17]. Authors argue that if children were present at medication collection, pharmacists could then make them feel comfortable with the information being provided and the setting [17]. Other literature also agrees that regular attendance of children at medication collection could improve adherence [28]. This combined with counselling of the children and distribution of relevant leaflets, can help reduce the rate of medication non-adherence in this population group [28]. Specifically for adolescents, it was found that they could be counselled on the interaction of medications with alcohol or other drugs, as this is both relevant to their lifestyle and can help build rapport with a 'non-judgmental' pharmacist [14].

Furthermore, to successfully manage chronic conditions in children, more could be done to facilitate communications between the hospital, community pharmacy, and primary care in order to improve continuity of care for children and parents [29]. This is especially because of the lack of information sharing between these three interfaces of care, regarding paediatric medication [29]. To ensure that parents remain committed and not frustrated with the care of their unwell child, there must be a greater deal of cohesion between the services [29].

3.2.3. Pregnancy and Antenatal Care

A study in the Netherlands set up a new, pharmacist-led service for women trying to conceive, which looked to increase the awareness of folic acid use in pregnancy. Following the programme, it was seen that the prevalence of NTD almost halved in just a year while 93% of the community approved of the initiative [30].

3.2.4. Pharmacovigilance

The literature identified the potential use of pharmacies for enhanced pharmacovigilance. The incidence of epilepsy in children under 18 is approximately 0.5% [31], while ADHD incidence in school-aged children is about 5% [32]. Management of these conditions involves medication that has a high rate of adverse events [33] and so there is a need here for medication monitoring especially in young children. Two separate studies in Scotland recommended wider pharmacist involvement in the UK Yellow Card scheme (YCS) for adverse events, to ensure that the proper side effect profiles of the drugs can be documented [34,35]. If uptake were to be increased in a sufficient number of pharmacists, this could be a very valuable source of adverse drug reaction reporting, as pharmacists are frequently the first port of call for medication issues [34,35].

Pharmacists could also improve their role in pharmacovigilance through increasing the number of medicines use reviews (MURs) performed on medications for chronic conditions. One English study found the level of pharmacists engaging in MURs to be as low as 23.7% when monitoring the experience of young children on medication for chronic conditions [36]. The importance was highlighted in a related UK trial study, which found an increase in the average asthma control by seven points when MURs and asthma counselling were routinely offered by pharmacists [37]. The increase in MURs however, would necessitate increased reimbursement and further training in order for pharmacists to be confident in carrying out such reviews [36].

3.2.5. OTC Drug Use in Children

There are varying levels of OTC medicine usage across Europe. Almost 50% of Finnish children use OTC self-medication, especially for treating asthma and fevers [38]. In an Italian study of over

1.5 million children and adolescents, it was reported that a similar proportion (48%) of children received at least one drug prescription every month [39]. Germany seemed to have a lower reported use of OTC drug use with only 31.6% of 15 year olds having consumed them in the last month [40]. However, it was found that 30% of all medication purchased by children in Germany, especially sedatives, were being used without prescription [41]. The use of OTC prescriptions in German children was attributed to a variety of factors including greater maternal education, families with higher household incomes, non-immigrants, and children that had long-term illness [42]. In the UK, it was found that there were 24 million episodes of cough medication being used in children [43] even though a Cochrane review found no good evidence for or against the effectiveness of these medications [44]. Furthermore, the 59 deaths attributed to cough medicines were related to accidental exposure (22%), intentional overdose (6%), and medication error (16%) with the manner of overdose undetermined in the remaining 56% of cases [43]. Children are not being educated on the risks of overusing OTC medication with a Swedish study indicating that adolescent behaviour towards OTC was 'careless and casual' [45].

3.2.6. Off-Label Drug Use

The literature gave insight into the use of off-label drugs by pharmacists, with a UK study showing that 40% of pharmacists had prescribed drugs in this way [46]. Pharmacists certainly had the highest level of concern (86%) among health care professionals, regarding off-label prescribing, with a majority arguing the need for urgent clinical trials to correct paediatric formulations [47]. They are willing to be flexible in prescribing appropriately for children although they mostly believed (66%) that they had a responsibility to warn parents about potential problems with off-label prescribing [46].

3.3. Further Training Needs

The literature reviewed the current practice of community pharmacists suggesting some possible improvements to ensure the standards of care were being met for children and young people.

3.3.1. Emergency Setting

Disease or treatment specific training in community pharmacists has been shown to be effective. One such example was in a study of pharmacist perceptions to anaphylaxis. It was found that 77% of pharmacists were aware of adrenaline auto-injector use as the first line management of paediatric food allergy anaphylaxis [48], while only 7% were confident in using the device. This suggests that further training in emergency scenarios would be a useful addition to the knowledge base possessed by pharmacists.

3.3.2. Community Pharmacists as Medication Advisers

The literature described how community pharmacists were averse to using corticosteroids in the management of chronic asthma in children. Due to their own beliefs and their position as trusted medication advisers, they dissuaded parents from using corticosteroids in asthma management leading to what one author described as a nationwide 'corticosteroid phobia' in France [48]. Improved training of pharmacists in asthma care, especially around appropriate corticosteroid usage, is certainly needed to avoid over emphasis of the 'dangerous' side effects [49].

3.3.3. Drug Safety

One of the issues that was evident in the literature review was the prevalence of safety incidents that occurred at community pharmacies. A study of about 3000 safety incidents in England and Wales alone revealed that medication errors occurred at a much higher rate in community pharmacies than general practice, dental surgeries, or even community nursing services [50]. Authors argued the case for a barcoding system that could reduce error potential from manual entry and act as a further safety check [50].

Other than technical errors in prescribing, pharmacists occasionally make mistakes in the choice of medication for acutely unwell children. A Swedish 'mystery-shopper' study indicated that pharmacists provided inappropriate medication to feverish children, up to 6% of the time [51] and a French study found that pharmacists were offering strictly contra-indicated drugs to children 12.9% of the time [52].

A Dutch study argued that these errors might be the result of a low use (14%) of up-to-date literature by pharmacists, while a large proportion of pharmacists (60%) were extremely dependent on the product monographs [53]. However, the poor choice of medication may also be explained by the history taking of pharmacists in acutely unwell children. A Belgian study showed that 84% of pharmacists did not enquire about dehydration symptoms in an eight-month-old with acute diarrhoea, while only 30% proceeded to prescribe an ORS [54]. Giving them the benefit of the doubt, some literature suggests that pharmacists' knowledge may not be applied adequately due to a lack of questioning, poor communication skills, and parental pressures [52]. One possible solution to this is increasing the frequency, and improving the quality, of training received by pharmacists, alongside their routine practice [50].

4. Discussion

This is the first major narrative review of community pharmacy use by parents, children, and young people in Europe. Overall, parents and young people have a high regard for local community pharmacists who are considered as authoritative sources of information and advice particularly for minor illness, chronic disease management, and medication review. Issues of communication with primary care and hospital pharmacy providers remain an area for further quality improvement to ensure both timely and consistent advice as well as safe prescribing. We have found that adolescents, in particular, value the confidentiality aspects of community pharmacists especially in relation to sexual health and vaccination advice. On the other hand, the high use of OTC products and off-label drugs by this age group is of concern and presents both opportunities for health education and a greater attention to pharmacovigilance.

Despite the fact that pharmacists may not be necessarily seen as first points of contact when compared to general practitioners or the internet from a parental perspective, there is potential for additional training and accreditation to support the needs of this age group. This would allow a broadening of the scope of services offered in a suitable physical environment. Infants and young children's health is very much determined by the health of the mother in pregnancy and pharmacies can provide a valuable service in identification of at risk women and optimization of infant health. This could be done through ensuring nutritional supplementation throughout pregnancy like in the Netherlands where there was a substantial reduction in the incidence of neural tube defects found in the intervention group [30]. With appropriate training and accreditation, many more services could be offered by community pharmacists including increased access to smoking cessation, weight management services, and drug or alcohol reduction services. These in turn could have a considerable impact on maternal and infant health. We hope to soon report on a paediatric–pharmacy joint training initiative scheme currently being piloted in three areas of London, which might provide a useful model for other countries.

5. Conclusions

Community pharmacists in Europe are an untapped resource for children, young people and their parents and further recognition of their important role could usefully support the demands made on other primary care services.

6. Limitations

There are a few limitations of the review that may have affected the results obtained. The main limitation was that only English language studies were included in the research due to the limited resources. Following on from this, only a small number of English language research articles were published in other EU countries. Of the articles used in the synthesis, 18 were papers from the UK, while the remainder originated from 11 different countries. This represents a bias in the results, as across countries, there are likely to be national and cultural differences with regards to community pharmacy practice. Inclusion of foreign language papers may have revealed pertinent work from the other countries that may have informed future practice and training recommendations. Furthermore, the results were screened by just one researcher and therefore, some relevant results may have been excluded based on the researchers' own selection bias of what was included in the synthesis. To mitigate this, any uncertainty was discussed by both authors who then agreed upon inclusion/exclusion. Moreover, time and resource limitations meant that the researchers were not able to obtain and confirm additional data from individual study investigators.

7. Further Research

This research could be used to support a periodic EU survey of parents and young people, which would ensure a more representative sampling of countries. Studies are clearly needed on the effectiveness of any pharmacy training initiatives which enhance safe prescribing practices or are designed to divert minor illnesses from emergency departments with appropriate safety netting.

Author Contributions: M.B. originated the idea and prepared the first draft while A.M. completed a systematic review, compiled the results, and refined the manuscript.

Acknowledgments: This project has received funding for dissemination from the European Union's Horizon 2020 research and innovation programme (MOCHA), grant agreement no. 634201.

References

1. Svarcaite, J. Overview of Community Pharmacy Services in Europe. 2016. Available online: https://www.oecd.org/els/health-systems/Item-2b-Overview-Community-Pharmacy-Services-Svarcaite%20.pdf (accessed on 18 December 2017).
2. OECD; EU. *Health at a Glance: Europe 2016*, 4th ed.; Organisation for Economic Co-Operation and Development: Paris, France, 2016.
3. EU. Living in the EU. 2017. Available online: https://europa.eu/european-union/about-eu/figures/living_en (accessed on 25 December 2017).
4. OECD; European Observatory on Health Systems. *State of Health in the EU. Slovak Republic: Country Health Profile 2017*; OECD: Paris, France; European Observatory on Health Systems: Brussels, Belgium, 2017.
5. Association, P. NHS Urges Parents to Use Pharmacies for Children's Illnesses. The Guardian Online 2018. Available online: https://read.oecd-ilibrary.org/social-issues-migration-health/slovak-republic-country-health-profile-2017_9789264283541-en#page1 (accessed on 12 February 2018).
6. Gill, P.; Goldacre, M.J.; Mant, D.; Heneghan, C.; Thomson, A.; Seagroatt, V.; Harnden, A. Increase in emergency admissions to hospital for children aged under 15 in England, 1999–2010: National database analysis. *Arch. Dis. Child.* **2013**, *98*, 328–334. [CrossRef] [PubMed]
7. Blair, M.; Oligbu, G.; EI Tokhy, O.; Levitan, M.; Goldstone, P.; Lathlean, P. G69 how do community pharmacies support children with minor illness. *Arch. Dis. Child.* **2018**, *103*, A28–A29.
8. Fraeyman, J.; Foulon, V.; Mehuys, E.; Boussery, K.; Saevels, J.; De Vriese, C.; Dalleur, O.; Housiaux, M.; Steurbaut, S.; Naegels, M.; et al. Evaluating the implementation fidelity of New Medicines Service for asthma patients in community pharmacists in Belgium. *Res. Soc. Adm. Pharm.* **2017**, *13*, 98–108. [CrossRef] [PubMed]

9.   Asthma UK. Asthma Facts and Statistics. 2016. Available online: https://www.asthma.org.uk/about/media/facts-and-statistics/ (accessed on 25 December 2017).

10.   Pharmaceutical Society of Ireland. *Guidance on the Provision of Vaccination Services by Pharmacists in Retail Pharmacy Businesses*; Pharmaceutical Society of Ireland: Dublin, Ireland, 2016; p. 4.

11.   Liberati, A.; Altman, D.G.; Tetzlaff, J.; Mulrow, C.; Gotzsche, P.C.; Ioannidis, J.P.A.; Clarke, M.; Devereaux, P.J.; Kleijnen, J.; Moher, D. The PRISMA statement for reporting systematic reviews and meta-analyses of studies that evaluate health care interventions: Explanation and elaboration. *PLoS Med.* **2009**, *6*, e1000100. [CrossRef] [PubMed]

12.   Hammond, T.; Clatworthy, J.; Horne, R. Patients' use of GPs and community pharmacists in minor illness: A cross-sectional questionnaire-based study. *Fam. Pract.* **2004**, *21*, 146–149. [CrossRef] [PubMed]

13.   Hodgson, C.; Wong, I. What do mothers of young children think of community pharmacists? A descriptive survey. *J. Fam. Health Care* **2004**, *14*, 73–74. [PubMed]

14.   Gray, N.J.; Boardman, H.F.; Symonds, B.S. Information sources used by parents buying non-prescription medicines in pharmacies for preschool children. *Int. J. Clin. Pharm.* **2011**, *33*, 842–848. [CrossRef] [PubMed]

15.   Bamford, S.; Kneale, D.; Wilson, J.; Watson, J. *A New Journey to Health—Health Infrormation Seeking Behaviour Across the Ages*; International Longevity Centre: London, UK, 2015; p. 1.

16.   Holappa, M.; Ahonen, R.; Vainio, K.; Hameen-Anttila, K. Information sources used by parents to learn about medications they are giving their children. *Res. Soc. Adm. Pharm.* **2012**, *8*, 579–584. [CrossRef] [PubMed]

17.   Gray, N.J.; Shaw, K.L.; Smith, F.J.; Burton, J.; Prescott, J.; Roberts, R.; Terry, D.; McDonagh, J.E. The Role of Pharmacists in Caring for Young People with Chronic Illness. *J. Adolesc. Health* **2017**, *60*, 219–225. [CrossRef] [PubMed]

18.   Plachouras, D.; Kavatha, D.; Antoniadou, A.; Giannitsioti, E.; Poulakou, G.; Kanellakopoulou, K.; Giamarellou, H. Dispensing of antibiotics without prescription in Greece, 2008: Another link in the antibiotic resistance chain. *Euro Surveill* **2010**, *18*, 15.

19.   Stakenborg, J.P.; de Bont, E.G.; Peetoom, K.K.; Nelissen-Vrancken, M.H.; Cals, J.W. Medication management of febrile children: A qualitative study on pharmacy employees' experiences. *Int. J. Clin. Pharm.* **2016**, *38*, 1200–1209. [CrossRef] [PubMed]

20.   Gidman, W.; Coomber, R. Contested space in the pharmacy: Public attitudes to pharmacy harm reduction services in the West of Scotland. *Res. Soc. Adm. Pharm.* **2014**, *10*, 576–587. [CrossRef] [PubMed]

21.   Parsons, J.; Adams, C.; Aziz, N.; Holmes, J.; Jawad, R.; Whittlesea, C. Evaluation of a community pharmacy delivered oral contraception service. *J. Fam. Plan. Reprod. Health Care* **2013**, *39*, 97–101. [CrossRef] [PubMed]

22.   Guegan, E. Infection prevention and management by community pharmacists. *J. Infect. Prev.* **2010**, *11*, 106–109. [CrossRef]

23.   Karamanidou, C.; Dimopoulos, K. Greek health professionals' perceptions of the HPV vaccine, state policy recommendations and their own role with regards to communication of relevant health information. *BMC Public Health* **2016**, *16*, 467. [CrossRef] [PubMed]

24.   Terry, D.; Petridis, K.; Aiello, M.; Sinclair, A.; Huynh, C.; Mazard, L.; Ubhi, H.; Terry, A.; Hughes, E. The Potential for Pharmacists to Manage Children Attending Emergency Departments. *Arch. Dis. Child.* **2016**, *101*, e2. [CrossRef] [PubMed]

25.   Carr, A.; Patel, R.; Jones, M.; Suleman, A. A pilot study of a community pharmacist intervention tp promote the effective use of emollients in childhood eczema. *Pharm. J.* **2007**, *278*, 319–322.

26.   Jacome, J.; Inesta Garcia, A. Prospective study about the impact of a community pharmaceutical care service in patients with asthma. *Rev. Esp. Salud Publica* **2003**, *77*, 393–403.

27.   Gay, C.L.; Chapuis, F.; Bendelac, N.; Tixier, F.; Treppoz, S.; Nicolino, M. Reinforced follow-up for children and adolescents with type 1 diabetes and inadequate glycaemic control: A randomized controlled trial intervention via the local pharmacist and telecare. *Diabetes Metab.* **2006**, *32*, 159–165. [CrossRef]

28.   Koster, E.S.; Philbert, D.; Winters, N.A.; Bouvy, M.L. Medication adherence in adolescents in current practice: Community pharmacy staff's opinions. *Int. J. Pharm. Pract.* **2015**, *23*, 221–224. [CrossRef] [PubMed]

29.   Terry, D.; Sinclair, A. Prescribing for children at the interfaces of care. *Arch. Dis. Child. Educ. Pract. Ed.* **2012**, *97*, 152–156. [CrossRef] [PubMed]

30.   De Jong-van den Berg, L.T. Monitoring of the folic acid supplementation program in The Netherlands. *Food Nutr. Bull.* **2008**, *29* (Suppl. 2), S210–S213. [CrossRef] [PubMed]

31. Deacon, K. *Epilepsy Prevalence, Incidence and Other Statistics*; Epilepsy Foundation: Landover, MD, USA, 2011; p. 1.

32. Bilbow, A. *ADHD: Paying Enough Attention*; ADDISS: Middlesex, UK, 2016; p. 1.

33. Perucca, E.; Meador, K.J. Adverse effects of antiepileptic drugs. *Acta Neurol. Scand. Suppl.* **2005**, *181*, 30–35. [CrossRef] [PubMed]

34. Tobaiqy, M.; Stewart, D.; Helms, P.J.; Bond, C.; Lee, A.J.; Bateman, N.; McCaig, D.; McLay, J. A pilot study to evaluate a community pharmacy-based monitoring system to identify adverse drug reactions associated with paediatric medicines use. *Eur. J. Clin. Pharmacol.* **2010**, *66*, 627–632. [CrossRef] [PubMed]

35. Stewart, D.; Helms, P.; McCaig, D.; Bond, C.; McLay, J. Monitoring adverse drug reactions in children using community pharmacies: A pilot study. *Br. J. Clin. Pharmacol.* **2005**, *59*, 677–683. [CrossRef] [PubMed]

36. Aston, J.; Wilson, K.A.; Terry, D.R. Children/young people taking long-term medication: A survey of community pharmacists' experiences in England. *Int. J. Pharm. Pract.* **2017**, *26*, 104–110. [CrossRef] [PubMed]

37. Lilley, A. Assessing the Benefits that Community Pharmacies can have on Childhood Asthma Outcomes. *Arch. Dis. Child.* **2016**, *101*, e2. [CrossRef] [PubMed]

38. Ylinen, S.; Hameen-Anttila, K.; Sepponen, K.; Lindblad, A.K.; Ahonen, R. The use of prescription medicines and self-medication among children—A population-based study in Finland. *Pharmacoepidemiol. Drug Saf.* **2010**, *19*, 1000–1008. [CrossRef] [PubMed]

39. Clavenna, A.; Sequi, M.; Bortolotti, A.; Merlino, L.; Fortino, I.; Bonati, M. Determinants of the drug utilization profile in the paediatric population in Italy's Lombardy Region. *Br. J. Clin. Pharmacol.* **2009**, *67*, 565–571. [CrossRef] [PubMed]

40. Italia, S.; Brand, H.; Heinrich, J.; Berdel, D.; von Berg, A.; Wolfenstetter, S.B. Utilization of self-medication and prescription drugs among 15-year-old children from the German GINIplus birth cohort. *Pharmacoepidemiol. Drug Saf.* **2015**, *24*, 1133–1143. [CrossRef] [PubMed]

41. Koelch, M.; Prestel, A.; Singer, H.; Keller, F.; Fegert, J.M.; Schlack, R.; Hoelling, H.; Knopf, H. Psychotropic medication in children and adolescents in Germany: Prevalence, indications, and psychopathological patterns. *J. Child Adolesc. Psychopharmacol.* **2009**, *19*, 765–770. [CrossRef] [PubMed]

42. Du, Y.; Knopf, H. Self-medication among children and adolescents in Germany: Results of the National Health Survey for Children and Adolescents (KiGGS). *Br. J. Clin. Pharmacol.* **2009**, *68*, 599–608. [CrossRef] [PubMed]

43. Smith, S.M.; Henman, M.; Schroeder, K.; Fahey, T. Over-the-counter cough medicines in children: Neither safe or efficacious? *Br. J. Gen. Pract.* **2008**, *58*, 757–758. [CrossRef] [PubMed]

44. Smith, S.M.; Schroeder, K.; Fahey, T. Over-the-counter medications for acute cough in children and adults in ambulatory settings. *Cochrane Database Syst. Rev.* **2008**, *23*, CD001831. [CrossRef]

45. Holmstrom, I.K.; Bastholm-Rahmner, P.; Bernsten, C.; Roing, M.; Bjorkman, I. Swedish teenagers and over-the-counter analgesics—Responsible, casual or careless use. *Res. Soc. Adm. Pharm.* **2014**, *10*, 408–418. [CrossRef] [PubMed]

46. Stewart, D.; Rouf, A.; Snaith, A.; Elliott, K.; Helms, P.J.; McLay, J.S. Attitudes and experiences of community pharmacists towards paediatric off-label prescribing: A prospective survey. *Br. J. Clin. Pharmacol.* **2007**, *64*, 90–95. [CrossRef] [PubMed]

47. Mukattash, T.; Hawwa, A.F.; Trew, K.; McElnay, J.C. Healthcare professional experiences and attitudes on unlicensed/off-label paediatric prescribing and paediatric clinical trials. *Eur. J. Clin. Pharmacol.* **2011**, *67*, 449–461. [CrossRef] [PubMed]

48. Hanna, H.J.; Emmanuel, J.; Naim, S.; Umasunthar, T.; Boyle, R.J. Community healthcare professionals overestimate the risk of fatal anaphylaxis for food allergic children. *Clin. Exp. Allergy* **2016**, *46*, 1588–1595. [CrossRef] [PubMed]

49. Raffin, D.; Giraudeau, B.; Samimi, M.; Machet, L.; Pourrat, X.; Maruani, A. Corticosteroid Phobia Among Pharmacists Regarding Atopic Dermatitis in Children: A National French Survey. *Acta Derm. Venereol.* **2016**, *96*, 177–180. [CrossRef] [PubMed]

50. Rees, P.; Edwards, A.; Powell, C.; Hibbert, P.; Williams, H.; Makeham, M.; Carter, B.; Luff, D.; Parry, G.; Avery, A.; et al. Patient Safety Incidents Involving Sick Children in Primary Care in England and Wales: A Mixed Methods Analysis. *PLoS Med.* **2017**, *14*, e1002217. [CrossRef] [PubMed]

51. Bardage, C.; Westerlund, T.; Barzi, S.; Bernsten, C. Non-prescription medicines for pain and fever—A comparison of recommendations and counseling from staff in pharmacy and general sales stores. *Health Policy* **2013**, *110*, 76–83. [CrossRef] [PubMed]

52. Lapeyre-Mestre, M.; Pin, M. Management of acute infantile diarrhoea: A study on community pharmacy counseling in the Midi-Pyrenees region. *Arch. Pediatr.* **2004**, *11*, 898–902. [CrossRef] [PubMed]

53. Venables, R.; Stirling, H.; Batchelor, H.; Marriott, J. Problems with oral formulations prescribed to children: A focus group study of healthcare professionals. *Int. J. Clin. Pharm.* **2015**, *37*, 1057–1067. [CrossRef] [PubMed]

54. Driesen, A.; Vandenplas, Y. How do pharmacists manage acute diarrhoea in an 8-month-old baby? A simulated client study. *Int. J. Pharm. Pract.* **2009**, *17*, 215–220. [CrossRef] [PubMed]

18

"Being in Control of My Asthma Myself" Patient Experience of Asthma Management: A Qualitative Interpretive Description

Damilola T. Olufemi-Yusuf [1], **Sophie Beaudoin Gabriel** [1], **Tatiana Makhinova** [1,2] and **Lisa M. Guirguis** [1,2,*] (iD)

[1] Faculty of Pharmacy and Pharmaceutical Sciences, University of Alberta, Edmonton, AB T6G 1C9, Canada; damiade@ualberta.ca (D.T.O.-Y.); sophie.beaudoin@gmail.com (S.B.G.); tatiana.makhinova@ualberta.ca (T.M.)

[2] Asthma Working Group of the Respiratory Health Strategic Clinical Network, Alberta Health Services, Calgary, AB T2W 1S7, Canada

* Correspondence: lisa.guirguis@ualberta.ca

Abstract: Asthma control can be achieved with effective and safe medication use; however, many patients are not controlled. Patients' perceptions of asthma, asthma treatment, and pharmacist roles can impact patient outcomes. The purpose of this study was to explore patients' experiences and patient–pharmacist relationships in asthma care. Qualitative Interpretive Description method guided the study. Semi-structured individual interviews were conducted with 11 patients recruited from personal contacts, pharmacies, and asthma clinics. Categories and themes were identified using inductive constant comparison. Themes indicated patients had a personalized common sense approach to asthma management, "go-to" health care provider, and prioritized patient–pharmacist relationships. Patients described their illness experiences and asthma control based on personal markers similar to the common sense model of self-regulation. Patients chose a family physician, asthma specialist, respiratory therapist, or pharmacist as an expert resource for asthma management. Patient perceived pharmacists' roles as information provider, adviser, or care provider. Pharmacists who develop a collaborative relationship with their asthma patients are better positioned to provide tailored education and self-management support. Inviting patients to share their perspective could increase patient engagement and uptake of personalised asthma action plans to achieve asthma control.

Keywords: asthma; patient experience; patient-centred care; communication; patient education; patient-pharmacist relationship; self-regulation; qualitative interpretive description

1. Introduction

Asthma is a significant public health problem all over the world and an everyday reality for the 2.4 million Canadians living with asthma [1]. Asthma control can be achieved with effective and safe medications and treatment guidelines [2]. However, level of asthma control has not improved over the last decade and currently 9 out of 10 Canadians with asthma are out of control [3]. Poor asthma control is burdensome to patients and increases emergency room visits, hospitalizations, and absence from work or school [4].

The reasons for poor asthma management are multifaceted including the disease itself, presence of comorbidities, patients' self-management, healthcare professionals' care, or the interaction among these factors [5,6]. Medication therapy is the primary intervention used in asthma highlighting asthma patients have needs that pharmacists can address [7,8]. Pharmacists frequently encounter asthma patients and are not only well placed to identify patients with poorly controlled asthma but also resolve medication problems, educate patients on inhaler technique, monitor therapy, and develop personalised asthma action plans [8–10].

Pharmacist-delivered interventions in asthma management have improved patient outcomes [11–15] but only few have explored the patient experience of pharmacist care as one of the factors contributing to positive outcomes [16–18]. Understanding the patient, their beliefs and experience about asthma and asthma treatment reduces barriers to effective asthma treatment [19,20]. Patients involved in their care are more likely to communicate their goals, preferences, and concerns, to seek support in adhering to their care plan, and to take more ownership of their treatment [20–22]. More so, effective communication between patients and pharmacists provides an enabling context for optimizing therapy and achieving asthma control for patients [17,23,24]. The patient's experience in managing asthma and how they are supported by pharmacists needs to be explored further.

With the shift toward patient-centred care in Canada and around the world, pharmacists have taken on an expanded role in providing patient care services to those living with chronic conditions including asthma [25]. In the province of Alberta, where the scope of pharmacy practice is the widest (pharmacists can prescribe for minor ailments, renew, adjust, initiate or substitute prescriptions, administer vaccinations, order and interpret laboratory tests, conduct medication reviews, and develop care plans), the experiences of those living with asthma are important in order to enhance care [26]. Given that the patient's perspective has not been examined in this patient-focused practice model, we sought to understand how asthma patients have experienced pharmacists' care. Our findings could have potential application in the design of patient-centred interventions in pharmacy care and improve care for asthma patients. Our study objectives were:

1. To identify how patients manage their asthma
2. To describe what resources patients need to access for asthma management
3. To understand how patients view and experience pharmacists' roles in ongoing management of asthma.

2. Methods

2.1. Research Team and Reflexivity

The research team consisted of three researchers, one patient with asthma (i.e., only research team member with asthma), and one pharmacy student, who were all invested in improving the quality of care for people with asthma. All three researchers were pharmacists; however, none was practicing. The pharmacy student conducted the interviews and was trained and supervised by one of the authors (L.G.). The patient was identified as a patient adviser with the Alberta Health Services Respiratory Health Strategic Clinical Network (RSCN) where two researchers were active members. The patient participated in one interview and reviewed a subset of interviews to provide insights on patient perspectives.

2.2. Study Design

Interpretive Description was the qualitative methodology used to frame the study [27,28]. Its constructivist paradigm formed the basis of our theoretical approach to knowing how patients perceived and interpreted meaning created through their asthma experiences [27,28]. The constructivist position recognizes that multiple perspectives exist and fit with our study objective of understanding the different perspectives of asthma patients' self-management in community pharmacy practice. As an applied qualitative approach, interpretive description focuses on thoughtful consideration of factors that could influence practice such as practice models, professional mandates, and biases of individuals and disciplines [29,30]. The orientation toward practice settings ensures that the creation of knowledge that is relevant to real-world clinical practice as well as theory development or expansion.

We used an inductive approach without the influence of a priori theories though we were open to theory to inform the analysis and discussion. We favoured the use of theory as an analytical tool rather than as a theoretical framework made explicit from the beginning to allow for the generation and interpretation of new themes that fit into broader contexts [31,32]. This study was driven by the need to better understand the experiences and perspectives of patients on managing their asthma and the role of community pharmacists in order to generate knowledge that could improve care practices for asthma patients. Ethics approval for the study was granted by the University of Alberta Health Research Ethics Board (study ID Pro00065978) prior to recruitment.

2.3. Recruitment and Sample

Adults between 18 and 70 years old were eligible if they or their children had asthma, took at least one asthma medication, spoke English, and were able to consent. Patients were ineligible if they had limited capacity to communicate. Purposive and convenience sampling were used to recruit 11 patient participants from three settings. The first five patients (i.e., Patients 1–5) were recruited from personal networks of members of the RHSCN. It was noted that these patients had positive experiences with pharmacists and thus we purposively sample two patients (Patients 6 and 7) from a community pharmacy with a known high level of care. Finally, four patients were purposively recruited from an asthma clinic to capture the voices of patients who may have more complex or severe asthma (Patients 8–11) than those in primary health care sites.

2.4. Data Collection

Data collection consisted of semi-structured individual interviews conducted by the trained pharmacy student who did not know the participants. Interviews occurred face to face and interviews occurred by telephone as participants lived out of Edmonton or they preferred to do so for scheduling or personal reasons. Seven interviews were conducted between July and August 2016. Additional four patients were recruited and interviewed in June 2017. Interviews were guided by a semi-structured interview guide lasted between 16 and 38 min. The questions in the interview guide were developed based on literature and knowledge of asthma care and community pharmacy practice (Appendix A). We explored the patient's experience of asthma, management strategies, and interactions with community pharmacists. As data collection and analysis occurred concurrently, areas of emerging interest were noted and included as probes in the next interview. Thus, the interview guide was modified as the interviews progressed to reflect additional questions.

During and after each interview, handwritten field notes were taken to record important observations made at the interview such as non-verbal behaviour, interpersonal disposition, and the researcher's impressions of the participant within the context of the interview. All interviews were audio recorded and transcribed verbatim.

2.5. Data Analysis

Interpretive description methods and thematic analysis shaped the data analysis [27,28,33,34]. First, researchers wrote a summary of each patient interview, included information about each patient and potential themes. Each transcript was open coded to identify main ideas and develop a taxonomy of related codes. Similar codes were sorted and collapsed together to create categories. Categories were then compared and contrasted across transcripts to generate themes that ran through the data. Constant comparison was used to compare between patients, provider preferences, type of pharmacist relationships to refine themes. Themes moved beyond clustering similar categories to develop a conceptual understanding of the patients' experiences with asthma [33,34]. We also used theory to create themes which contributed to making sense of the data and contextualizing study findings within the body of knowledge. Without the use of theory and thematic analysis, the results of the research will have little meaning and application in real world practice [31,35,36]. We involved one patient participant in the data analysis to draw on her patient experiences in the interpretation of a subset of interview transcripts. This helped improve the study's transparency and trustworthiness.

2.6. Rigour

Rigour was ensured throughout the study. First, the study was designed to achieve congruence between the research question and the theoretical position. Recruitment was adapted to capture patients with varying levels of asthma control and types of pharmacist relationships. Data collection and analysis were conducted concurrently to ensure our ongoing interview explored both new and evolving ideas introduced by participants. Analysis involved interview summaries including field notes, four coders, and iterative coding process. The recognition of three types of patient–pharmacist relationships allowed for multi-faceted comparisons between patients. A patient who was interviewed also participated in the data analysis to bring her experiences and improve the study's transparency and trustworthiness.

3. Results

The sample was predominantly female (n = 8, 73%) with a mean age of 42 years (range = 24 to 56 years). Patients recruited by the members of the RHSCN formed the largest group followed by the asthma clinics and then the community pharmacy. Within two groups sampled from the RSCN and asthma clinics, we observed variation in patients' experiences of interacting with pharmacists. Four patients visited family physician clinics, another four saw an asthma specialist, and one patient used a respiratory therapist for routine asthma care. One patient used both a respiratory a family physician and pharmacist and another an asthma specialist and pharmacist. The characteristics of patients are shown in Table 1.

Table 1. Patients' demographics and provider relationships associated with asthma care.

Patient Identifier	Age	Gender	Recruitment Strategy	"Go-To" Healthcare Provider	Type of Pharmacist Relationship
Patient 1	24	F	RSCN	Family physician	Valuable
Patient 2	43	M	RSCN	Family physician	Information
Patient 3	41	M	RSCN	Family physician	Information
Patient 4	51	M	RSCN	Asthma specialist	Information
Patient 5 [a]	45, 18, 14	F, M, M	RSCN	Respiratory therapist	Valuable
Patient 6 [b]	54	F	Community Pharmacy	Pharmacist and Family physician	Collaboration
Patient 7 [b]	56	F	Community Pharmacy	Pharmacist and Asthma specialist	Collaboration
Patient 8	30	F	Asthma Clinic	Family physician	Valuable
Patient 9	56	F	Asthma Clinic	Asthma specialist	Information
Patient 10	30	F	Asthma Clinic	Asthma specialist	Information
Patient 11	36	F	Asthma Clinic	Asthma specialist	Information

[a] Patient has two teenage sons who have asthma; [b] Patients have the same pharmacist who is a Certified Asthma Educator.

3.1. Theme 1: Personalized Common Sense Approach to Asthma Management

The patients described their illness experiences in a personal way. Similar to Leventhal's Common sense model of self-regulation [37], their perceptions of asthma symptoms, level of control and emotions were modifiable based on their knowledge and feelings of what they experienced over time. Patients discussed how they made sense of asthma symptoms, came up with their own individual non-medical strategies for coping and monitoring improvements or worsening of symptoms. What was most striking is that the patients constructed representations of their asthma from their everyday experiences but these narratives were not always discussed in medical visits. Patient ideas were considered non-medical and diverged from biomedical conversations that predominantly occur in medical settings.

3.1.1. Sub-Theme 1: Personalized Markers for Self-Monitoring

Patients determined if their asthma was under control based on personal markers of control and severity. Patients regularly made connections between symptoms and severity of their condition, relying on these subjective experiences as an early warning of an impending attack. Here are three individual examples of patient symptoms:

As soon as I start coughing, I know this is going to be a three-month adventure, trying to figure out why. (Patient 1)

So as soon as I start to get a tickle in my throat, and kind of that feeling that there's feathers in there . . . then I make sure that I take my Advair® at night time as well, (Patient 6)

I know if I can't make it up the stairs without wheezing, or a problem with my breath, that's when I go to my primary care doc. (Patient 3)

After recognizing the seriousness of the condition, patients knew what steps to take to address symptoms. Patients' self-management practices combined both medical (e.g., mainly medications) and non-medical lifestyle strategies to control current symptoms and prevent future problems.

3.1.2. Sub-Theme 2: Personalized Non-Medical Measures

Mostly, non-medication related strategies were seen to be as beneficial as medications for day to day management. One patient took preventative measures.

So probably lifestyle wise is my biggest thing—like, you know, I try and exercise, get my cardiovascular as much as I can, make sure that my core is strong and strengthen everything around there. (Patient 4)

Other patients had non-medication strategies for asthma attacks

What I used to do was just to try to lay [sic] down, relax my muscles—there are a lot of times when you have an asthma attack, your core muscles are kind of working overtime to force air in and out of your lungs. Um, so, just the more relaxed I can make myself, the better. (Patient 2)

3.1.3. Sub-Theme 3: Personalized Access to Medication

Patients figured ways to obtain cheaper medications and avoid the hikes in travel health insurance premiums that result from asthma attacks and their association use of oral emergency medications. With insights into the ease of getting medications in less regulated markets outside of Canada (e.g., Mexico), Patient 3 and 9 were sensible to proactively stock up on asthma medications to ensure they always had sufficient supply to meet asthma needs. It was clear that these patients knew what they needed and actively pursued practical solutions.

Now, the fun part about prednisone is, for some insurance companies, it's an indicator of disease severity—especially if you've taken it in the last six months and all that, and they won't insure you for travel. So, like I said, I handle my asthma, and I know when I need to hit it hard and hit it quick. And, so, what you end up doing too is you have some patients—such as maybe myself—going down to Mexico, getting prednisone. Because they know that, number one, it's an insurance flag if you take it. (Patient 3)

3.2. Theme 2: Patients Identify Their "Go-To" Health Care Provider

Although patients apply a common sense view to manage and monitor asthma symptoms, the chronic nature of asthma implies frequent contact with the health care system. In our study, all patients used their common sense approach to choose one or more healthcare providers for routine asthma care. This "go-to" person was a family doctor, asthma specialist, respiratory therapist or pharmacist whom they recognized as an expert resource for asthma management. The patients described benefits of the encounter such as prescribing new medication or refills, a demonstration of proper inhaler technique, monitoring asthma medications.

Would I have booked an appointment to come in, and sit down, and do this [asthma action plan] with them? Probably not. I think that's probably—you know, that's something again that I would reserve for my family doctor, but, (I) would appreciate that. (Patient 2)

When I go to [name of Asthma specialist] for the respiratory end of things, she'll ask if I need any prescriptions. (Patient 9)

The choice of provider was informed by their perceived needs and expertise of the healthcare provider. Four patients saw their family physician (Patients 1, 2, 3, and 8) as the go-to-healthcare provider. Patients 4, 9, 10, and 11 that did not trust their family physician to provide expert advice on asthma preferred to seek help from an asthma specialist who focuses on asthma patients. Another patient (Patient 5) saw a respiratory therapist. Patients 6 and 7 had positive relationships with their pharmacist thus listed the pharmacists and either their family physician or asthma specialist respectively. The preferred provider(s) for each patient is outlined in Table 1.

3.3. Theme 3: Patient–Pharmacist Relationship Comes First

Patient and pharmacist relationships ranged from non-existent to an ideal situation where the pharmacist partnered with the patient. These relationships influenced care and how their asthma needs were met (Figure 1). For instance, Patients 6 and 7 had the only collaborative relationship with their pharmacist and correspondingly were the sole patients to consider their pharmacist a "go-to" provider. Patient 4 aptly described how relationships are important to patient care.

I think it takes some time to build trust, that sometimes is built in that patient-physician, that's important . . . But if you're comfortable, I think a pharmacist is well within their scope of practice to help create an action plan, for sure. (Patient 4)

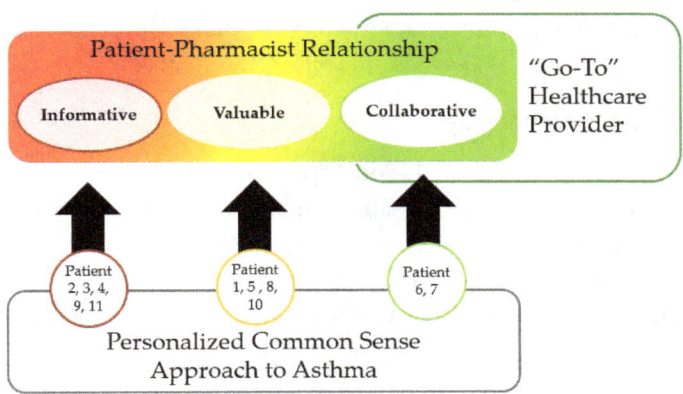

Figure 1. Relation of Spectrum of Patient–Pharmacist Relationships to Study Themes. Pharmacists were only considered the go-to healthcare providers when there was a collaborative relationship.

3.3.1. Sub-Theme 1: Information-Focused Relationship

Majority of the patient–pharmacist relationships clustered toward the bottom end of the spectrum where there is little existing positive relationship or a negative relationship. A group of patients described pharmacist interactions as "impersonal" and transactional. In such cases, they felt the relationship with the pharmacist was limited to dispensing without actively engaging the person behind the prescription.

It's [the interaction] very brief. It's just because I've had it for so long, that they know that I know what I'm doing with it. Um, but yeah, there's no real discussion regarding the medication. (Patient 2)

Generally, patients seemed to have low expectations of the pharmacist because they were satisfied with brief straightforward conversations and minimal interaction with the pharmacist.

The challenge is, it's [role of pharmacist] only appropriate in what's asked, right—I mean, nobody really wants anything forced on them, so, um . . . I imagine a pharmacist who is a certified respiratory educator would be a great thing, and [inaudible] lean on that background and work with them . . . But essentially in the end, I just want to know about the drug, interactions, possible side effects, and how to do it properly. (Patient 4)

Similar experiences evoked different reactions in patients. One patient explained that being disappointed by their pharmacist's inability to renew prescriptions for asthma medications in an emergency caused expectations to drop very low.

Didn't engage me on, yeah, "How well is he controlled? What is he doing about it? Does he know what he's doing?" Right? I rarely get that question. But once again, I think that's because in the last few years, I just . . . I just see that pharmacy as a dispensing outlet. (Patient 3)

The type of patient–pharmacist relationship can be also understood from the perspective of trust. People may have an inherent distrust in the involvement of pharmacists in the health care system. Those who hold this view believe that any advice beyond filling a prescription and drug interaction information is unsolicited and out of professional boundaries. Our study revealed one patient with such view. The patient opposed pharmacists monitoring asthma drug therapy, developing an asthma action plan and preferred to stick to her asthma specialist who has the specialised knowledge and expertise to assess and manage asthma.

"Well it's a nightmare to be honest with you. I find that whenever I've gone to a pharmacy in [city name] I have either had a pharmacist try to tell me what my asthma medication should be or they try to ask you tons of questions because you have asthma, but they don't know the whole picture. They only see the prescription that you're bringing in, they don't have your medical file, they don't know how many doctors you've been to or what steps you've taken so far. They just assume that because you have asthma, it's not under control and they can provide additional advice that is actually unsolicited. It's really irritating to be honest with you". (Patient 11)

3.3.2. Sub-Theme 2: Valuable Relationship

The middle group of patients had a relationship with their pharmacists where the pharmacist knew them by name and supported technical skills by demonstrating inhaler technique. These patients attested to the value of pharmacist-provided patient education since many patients have poor inhaler technique. For example, one patient alluded to the fact that using the Aerosol holding chamber recommended by a pharmacist eased taking her rescue medication and improved its effectiveness.

I do [use the AeroChamber®] yeah. Yeah I don't even see that as a concern because I've always used it. It was actually a pharmacist who told me about that, not my family doctor. Which is part of why I wanted to participate in this because they play such an important role and that's made such a difference for me. (Patient 8)

Patients in this category demonstrated curiosity and desired additional care that might improve their asthma condition beyond filling prescriptions. They wanted to ask questions on medication effectiveness, user-friendly devices, and latest advancements in asthma therapy. Patients hoped to involve the pharmacist in their care to a greater extent but felt the pharmacists was responsible for initiating conversations and creating more awareness of patient care services. Though the patients have not experienced pharmacist prescribing or care plans, they indicated these would be helpful if done in collaboration with their family physician who has more knowledge of the patient's medical history.

Or maybe even like when I get to a pharmacist, having an appointment with them when I go to pick it up, to go over things and maybe decide if this even going to help me, instead of spending three months trying to figure it out with my doctor, who maybe not as knowledgeable on that kind of stuff. So yeah, it'd be nice—I mean, I know they offer that kind of stuff, so maybe making it more known (Patient 1)

Reflecting on previous challenges in obtaining medications, some patients gave suggestions on ways to enhance access to pharmacy services. For example, relocating the pharmacy to the front of the building would facilitate access for urgent medication pickups. Additionally, pharmacists should have the mandate to refill medications for patients with controlled asthma in order to free up time for doctors to attend to sicker patients with greater medical needs.

I understand that there might be insurance stuff involved in that but I do believe that I should not have to make an appointment with my doctor just to get medication refills. I think that is ridiculous and it's a waste [of time]. There is legitimate sick people out there that really need to see the doctor and all that does is put stress on an already stressful system. So I really think the doctor should just be able to push a button to refill the prescriptions at the pharmacist or something. The pharmacy should be able to refill your medication without your doctor. (Patient 10)

3.3.3. Sub-Theme 3: Collaborative Relationship

Two Patients (6 and 7) credited their ability to take control of their asthma to the written asthma action plan co-created with their pharmacist. They visited the same pharmacist who is a Certified Asthma Educator (CAE) and spoke very highly of the pharmacist's commitment and advocacy in helping them become empowered in managing their asthma and monitoring the effectiveness of medications.

Her [the CAE pharmacist's] role is to advocate for being in control of my asthma myself, and making sure that the things she or my doctor are prescribing are actually benefitting me in the way they're supposed to, because I have the right knowledge to use them properly". (Patient 6)

These two patients valued the one-to-one consultation that could have with the pharmacist saying that these were helpful in reviewing and reinforcing the patients' knowledge of asthma and monitoring asthma goals. One patient specifically said that her pharmacist keeps encouraging her to be symptom-free and that goal motivates her to know all aspects of her condition and maintain control of symptoms.

You know, she's really, really educated me on all aspects of asthma—it's been a real eye opener. Because I've had it for so long, and for probably at least the first fifteen years or so, I was just ... Kind of on my own. You know, I'd go to the doctor. "Oh hi, how you doing?" "Um yeah, kind of coughing." You know, he was pretty good, but he didn't help me understand why I was coughing, and why I was having these symptoms. Whereas she sits me down and says, "Okay, look. This is why you're doing this, this, and this. And this is what you need to do. And you should not cough, period." [laugh]. (Patient 7)

Apart from providing a better understanding of the illness and medications, the patients acknowledged their relationship with the pharmacist was immensely supportive. One patient in particular worried and felt she had to tough it out on her own before having an action plan. Now she felt supported to change her medication-taking behaviour and successfully monitor symptoms. Being able to know when control is worsening and what specific actions to take to tackle asthma exacerbations were important benefits of the asthma action plan for these patients.

And I've always wanted one. I would ask the doctor, and ... They either didn't know about it or didn't have time. But she [the pharmacist] will sit down with me every month or two and go through it and do any changes .... So the action plan gives me specific things to do when my chest gets tight, when I get short of breath—then I can be flexible with the Symbicort. And I don't have to be afraid to take more Ventolin, or take even less than, like, one an hour. If it gets bad, I can do more. (Patient 7)

The pharmacist was described as being non-judgmental, caring, personable, attentive, and listening deeply to understand the patient's situation and encourage them toward their asthma goals. The two patients who had a positive and trusting relationship with their pharmacist have experienced comprehensive asthma care.

[Speaking about pharmacist] "*and be very caring and personable during the process*" *(Patient 6)*

And [the pharmacist] is so good that way, she's always encouraging me to, you know—by the time the next action plan comes up, 'Oh yeah, I was supposed to do that, okay'. So she doesn't judge, she doesn't criticize, she just (says), 'Okay, well let's work on that'. (Patient 7)

4. Discussion

This study extends the knowledge in pharmacy literature by exploring patients' experiences of asthma within the movement toward patient-centred care in pharmacy practice. Previous studies that examined pharmacists' contribution to asthma care found that pharmacists possess the skills and competencies required to support patients with self-management education, demonstrating inhaler technique, and monitoring asthma therapy and could do more for patients in therapy monitoring and follow-up [7,8,38]. Findings from prior studies highlight the need for community pharmacists to work together with patients to attain control of their asthma. This study adds to earlier work by privileging the patient's perspectives on how they experienced the community pharmacist's delivery of asthma care. We found three themes namely: patients had a personalized common sense approach to asthma management, had a "go-to" health care provider to address asthma needs, and considered patient–pharmacist relationships important in asthma care (Figure 1).

Patients mostly evaluate their level of asthma control based on personally defined parameters and represent and manage asthma in a way that is consistent with the common sense model of self-regulation [37]. This model describes how patients rely on a mentally constructed approach to assign meaning to their illness symptoms (or lack thereof) and how this affects care seeking and self-management behaviours. Previous studies have demonstrated the relationships between asthma patients' representation of illness and medication adherence [21,39]. Our study adds to prior knowledge that caring for asthma patients goes beyond understanding the disease, clinical presentation, or providing medications to understanding the patient. The study points to the need to develop a shared understanding with the person living with asthma including their perceptions of asthma and asthma treatment as well as shared goals of asthma control [19,40]. Knowing that many patients' representations are dynamic and based on experiences, pharmacists, and other healthcare professionals could employ patient-centred communication [41,42]. Patient-centred communication involves inviting the patient to share their perspective, addressing concerns about treatment, regularly monitoring asthma medications and level of control in individual patients [20,43,44]. Patients knowledge and experiences should be recognized as valid during routine encounters to make interactions more meaningful and patient-focused [45].

In addition to adopting personal definitions of asthma, patients with asthma drew on a variety of resources within the healthcare system to manage their condition [46]. This was also reflected in the range of preferred healthcare providers for patients in our study. This "go-to" person included a family physician, asthma specialist, respiratory therapist, or pharmacist, or at least two of these providers, who they recognized as an expert resource for asthma information, advice and support. The nature and development of relationships with the health care provider is influenced by the perceived asthma needs and perceived role of the health care provider as being able to provide good asthma care, level of trust, convenience, and ease of access [19]. It may be that patients who had at least two "go-to" health care providers may have had complex needs or reasoned that they need more than one healthcare professional to address their needs. While it is desirable for asthma specialists to care for people with complex asthma, they are neither sufficient in number nor accessible to patients when needed. More so, patients with chronic obstructive pulmonary disease receiving both care specialist and primary care were not shown to have better outcomes than those receiving primary care only, though the case for asthma may be different [47]. Patients mentioned the benefits of having a regular health care provider was to prescribe new medication or refills, check and demonstrate proper inhaler technique, monitor asthma medications. Patient can access these services in a community pharmacy in Alberta where a government funded model supports all pharmacists to extend prescriptions and provide care plans as well as approved pharmacists to initiate new medications [48]. The reliance of patients on different healthcare providers would be an important factor to consider if a shift to multidisciplinary team care delivery were to occur. Another factor would be if patients' choice of healthcare provider changes with time though our study did not examine this possibility.

Patients' expectations of pharmacist roles and the type of patient-pharmacist relationship influences perceptions on the quality of care and this was supported by our findings [49,50]. Majority of the patient-pharmacist relationships clustered toward the bottom end of the spectrum where there is little positive relationship or even a negative relationship. On the other end, two patients had positive relationships with their pharmacists that impacted their asthma care. Our study conceptualises patient–pharmacist relationship (Figure 1) as a continuum of information-focused, valuable, and collaborative relationships similar to patient's perceptions of pharmacist roles as retailers, medication experts, and care providers [49–57]. While policy changes to enhance care for people with chronic conditions has been a significant driver of pharmacists expanded role, every patient encounter is an opportunity to build the relationship and support the uptake of patient care services [58]. The use of patient-centred communication strategies are linked to higher therapy monitoring and the use of asthma action plans, an important self-management tool [23]. Compared with patients with a low engagement with pharmacists, those who had valuable and collaborative relationships reported they not only had better understanding of asthma and asthma treatment but also more confidence and skill in managing their asthma.

The themes in our study reflect that asthma patients value patient-centred communication in their encounter with pharmacists which has the potential to increase patient acceptance of professional roles [59,60]. This implies pharmacists could invite patients to share their perspective asthma and common sense approaches to achieving control. This could increase patient engagement and tailoring of asthma education focused on patient needs. The practice of pharmacy has expanded beyond traditional dispensing roles to a more collaborative relationship and pharmacists should become competent in incorporating specific markers of asthma control into personalized asthma action plans. What matters to patients in their asthma management is just as important as telling patients what to monitor.

Limitations

Our study focused on patients' perspectives only which are different from providers' perspectives [19]. Future work could compare the experiences of patients and pharmacists to provide a complete understanding on the dynamics of the patient–pharmacist interaction and how it influences the quality of asthma care. Another limitation was that all the patients were experienced, had an asthma diagnosis for a long period of time and mostly likely learned how to navigate the health system and adequately manage their asthma. Since their views may be different from newly diagnosed patients where pharmacists have been known to spend more time with patients, more research is needed to explore the initial interactions between new asthma patients and pharmacist in the era of higher public and patient interest in pharmacist roles. Although the patient and pharmacist relationships have been the focus in the patient-centred care, a broader range of "system" factors may affect the patient experience care but our study did not investigate how structural and political factors influence patient attitudes and experience of asthma care [61]. Further research is necessary to evaluate strategies at the organization and policy level that could foster the patient-centredness of care within pharmacy practice.

5. Conclusions

Patients had a personalized common sense approach to asthma management, a "go-to" health care provider to address asthma needs and considered patient-pharmacist relationships important in asthma care. Our study indicated that asthma patients viewed pharmacists as retailers, medication experts, or care providers and their perceptions were shaped by their beliefs and experience of the pharmacist role. Pharmacists routinely encounter asthma patients and would be better positioned to provide tailored education and self-management support if they developed a collaborative relationship with patients and invited patients to share their common sense approaches to asthma. This starting point could increase patient engagement and uptake of personalised asthma action plans to achieve asthma control.

Author Contributions: L.G. conceived the study; S.B.G. performed the data collection; S.B.G., L.G., D.A. and T.M. analysed the data; D.A. wrote the initial draft. All authors reviewed and approved the final draft of the paper.

Funding: This research received no external funding.

Acknowledgments: We thank the participating patients, pharmacists, asthma specialists, physicians and the Asthma Working Group of the Alberta Health Services (AHS) Respiratory Health Strategic Clinical Network. We appreciate the contribution of Mindy Tindall who participated in data analysis and interpretation.

References

1.   Statistics Canada. Asthma, by Age Group. Available online: https://www150.statcan.gc.ca/t1/tbl1/en/tv.action?pid=1310009608 (accessed on 24 August 2018).

2.   Papaioannou, A.I.; Kostikas, K.; Zervas, E.; Kolilekas, L.; Papiris, S.; Gaga, M. Control of asthma in real life: Still a valuable goal? *Eur. Respir. Rev.* **2015**, *24*, 361–369. [CrossRef] [PubMed]

3.   The Canadian Lung Association. Asthma Control in Canada Survey 2016. Available online: https://www.lung.ca/news/latest-news/survey-asthma-not-well-controlled-most-canadians (accessed on 24 August 2018).

4.   Sawicki, G.S.; Vilk, Y.; Schatz, M.; Kleinman, K.; Abrams, A.; Madden, J. Uncontrolled asthma in a commercially insured population from 2002 to 2007: Trends, predictors, and costs. *J. Asthma* **2010**, *47*, 574–580. [CrossRef] [PubMed]

5.   Braido, F. Failure in asthma control: Reasons and consequences. *Scientifica* **2013**, *2013*, 1–15. [CrossRef] [PubMed]

6.   Pinnock, H.; Parke, H.L.; Panagioti, M.; Daines, L.; Pearce, G.; Epiphaniou, E.; Bower, P.; Sheikh, A.; Griffiths, C.J.; Taylor, S.J.C.; et al. Systematic meta-review of supported self-management for asthma: A healthcare perspective. *BMC Med.* **2017**, *15*, 64. [CrossRef] [PubMed]

7.   Saini, B.; Krass, I.; Smith, L.; Bosnic-Anticevich, S.; Armour, C. Role of community pharmacists in asthma —Australian research highlighting pathways for future primary care models. *Australas. Med. J.* **2011**, *4*, 190–200. [CrossRef] [PubMed]

8.   Watkins, K.; Bourdin, A.; Trevenen, M.; Murray, K.; Kendall, P.A.; Schneider, C.R.; Clifford, R. Opportunities to develop the professional role of community pharmacists in the care of patients with asthma: A cross-sectional study. *NPJ Prim. Care Respir. Med.* **2016**, *26*, 1–10. [CrossRef] [PubMed]

9.   Armour, C.L.; Lemay, K.; Saini, B.; Reddel, H.K.; Bosnic-Anticevich, S.Z.; Smith, L.D.; Burton, D.; Song, Y.J.; Alles, M.C.; Stewart, K.; et al. Using the community pharmacy to identify patients at risk of poor asthma control and factors which contribute to this poor control. *J. Asthma* **2011**, *48*, 914–922. [CrossRef] [PubMed]

10. Apikoglu-Rabus, S.; Yesilyaprak, G.; Izzettin, F.V. Drug-related problems and pharmacist interventions in a cohort of patients with asthma and chronic obstructive pulmonary disease. *Respir. Med.* **2016**, *120*, 109–115. [CrossRef] [PubMed]

11. Saini, B.; Krass, I.; Armour, C. Development, Implementation, and Evaluation of a Community Pharmacy–Based Asthma Care Model. *Ann. Pharmacother.* **2004**, *38*, 1954–1960. [CrossRef] [PubMed]

12. Manfrin, A.; Tinelli, M.; Thomas, T.; Krska, J. A cluster randomised control trial to evaluate the effectiveness and cost-effectiveness of the Italian medicines use review (I-MUR) for asthma patients. *BMC Health Serv. Res.* **2017**, *17*, 9. [CrossRef] [PubMed]

13. Anum, P.O.; Anto, B.P.; Forson, A.G. Structured pharmaceutical care improves the health-related quality of life of patients with asthma. *J. Pharm. Policy Pract.* **2017**, *10*, 8. [CrossRef] [PubMed]

14. Benavides, S.; Rodriguez, J.C.; Maniscalco-Feichtl, M. Pharmacist involvement in improving asthma outcomes in various healthcare settings: 1997 to present. *Ann. Pharmacother.* **2009**, *43*, 85–97. [CrossRef] [PubMed]

15. Armour, C.; Bosnic-Anticevich, S.; Brillant, M.; Burton, D.; Emmerton, L.; Krass, I.; Saini, B.; Smith, L.; Stewart, K. Pharmacy Asthma Care Program (PACP) improves outcomes for patients in the community. *Thorax* **2007**, *62*, 496. [CrossRef] [PubMed]

16. Naik Panvelkar, P.; Armour, C.; Saini, B. Community Pharmacy-Based Asthma Services—What Do Patients Prefer? *J. Asthma* **2010**, *47*, 1085–1093. [CrossRef] [PubMed]

17. Onda, M.; Sakurai, H.; Hayase, Y.; Sakamaki, H.; Arakawa, Y.; Yasukawa, F. Effects of patient-pharmacist communication in the treatment of asthma. *Yakugaku Zasshi* **2009**, *129*, 427–433. [CrossRef] [PubMed]

18. Street, R.L.; Mazor, K.M. Clinician–patient communication measures: Drilling down into assumptions, approaches, and analyses. *Patient Educ. Couns.* **2017**, *100*, 1612–1618. [CrossRef] [PubMed]

19. Sapir, T.; Moreo, K.F.; Greene, L.S.; Simone, L.C.; Carter, J.D.; Mateka, J.J.L.; Hanania, N.A. Assessing Patient and Provider Perceptions of Factors Associated with Patient Engagement in Asthma Care. *Ann. Am. Thorac. Soc.* **2017**, *14*, 659–666. [CrossRef] [PubMed]

20. Horne, R.; Price, D.; Cleland, J.; Costa, R.; Covey, D.; Gruffydd-Jones, K.; Haughney, J.; Henrichsen, S.H.; Kaplan, A.; Langhammer, A.; et al. Can asthma control be improved by understanding the patient's perspective? *BMC Pulm. Med.* **2007**, *7*, 8. [CrossRef] [PubMed]

21. Horne, R.; Weinman, J. Self-regulation and self-management in asthma: Exploring the role of illness perceptions and treatment beliefs in explaining non-adherence to preventer medication. *Psychol. Health* **2002**, *17*, 17–32. [CrossRef]

22. Driesenaar, J.A.; De Smet, P.A.; van Hulten, R.; Noordman, J.; van Dulmen, S. Cue-Responding Behaviors During Pharmacy Counseling Sessions With Patients With Asthma About Inhaled Corticosteroids: Potential Relations With Medication Beliefs and Self-Reported Adherence. *Health Commun.* **2016**, *31*, 1266–1275. [CrossRef] [PubMed]

23. Berry, T.M.; Prosser, T.R.; Wilson, K.; Castro, M. Asthma Friendly Pharmacies: A Model to Improve Communication and Collaboration among Pharmacists, Patients, and Healthcare Providers. *J. Urban Health* **2011**, *88*, 113–125. [CrossRef] [PubMed]

24. Cole, A.; Shaw, M.; Wright, H. How you can encourage medicines optimisation for patients with asthma. *Pharm. J.* **2014**, *292*, 125. [CrossRef]

25. Canadian Pharmacists Association. Pharmacists' Scope of Practice in Canada. Available online: https://www.pharmacists.ca/pharmacy-in-canada/scope-of-practice-canada (accessed on 20 September 2018).

26. Morrison, J. Expanded pharmacy practice: Where are we, and where do we need to go? *Can. Pharm. J.* **2013**, *146*, 365–367. [CrossRef] [PubMed]

27. Thorne, S. *Interpretive Description*; Routledge: New York, NY, USA, 2016.

28. Thorne, S.; Kirkham, S.R.; MacDonald-Emes, J. Interpretive description: A noncategorical qualitative alternative for developing nursing knowledge. *Res. Nurs. Health* **1997**, *20*, 169–177. [CrossRef]

29. Hunt, M.R. Strengths and Challenges in the Use of Interpretive Description: Reflections Arising from a Study of the Moral Experience of Health Professionals in Humanitarian Work. *Qual. Health Res.* **2009**, *19*, 1284–1292. [CrossRef] [PubMed]

30. Kahlke, R.M. Generic Qualitative Approaches: Pitfalls and Benefits of Methodological Mixology. *Int. J. Qual. Meth.* **2014**, *13*, 37–52. [CrossRef]

31. Lau, S.R.; Traulsen, J.M. Are we ready to accept the challenge? Addressing the shortcomings of contemporary qualitative health research. *Res. Soc. Adm. Pharm.* **2017**, *13*, 332–338. [CrossRef] [PubMed]

32. Collins, C.S.; Stockton, C.M. The Central Role of Theory in Qualitative Research. *Int. J. Qual. Meth.* **2018**, *17*. [CrossRef]

33. Braun, V.; Clarke, V. What can "thematic analysis" offer health and wellbeing researchers? *Int. J. Qual. Stud. Health* **2014**, *9*. [CrossRef] [PubMed]

34. Braun, V.; Clarke, V. Using thematic analysis in psychology. *Qual. Res. Psychol.* **2006**, *3*, 77–101. [CrossRef]

35. Green, J.; Karen, W.; Emma, H.; Small, R.; Welch, N.; Lisa, G.; Daly, J. Generating best evidence from qualitative research: The role of data analysis. *Aust. N. Z. J. Public Health* **2007**, *31*, 545–550. [CrossRef] [PubMed]

36. Morse, J.M. Confusing categories and themes. *Qual. Health Res.* **2008**, *18*, 727–728. [CrossRef] [PubMed]

37. Leventhal, H.; Phillips, L.A.; Burns, E. The Common—Sense Model of Self-Regulation (CSM): A dynamic framework for understanding illness self-management. *J. Behav. Med.* **2016**, *39*, 935–946. [CrossRef] [PubMed]

38. Guirguis, L.M. Assessing the knowledge to practice gap: The asthma practices of community pharmacists. *Can. Pharm. J.* **2018**, *151*, 62–70. [CrossRef] [PubMed]

39. McAndrew, L.M.; Musumeci-Szabo, T.J.; Mora, P.A.; Vileikyte, L.; Burns, E.; Halm, E.A.; Leventhal, E.A.; Leventhal, H. Using the common sense model to design interventions for the prevention and management of chronic illness threats: From description to process. *Br. J. Health Psychol.* **2008**, *13*, 195–204. [CrossRef] [PubMed]

40. Bodenheimer, T.; Lorig, K.; Holman, H.; Grumbach, K. Patient self-management of chronic disease in primary care. *JAMA* **2002**, *288*, 2469–2475. [CrossRef] [PubMed]

41. Naughton, A.C. Patient-Centered Communication. *Pharmacy* **2018**, *6*, 1–8. [CrossRef] [PubMed]

42. King, A.; Hoppe, R.B. "Best practice" for patient-centered communication: A narrative review. *J. Grad. Med. Educ.* **2013**, *5*, 385–393. [CrossRef] [PubMed]

43. Phillips, L.A.; Leventhal, H.; Leventhal, E.A. Physicians' communication of the common-sense self-regulation model results in greater reported adherence than physicians' use of interpersonal skills. *Br. J. Health Psychol.* **2012**, *17*, 244–257. [CrossRef] [PubMed]

44. de Oliveira, D.R.; Shoemaker, S.J. Achieving Patient Centeredness in Pharmacy Practice: Openness and the Pharmacist's Natural Attitude. *J. Am. Pharm. Assoc.* **2006**, *46*, 56–66. [CrossRef]

45. Houben-Wilke, S.; Augustin, I.M.L.; Wouters, B.B.; Stevens, R.A.H.; Janssen, D.J.A.; Spruit, M.A.; Vanfleteren, L.E.G.W.; Franssen, F.M.E.; Wouters, E.F.M. The patient with a complex chronic respiratory disease: A specialist of his own life? *Expert Rev. Respir. Med.* **2017**, *11*, 919–924. [CrossRef] [PubMed]

46. Cheong, L.H.; Armour, C.L.; Bosnic-Anticevich, S.Z. Patient asthma networks: Understanding who is important and why. *Health Expect.* **2015**, *18*, 2595–2605. [CrossRef] [PubMed]

47. Gershon, A.S.; Macdonald, E.M.; Luo, J.; Austin, P.C.; Gupta, S.; Sivjee, K.; Upshur, R.; Aaron, S.D. Concomitant pulmonologist and primary care for chronic obstructive pulmonary disease: A population study. *Fam. Pract.* **2017**, *34*, 708–716. [CrossRef] [PubMed]

48. Alberta Health. Pharmacy Services and Prescription Drugs. Available online: http://www.health.alberta.ca/services/pharmacy-services.html (accessed on 28 September 2018).

49. Assa-Eley, M.; Kimberlin, C.L. Using interpersonal perception to characterize pharmacists' and patients' perceptions of the benefits of pharmaceutical care. *Health Commun.* **2005**, *17*, 41–56. [CrossRef] [PubMed]

50. Tarn, D.M.; Paterniti, D.A.; Wenger, N.S.; Williams, B.R.; Chewning, B.A. Older patient, physician and pharmacist perspectives about community pharmacists' roles. *Int. J. Pharm. Pract.* **2012**, *20*, 285–293. [CrossRef] [PubMed]

51. Guirguis, L.M.; Chewning, B.A. Role theory: Literature review and implications for patient-pharmacist interactions. *Res. Soc. Adm. Pharm.* **2005**, *1*, 483–507. [CrossRef] [PubMed]

52. Shah, B.; Chewning, B. Conceptualizing and measuring pharmacist-patient communication: A review of published studies. *Res. Soc. Adm. Pharm.* **2006**, *2*, 153–185. [CrossRef] [PubMed]

53. Worley, M.M.; Schommer, J.C.; Brown, L.M.; Hadsall, R.S.; Ranelli, P.L.; Stratton, T.P.; Uden, D.L. Pharmacists' and patients' roles in the pharmacist-patient relationship: Are pharmacists and patients reading from the same relationship script? *Res. Soc. Adm. Pharm.* **2007**, *3*, 47–69. [CrossRef] [PubMed]

54. Antunes, L.P.; Gomes, J.J.; Cavaco, A.M. How pharmacist–patient communication determines pharmacy loyalty? Modeling relevant factors. *Res. Soc. Adm. Pharm.* **2015**, *11*, 560–570. [CrossRef] [PubMed]

55. Mossialos, E.; Courtin, E.; Naci, H.; Benrimoj, S.; Bouvy, M.; Farris, K.; Noyce, P.; Sketris, I. From "retailers" to health care providers: Transforming the role of community pharmacists in chronic disease management. *Health Policy* **2015**, *119*, 628–639. [CrossRef] [PubMed]

56. McCullough, M.B.; Petrakis, B.A.; Gillespie, C.; Solomon, J.L.; Park, A.M.; Ourth, H.; Morreale, A.; Rose, A.J. Knowing the patient: A qualitative study on care-taking and the clinical pharmacist-patient relationship. *Res. Soc. Adm. Pharm.* **2016**, *12*, 78–90. [CrossRef] [PubMed]

57. Schindel, T.J.; Yuksel, N.; Breault, R.; Daniels, J.; Varnhagen, S.; Hughes, C.A. Perceptions of pharmacists' roles in the era of expanding scopes of practice. *Res. Soc. Adm. Pharm.* **2017**, *13*, 148–161. [CrossRef] [PubMed]

58.   Kelly, D.V.; Young, S.; Phillips, L.; Clark, D. Patient attitudes regarding the role of the pharmacist and interest in expanded pharmacist services. *Can. Pharm. J.* **2014**, *147*, 239–247. [CrossRef] [PubMed]

59.   Mead, N.; Bower, P. Patient-centredness: A conceptual framework and review of the empirical literature. *Soc. Sci. Med.* **2000**, *51*, 1087–1110. [CrossRef]

60.   Tinelli, M.; Bond, C.; Blenkinsopp, A.; Jaffray, M.; Watson, M.; Hannaford, P. Patient Evaluation of a Community Pharmacy Medications Management Service. *Ann. Pharmacother.* **2007**, *41*, 1962–1970. [CrossRef] [PubMed]

61.   Greene, S.M.; Tuzzio, L.; Cherkin, D. A Framework for Making Patient-Centered Care Front and Center. *Perm. J.* **2012**, *16*, 49–53. [CrossRef] [PubMed]

19

Women's Beliefs on Early Adherence to Adjuvant Endocrine Therapy for Breast Cancer: A Theory-Based Qualitative Study to Guide the Development of Community Pharmacist Interventions

Brittany Humphries [1,2,3], Stéphanie Collins [1,4] (ID), Laurence Guillaumie [1,5] (ID), Julie Lemieux [6,7], Anne Dionne [2,6,7], Louise Provencher [6,7], Jocelyne Moisan [1,2] and Sophie Lauzier [1,2,7,*]

[1] Population Health and Optimal Health Practices, CHU de Quebec–Université Laval Research Centre, Hôpital du Saint-Sacrement, 1050 chemin Ste-Foy, Quebec, QC G1S 4L8, Canada; humphrib@mcmaster.ca (B.H.); steph1collins@hotmail.com (S.C.); laurence.guillaumie@fsi.ulaval.ca (L.G.); jocelyne.moisan@pha.ulaval.ca (J.M.)

[2] Faculty of Pharmacy, Université Laval, 1050 avenue de la Médecine, Quebec, QC G1V 0A6, Canada; Anne.Dionne@pha.ulaval.ca

[3] Department of Health Research Methods, Evidence and Impact, McMaster University, 1280 Main Street West, Hamilton, ON L8S 4K1, Canada

[4] Faculty of Pharmacy, Université de Montréal, 2940 Chemin de Polytechnique, Montréal, QC H3T 1J4, Canada

[5] Faculty of Nursing, Université Laval, Quebec, 1050 avenue de la Médecine, Quebec, QC G1V 0A6, Canada

[6] Oncology Research Unit, CHU de Quebec–Université Laval Research Centre, Hôpital du Saint-Sacrement, 1050 chemin Ste-Foy, Quebec, QC G1S 4L8, Canada; Julie.Lemieux@crchudequebec.ulaval.ca (J.L.); louise.provencher.cha@ssss.gouv.qc.ca (L.P.)

[7] Centre des maladies du sein Deschênes-Fabia, CHU de Quebec–Université Laval, Hôpital du Saint-Sacrement, 1050 chemin Ste-Foy, Quebec, QC, G1S 4L8, Canada

* Correspondence: sophie.lauzier@pha.ulaval.ca

Abstract: Adjuvant endocrine therapy (AET) taken for a minimum of five years reduces the recurrence and mortality risks among women with hormone-sensitive breast cancer. However, adherence to AET is suboptimal. To guide the development of theory-based interventions to enhance AET adherence, we conducted a study to explore beliefs regarding early adherence to AET. This qualitative study was guided by the Theory of Planned Behavior (TPB). We conducted focus groups and individual interviews among women prescribed AET in the last two years (n = 43). The topic guide explored attitudinal (perceived advantages and disadvantages), normative (perception of approval or disapproval), and control beliefs (barriers and facilitating factors) towards adhering to AET. Thematic analysis was conducted. Most women had a positive attitude towards AET regardless of their medication-taking behavior. The principal perceived advantage was protection against a recurrence while the principal inconvenience was side effects. Almost everyone approved of the woman taking her medication. The women mentioned facilitating factors to encourage medication-taking behaviors and cope with side effects. For adherent women, having trouble establishing a routine was their main barrier to taking medication. For non-adherent women, it was side effects affecting their quality of life. These findings could inform the development of community pharmacy-based adherence interventions.

Keywords: oncology; breast cancer; medication adherence; tamoxifen; aromatase inhibitors; qualitative research

1. Introduction

Adjuvant endocrine therapy (AET) (tamoxifen or aromatase inhibitors) is prescribed to women with hormone-sensitive breast cancer, approximately 75% of breast cancers [1,2]. AET has to be taken daily for five [3] or 10 years [4] to reduce the risks of recurrence and mortality. However, adherence to AET is suboptimal [5–8] as it is estimated that 28–59% of women do not take their medication on a daily basis [6,9] and 31–47% do not persist with treatment for the minimum recommended 5 years [7]. Taking <80% of AET doses has been associated with a 20% increased mortality risk [10,11].

Few interventions designed to enhance AET adherence have been developed and their evaluation in randomized controlled trials has provided inconclusive results [12–17]. Most of these interventions were limited to the provision of information and reminders by mail or telephone. None of the interventions systematically identified and addressed psychosocial factors from their target population [18]. In addition, baseline adherence was generally high among intervention and control groups. This limited the possibility of observing improvements in AET adherence following the intervention. Finally, no AET adherence-enhancing intervention has been developed and evaluated in community pharmacies [19]. Community pharmacies are a promising setting for this type of intervention since pharmacists have frequent encounters with women prescribed an AET. They also have the expertise to detect non-adherence and implement strategies to optimize medication use.

Identifying psychosocial factors that influence AET adherence is a crucial step in developing interventions with a potential to improve adherence. Previous qualitative studies [20–29] have furthered our understanding of the subjective experience of AET. An integrative review of the findings from these studies indicates that non-adherence to AET is multifaceted and influenced by several psychosocial factors, such as the experience of side effects, negative attitudes towards AET or medication in general, lack of a routine, and unsatisfactory relationships with healthcare professionals [30]. This review highlights how some of the factors influencing non-adherence to AET (e.g., side effects, patient-provider communication) are similar to those for non-adherence to medications prescribed for other chronic conditions [31,32]. However, other factors (e.g., fear of a breast cancer recurrence, conflicting representations about the (anti)hormonal effect of AET and the necessity of treatment) pertain specifically to the experience of AET.

Although these qualitative studies provide valuable insight into women's experiences with AET, only one study was based on a psychosocial theory [28]. This study conducted 31 individual interviews among women with various AET-taking behaviors. It was based on the Theoretical Domains Framework, which maps constructs from many psychosocial theories [33]. The authors identified a range of barriers and facilitating factors towards AET adherence that were primarily related to the domains of beliefs about consequences, intention and goals, and behavior regulation. The relative importance of these domains varied depending on the woman's AET-taking behavior.

There are several advantages in using psychosocial theories to inform the development and evaluation of an intervention [34]. First, they facilitate a systematic approach to identifying the potentially modifiable psychosocial factors that influence a health behavior. Second, they inform the selection of the best methods to influence these factors. This is essential to increase the potential for an effective behavioral intervention [35]. Third, they assist in the evaluation of the intervention since it is possible to describe how and to what extent the intervention affected these psychosocial factors as well as the health behavior of interest.

Among existing psychosocial theories, the Theory of Planned Behavior (TPB) has been widely used to identify the main psychosocial factors influencing health-related behaviors in quantitative [36–38] and qualitative studies [39]. It is considered as one of the most effective psychosocial theories to predict a behavior [36,37], such as medication adherence. The TPB postulates that an individual's intention to adopt a behavior is influenced by three constructs: attitude, subjective norm, and perceived behavioral control [40]. Each construct is influenced by a set of beliefs that are specific to the behavior and population under study. In the context of AET adherence, these are: (1) attitudinal beliefs, which are the perceived advantages and disadvantages of taking AET as prescribed; (2) normative beliefs, which are the perception of the extent that people important to the woman approve or disapprove of her taking AET as prescribed; and (3) control beliefs, which are factors perceived to hinder or facilitate taking AET as prescribed. The TPB authors recommend documenting these beliefs among the target population using qualitative methods since the beliefs and their importance may vary depending on the behavior and population of interest [40].

Given the extent of non-adherence to AET and the lack of theory-based studies that could be used to guide the development of an adherence-enhancing intervention, we conducted a qualitative study using the TPB among women prescribed AET within the last two years. The aim was to identify women's attitudinal, normative, and control beliefs regarding AET adherence that could be targeted by an intervention offered in the community pharmacy setting. This study was a crucial first step in addressing research gaps regarding interventions to enhance adherence to AET.

2. Materials and Methods

2.1. Design

This qualitative descriptive study was guided by the TPB. It was conducted from November 2013 to February 2014 using focus groups and individual interviews. We selected focus groups because interactions with others are likely to deepen participants' reflections on their experience [41]. Based on the analysis of focus groups, which comprised women who were mostly adherent at the time of the study, we conducted individual interviews [42] targeting specifically non-adherent women. Individual interviews were selected because we judged that women would be more comfortable discussing this experience privately.

2.2. Subjects

Women were eligible to participate in the study if they were aged 18 years or older, diagnosed with hormone receptor-positive breast cancer, had a first AET prescription for early breast cancer within the last two years and sufficient fluency in French. For individual interviews, women had to self-report difficulties adhering to AET (i.e., treatment non-initiation, cessation, or suboptimal adherence on a daily basis).

Potential participants for focus group were identified by the medical team of the *Centre des maladies du sein Deschênes-Fabia* (CMS), *CHU de Québec–Université Laval*. Participants for individual interviews were identified by the CMS team, an email sent to *Université Laval* employees, and advertisements placed in Quebec City pharmacies. If a potentially eligible woman identified by the CMS team expressed interest in participating in the study, the CMS team transmitted her contact information to the research team. If the woman was informed about the study by email or advertisement, she contacted the research team herself. In both instances, a member of the research team would follow up with the woman to explain the study, verify eligibility, and solicit consent. Potential participants had no contact with the research team prior to this study.

2.3. Data Collection

A topic guide comprised of questions recommended by the authors of the TPB to elicit attitudinal, normative, and control beliefs regarding AET was used for the group and individual interviews [40] (Figure 1). At the beginning of each group and individual interview, participants were reminded that researchers from *Université Laval* were interested in understanding their experience with AET. A (male) professional moderator conducted the focus groups while two members of the research team observed behind a one-way mirror (Sophie Lauzier [SL], Ph.D., Assistant Professor, trained in social and cultural anthropology and epidemiology, and Marjolaine Roy [MR], M.Sc., Research Professional, trained in psychology). The women were informed that the moderator was not part of the research team. Individual interviews were conducted by two (female) members of the research team (MR and Stephanie Collins, B.A., research assistant, trained in social and cultural anthropology). All focus group and individual interviews were tapped. In addition, each participant completed a questionnaire on their sociodemographic and treatment characteristics. They received $50 for their participation.

Part 1: General experience with adjuvant endocrine therapy (AET)
1. What was your reaction after your doctor prescribed you AET?
2. How did the initiation of this treatment go?
3. As of now, what is your experience with this treatment?

Part 2: Personal beliefs related to taking AET as prescribed
I'd like to now ask you questions about taking your AET, as prescribed by your doctor.

Theme 1: Attitudinal beliefs
1. During the next month, what are the benefits for you to take your AET as prescribed?
2. During the next month, what are the disadvantages for you to take your AET as prescribed?

Theme 2: Normative beliefs
1. What person(s) or group(s) of people do you think would approve of you taking your AET as prescribed for the next month?
2. What person (s) or group (s) of person (s) do you think would disapprove of you taking your AET as prescribed for the next month?

Theme 3: Control beliefs
1. What would prevent you from taking your AET as prescribed for the next month?
2. What would help you take your AET as prescribed for the next month?

Figure 1. Topic guide for focus groups and individual interviews.

2.4. Analysis

The principal investigator (SL) met with team members who attended the group or individual interviews to debrief after each data collection activity. Based on this preliminary analysis, it was estimated that data saturation was reached after three group and eight individual interviews. In total, five group and nine individual interviews were conducted. The transcripts were thematically analyzed [43,44] using a codebook developed through a validation process inspired by continuous thematic analysis [45]. Three team members (MR, SC, SL) developed a first version of the codebook. Codes were issued from the topic guide and also emerged from the data. The team members then independently coded transcripts from the first focus group before debriefing. This process was repeated for subsequent groups until consensus on the codebook was reached. Two team members (SC, Brittany Humphries [BH], B.A., Research Assistant, trained in social and cultural anthropology) used the final version to code remaining data, adding new codes if necessary. Codification was assisted by Microsoft WORD. Group and individual interviews were analyzed separately and then systematically compared for each code.

2.5. Ethical Considerations

All participants gave informed written consent before participating in the study. The study was conducted in accordance with the Declaration of Helsinki, and the protocol was approved by the ethics committee of the *CHU de Québec–Université Laval* (DR-002-1425).

3. Results

3.1. Participants

For the focus groups, 72 eligible women were referred to the research team by the CMS team. Among them, 37 refused to participate and one woman could not be reached by the research team. Thus, a total of 34 women participated in five focus groups. For the individual interviews, 30 women contacted the research team. Among them, 21 were ineligible to participate. Thus, nine individual interviews were conducted (Table 1). The focus groups were conducted at *Université Laval* while the individuals interviews were conducted in a location that suited the preferences of the women (i.e., *Université Laval*, *Hôpital du Saint-Sacrement*, a medical clinic or at the woman's home). The group and individual interviews lasted an average of 90 and 45 minutes, respectively.

Table 1. Sociodemographic and treatment characteristics of participants.

	Focus Groups	Individual Interviews	Total
	(*n* = 34)	(*n* = 9)	(*n* = 43)
Age (years)			
≤49	5	1	6
50–59	13	4	17
60–69	8	2	10
≥70	8	2	10
Level of education			
Primary school	1	1	2
Secondary school	7	1	8
College	11	3	14
University	15	4	19
Time since breast cancer diagnosis (months) [1]			
mean (range)	16.5 (5–30)	20.3 (6–32)	17.3 (5–32)
Breast surgery			
Yes	34	9	43
No	0	0	0
Other breast cancer treatments received			
Chemotherapy	14	4	18
Radiotherapy	32	6	38
Trastuzumab	5	1	6
Number of adjuvant treatments received in addition to AET [1]			
0	2	3	5
1	18	2	20
2	10	2	12
3	4	1	5
Adjuvant endocrine treatment prescribed at time of the study			
Tamoxifen	14	5	19
Letrozole	2	1	3
Anastrozole	18	3	21
Exemestane	0	0	0
Time since first AET prescription (months)			
mean (range)	10.9 (2–21)	12.6 (2–24)	11.2 (2–24)

[1] Information not provided for *n* = 1.

3.2. Medication-Taking Behaviors

Focus group participants identified mainly as adherent. These women had initiated treatment, intended to persist with AET for the recommended duration and took their medication daily with few (often unintentional) missed doses. Some women had temporarily stopped taking their medication but only if recommended by a healthcare professional. Participants in the individual interviews identified to some degree as non-adherent. These women did not initiate treatment, had definitively stopped taking AET, or did not take their medication as prescribed (intentionally missing doses for days or weeks at a time).

3.3. Attitudinal Beliefs

The principal perceived advantage of adhering to AET was prevention of a recurrence of cancer, although women from both the group and individual interviews understood it did not offer complete protection. Some participants expressed their fears of stopping AET, whether it was during treatment or at the end of prescription. These participants explained how taking AET afforded them a sense of security and peace of mind. In addition, several women felt a responsibility towards themselves, relatives, and their healthcare team. By not taking AET, the women felt they were betraying everyone's efforts to get them this far.

"The advantage they told me, was that it could save me. [...] I saw this as prevention against a recurrence."

Individual Interview, Participant E.

" ... All the effort made by everyone around us to support us. What's taking a pill? We owe them that."

Focus Group 1, Participant C.

Side effects were the main inconvenience perceived by the vast majority of participants (group and individual interviews). They ranged from hot flashes to vaginal dryness, depression, alopecia, and musculoskeletal pain. Side effects caused some women to change their daily habits (e.g., stop going to the gym because of musculoskeletal pain) and long-term goals (e.g., delay having children). Women's experiences with other breast cancer treatments also affected how they perceived side effects. Some women who experienced side effects from other treatments affirmed they were prepared to face anything, while others rejected the possibility of feeling poorly again. Adherent women were more inclined to accommodate them. For non-adherent women, the perceived advantages of AET did not justify the inconveniences they were experiencing. Another inconvenience was how AET became a daily reminder that the women were not finished with cancer.

"If the hot flashes are to help me stay alive, then I'll just turn down the heating system."

Focus Group 3, Participant Z.

"It's like a trace of what we've experienced, like a passport that you always have on you."

Focus Group 4, Participant M.

3.4. Normative Beliefs

Although everyone approved that they take AET, most women in the group and individual interviews stated that the opinions of others did not influence any decision regarding adherence. They did, however, explain how social support helped them take their medication as prescribed.

At the moment of prescription, the women discussed how the frantic pace of the treatments and the urgency of the situation left them with little space to reflect on what was happening. As a result, most of them relied on the judgement of their oncologist. During the treatment period, women received support from healthcare professionals such as oncologists, family doctors, oncology nurses and community pharmacists. These professionals reminded them of the benefits of AET, affirmed that the side effects they were experiencing were normal, answered their questions and informed them of the possibility of trying a different medication to reduce side effects. For women struggling with side effects, this support was a major factor in their decision to continue with treatment. Non-adherent women were more likely to have not found a healthcare professional with whom they could consult.

"Yes the doctor prescribed it to you, you trust him. It's like chemo treatment. It's preferable to not have it but you are told that you must."

Focus Group 3, Participant J.

"I had tons of questions and I wasn't able ask them because she [oncologist] was, I felt that she was anxious, busy, it seemed as though I had to go quickly. So I was left with my questions."

Individual Interview, Participant K.

Support from relatives often came in the form of reminders. However, certain women chose not to speak of AET. Reasons include an inability to talk about AET because it references the trauma of cancer, not wanting to worry their relatives, and a desire to avoid being pitied. Several women sought out support from breast cancer survivors. Discussing this shared experience provided these women with the emotional and informational support they needed.

"I don't talk because I'm not able to talk about it."

Individual Interview, Participant C.

"We were twelve and twice a day, morning group and evening [discussion] group, I received all the information from them because they had gone through it before me."

Focus Group 5, Participant S.

3.5. Control Beliefs

A list of facilitating factors and barriers reported by the women is presented in Figure 2. Important facilitating factors were strategies to establish a routine. The women spoke of leaving the medication somewhere visible, taking AET at the same time, setting an alarm and using a pill box. Other facilitating factors were strategies to mitigate side effects. Several women had tried natural products, meditation, and sports while others changed the type of medication or lowered doses. Finally, women in both the group and individual interviews were unanimous in saying that obtaining answers to their questions would facilitate their adherence. To find answers, they consulted several sources of information. Participants made a distinction between blogs and "official" sources, and wanted access to scientific information in a more approachable format.

"I asked myself what do I do everyday of my life? At breakfast, my jar of peanut butter . . . Every morning, it is there."

Focus Group 3, Participant F.

"She [nurse navigator] said "well, we will try another molecule. Maybe that one will serve you better than the other." [. . .] For me, it was like a door had opened and there could be something else that is more comfortable for five years."

Individual Interview, Participant J.

Facilitating Factors
• Having had previous cancer treatments that were well tolerated
• Having confidence in the healthcare team
• Receiving empathy and information from healthcare professionals
• Interacting with a helpful and available community pharmacist
• Consulting with a nurse
• Receiving information from a cancer foundation
• Being accompanied by a family member to appointments
• Receiving reminders to take medication from family and friends
• Leaving the pill box somewhere visible (e.g. beside table, beside the coffee machine, on the vanity in the bathroom, by the vitamins)
• Taking the medication at the same time everyday
• Taking other medications
• Setting up reminders by email, electronic calendar or cell phone alarm
• Trying alternative therapies to help cope with side effects
• Switching to a different type of AET with the goal of reducing side effects

Barriers
• Feeling as though the introduction to the medication was unexpected
• Having unanswered questions about AET (e.g.. air travel or dietary restrictions)
• Having unanswered questions about AET and changes to the body
• Not having enough information before treatment begun
• Not having personalized information on AET efficacy
• Not understanding the hormonal nature of AET
• Not understanding the difference between tamoxifen and aromatase inhibitors
• Not understanding medical terms
• Receiving different information from healthcare professionals
• Perceiving the doctor as being too busy to approach
• Feeling uneasy about discussing sensitive issues with a male pharmacist
• Having unreturned phone calls to healthcare professionals
• Lacking access to a healthcare professional for psychological issues
• Experiencing problems with side effects
• Lacking strategies to cope with side effects
• Travelling and the disruption of a routine
• Forgetting to take the medication
• Being unused to taking pills daily
• Taking too many medications
• Trying to take AET medication when outside the house
• Feeling alone in the decision to stop treatment

Figure 2. Facilitating factors and barriers to adherence to adjuvant endocrine therapy (AET).

The main barrier for adherent women was difficulty establishing a routine and forgetting their medication. For non-adherent women, it was side effects and a diminished of quality of life. A barrier common to all participants concerned the moment and quantity of information received. Most women were presented with their AET treatment plan when the pathology report was explained. Often, this information was not properly understood or retained because of the emotional charge of the meeting. In addition, women explained how their information needs varied with time. Some women had questions before they took their medication and others after they started treatment when a healthcare professional was not always accessible. Many women felt unprepared for side effects; namely that they were not warned of their severity or of potential psychological issues. Other women did not have enough information about how to incorporate AET into daily life; if they could travel by plane or eat foods containing phytoestrogens (e.g., soy, flax).

" ... *the hot flashes. I would wake up during the night and be drenched. I skipped one month [of AET].*"

Focus Group 3, Participant F.

3.6. Additional Constructs

In addition to the TPB, our results indicate that the following constructs are also important for AET adherence.

3.6.1. Perceived Risk

Perceived risk is an individual's assessment of their chance to develop a health problem if they adopt a behavior [46]. Although healthcare professionals presented AET as an important preventative treatment, they often did not offer information about its efficacy specific to each woman's medical characteristics. This was important for women suffering from side effects as it would enable them to make an informed decision about whether to continue with treatment.

"It [AET] was strongly recommended because I was in a risky age group. I had just turned 40. And then, because my cancer was hormone sensitive and very reactive . . . "

Individual Interview, Participant B.

3.6.2. Anticipated Regret

Anticipated regret is the feeling an individual would have if the behavior was not adopted [47]. In the context of AET, several women explained that they took their medication because they would experience guilt or regret if they did not and had a recurrence.

"If I don't take it I feel a bit guilty. I mean to say that if my cancer comes back, I'll say well there, you didn't follow it."

Individual Interview, Participant H.

3.6.3. Moral Standards

Moral standards are an individual's sense of obligation towards adopting a behavior [48]. Many women felt that they had no choice but to take AET. Some felt obligated because of their role as a patient or mother, others because AET was their only adjuvant treatment.

"It is THE treatment, that's it. I did not have anything else. I didn't have any treatment besides this. So it was awful, but I was obligated."

Individual Interview, Participant C.

3.6.4. Self-Identity

Self-identity is the extent that an individual identifies the behavior as part of their personality [49]. In the context of AET, women indicated that character had influenced their attitude towards AET.

"I have to say that I was never a person who is very pro-medication. I was very annoyed that I had to take it."

Individual Interview, Participant B.

4. Discussion

This is the first qualitative study to use the TPB to explore women's experience with AET. Our results indicate that most women had a positive attitude towards AET regardless of their medication-taking behavior. The principal advantage perceived by participants was protection against a recurrence while the principal inconvenience was side effects. With regards to normative beliefs, almost everyone approved of the woman taking her medication and women particularly valued the support of the health care team, their relatives, and cancer survivors. The women mentioned a diversity of barriers and facilitating factors to encourage AET adherence and cope with side effects.

For adherent women, having trouble establishing a routine was the main barrier to taking their medication. For non-adherent women, it was side effects and a diminished quality of life.

The main contribution of this study lies in the strength of TPB, which is considered to be one of the most effective psychosocial theories in predicting a health-related behavior [36,37]. The TPB provides a structured and comprehensive approach to investigating how three main factors (attitude, subjective norm, and perceived behavioral control) and related beliefs influence an individual's intention and, ultimately, their health behavior. Our objective for this study was to identify women's beliefs regarding AET adherence to guide the development of adherence-enhancing interventions . The following paragraphs will discuss our results and how they can be applied to the development of an intervention to be offered in the community pharmacy setting.

Attitudinal beliefs: Our findings are in line with those of previous quantitative [50,51] and qualitative studies [20–28]. These studies indicate that the perceived advantages of AET adherence include protection against a recurrence [21], feelings of guilt [22], and anxiety about a recurrence [25, 50,51]. Interventions developed for the community pharmacy setting should therefore emphasize the advantages of taking AET medication in relation to the risk of a breast recurrence. The fact that perceived risk and anticipated regret were identified as supplementary factors in our study indicates that pharmacists should also discuss advantages related to avoiding feelings of guilt and anxiety about a recurrence. These advantages should be reiterated throughout the course of treatment to help women maintain their motivation. In addition to reinforcing the benefits of AET, pharmacists could also discuss the potential inconveniences of taking this medication. Despite the fact that most women understand the therapeutic benefits of AET, the impact of side effects on their quality of life can be so great as to outweigh any perceived advantages [20,22,50]. In a previous study, women who were informed in advance of potential side effects were more likely to be adherent [52]. Interventions should therefore address potential side effects, which were the main inconvenience identified in our study.

Normative beliefs: Women who participated in our study reported that the opinion of others did not directly affect their intention to be adherent to AET. They did, however, explain how social interactions influenced their medication-taking behavior. Previous studies have acknowledged that support from healthcare professionals can influence AET adherence [20,21,23,24]. In our study, women mentioned that oncologists, nurse navigators, family physicians and community pharmacists were an essential source of guidance and information. Relatives were perceived as a source of emotional and practical support while cancer survivors provided an opportunity to share the experience of taking AET with others who can understand and offer advice. Interventions for the community pharmacy setting should therefore target these three sources of social support. The intervention could raise pharmacists' awareness of their potential to influence AET adherence. Relatives could be provided with additional resources about AET and encouraged to participate in consultations at the pharmacy, if desired by the woman. Relationships with other cancer survivors could be promoted by providing information about community-based organizations for cancer survivors and using survivors' testimonies in the documentation given to women.

Control beliefs: We identified similar barriers and facilitating factors towards AET adherence as other qualitative studies [20,23,24]. These touch on information about AET, side effects and routine. With regard to information about AET, participants in our study reported that having access to timely information and answers to their questions would facilitate adherence. Information about AET was generally presented for the first time by the oncologist when pathology report was discussed. Since the retention of information may not optimal at this time, community pharmacy interventions should be designed to ensure that essential information is recapitulated when the first prescription of AET is filled. In addition, information needs vary with time. This indicates that community pharmacists should reach out to women throughout the course of treatment (e.g., at renewals). With regard to side effects, community pharmacists are at the frontline for their detection and have the potential to play an important role in helping women overcome this barrier. In our study, women who were significantly affected by side effects explained how support from healthcare professionals was an important factor in their decision to continue with treatment. Interventions should therefore ensure that community pharmacists offer some form of counselling that provides women with coping strategies. With regard to the establishment of a routine, more guidance on incorporating AET into daily life is required for some women. This includes recommendations on the timing of medication to avoid missing doses or what to do in the event of a missed dose. Pharmacists should aim to proactively detect and address practical difficulties related to taking AET on a daily basis. Their interventions could be inspired by the practical strategies mentioned by women in our study.

Our study has several strengths. First, to our knowledge, it is the first qualitative study to use the TPB to explore the experiences of women with an AET prescription. The use of the TPB contributed to our understanding of beliefs that should be targeted in a community pharmacy-based intervention aimed at enhancing AET adherence. The identification of priority targets is especially important when designing brief interventions, such as those offered in the community pharmacy setting. Second, focus groups allowed for a general portrait of the experience of women with AET while individual interviews offered a deeper understanding of non-adherence. Few of the previous qualitative studies on AET have made an explicit effort to sample women with different medication-taking behaviors [28]. This supplementary effort to meet with women who were less adherent provided unique insights into the experience of non-adherence, which can happen to varying degrees and for different reasons throughout the treatment trajectory [53].

This study also has limitations. First, our sample was restricted to women prescribed AET within the last two years. This decision was made because our team aims to develop adherence-enhancing interventions to be offered during the first years of treatment, which represents a critical opportunity to influence the entire course of treatment. However, medication-taking behaviors can change over time [53] and more theory-based qualitative research is required to understand the long-term needs of women prescribed AET. Second, we used different methods to recruit women for group and individual interviews. It is generally more difficult to recruit patients with non-adherent behaviors because they are less inclined to share their experience. Given that most of the previous qualitative studies include few non-adherent women, supplementary efforts were required to ensure that we captured this experience. We accounted for the difference between group and individual interviews in our analyses.

5. Conclusions

The results from this theory-based study demonstrate how qualitative data on women's experience with AET can be used to inform the development of adherence-enhancing interventions delivered in the community pharmacy setting. Although it is within the scope of community pharmacists' practice to inform women of advantages and inconveniences of AET (behavioral beliefs), strengthen social support (normative beliefs), and address barriers and facilitating factors (control beliefs), several considerations have to be taken into account in the design and implementation of this type of intervention. First, community pharmacists may need additional training regarding AET counselling and monitoring. A survey conducted among Canadian pharmacists indicated that they did not have sufficient knowledge or training on oral oncology treatments [54]. Second, it may be challenging for community pharmacists to perform drug monitoring throughout the 5 or 10 years of AET treatment. Studies indicate that community pharmacist's monitoring of other long-term drug therapies is suboptimal mainly due to organizational constraints (e.g., lack of time or incentive, high workload) [55–59]. Given these considerations, an assessment of community pharmacists' ability, needs and attitudes toward performing these interventions should be conducted to complement results from the present study. This would optimize the potential success of AET adherence-enhancing interventions [34].

Reference

Author Contributions: S.L. and L.G. designed the study and supervised each study steps. J.L. and L.P. contributed to patient recruitment. A.D. and J.M. provided comments for each step of the study. B.H. and S.C. did the analyses and wrote the manuscript. All authors commented on the manuscript and approved the submitted version for publication.

Acknowledgments: The authors would like to thank the women who shared their experiences during focus groups and individual interviews. The authors also thank Marjolaine Roy who coordinated the study. This work was supported by the Fondation du CHU de Québec-Université Laval. B. Humphries had scholarships from the Canadian Institutes of Health Research (CIHR) and the *Fonds d'enseignement et de recherche de la Faculté de pharmacie de l'Université Laval*. S. Lauzier was a research scholar with funding from the *Fonds de recherche du Québec–Santé* (Quebec Health Research Fund) in partnership with the *Institut national d'excellence en santé et en services sociaux* (National Institute for Excellence in Health and Social Services).

References

1. Jatoi, I.; Chen, B.E.; Anderson, W.F.; Rosenberg, P.S. Breast cancer mortality trends in the united states according to estrogen receptor status and age at diagnosis. *J. Clin. Oncol.* **2007**, *25*, 1683–1690. [CrossRef] [PubMed]

2. Huang, H.J.; Neven, P.; Drijkoningen, M.; Paridaens, R.; Wildiers, H.; Van Limbergen, E.; Berteloot, P.; Amant, F.; Vergote, I.; Christiaens, M.R. Association between tumour characteristics and her-2/neu by immunohistochemistry in 1362 women with primary operable breast cancer. *J. Clin. Pathol.* **2005**, *58*, 611–616. [CrossRef] [PubMed]

3. Burstein, H.J.; Prestrud, A.A.; Seidenfeld, J.; Anderson, H.; Buchholz, T.A.; Davidson, N.E.; Gelmon, K.E.; Giordano, S.H.; Hudis, C.A.; Malin, J.; et al. American society of clinical oncology clinical practice guideline: Update on adjuvant endocrine therapy for women with hormone receptor-positive breast cancer. *J. Clin. Oncol.* **2010**, *28*, 3784–3796. [CrossRef] [PubMed]

4. Burstein, H.J.; Temin, S.; Anderson, H.; Buchholz, T.A.; Davidson, N.E.; Gelmon, K.E.; Giordano, S.H.; Hudis, C.A.; Rowden, D.; Solky, A.J.; et al. Adjuvant endocrine therapy for women with hormone receptor-positive breast cancer: American society of clinical oncology clinical practice guideline focused update. *J. Clin. Oncol.* **2014**, *32*, 2255–2269. [CrossRef] [PubMed]

5. Gotay, C.; Dunn, J. Adherence to long-term adjuvant hormonal therapy for breast cancer. *Expert Rev. Pharmacoecon. Outcomes Res.* **2011**, *11*, 709–715. [CrossRef] [PubMed]

6. Chlebowski, R.T.; Geller, M.L. Adherence to endocrine therapy for breast cancer. *Oncology* **2006**, *71*, 1–9. [CrossRef] [PubMed]

7. Huiart, L.; Ferdynus, C.; Giorgi, R. A meta-regression analysis of the available data on adherence to adjuvant hormonal therapy in breast cancer: Summarizing the data for clinicians. *Breast Cancer Res. Treat.* **2013**, *138*, 325–328. [CrossRef] [PubMed]

8. Murphy, C.C.; Bartholomew, L.K.; Carpentier, M.Y.; Bluethmann, S.M.; Vernon, S.W. Adherence to adjuvant hormonal therapy among breast cancer survivors in clinical practice: A systematic review. *Breast Cancer Res. Treat.* **2012**, *134*, 459–478. [CrossRef] [PubMed]

9. Dunn, J.; Gotay, C. Adherence rates and correlates in long-term hormonal therapy. *Vitam. Horm.* **2013**, *93*, 353–375. [PubMed]

10. Makubate, B.; Donnan, P.T.; Dewar, J.A.; Thompson, A.M.; McCowan, C. Cohort study of adherence to adjuvant endocrine therapy, breast cancer recurrence and mortality. *Br. J. Cancer* **2013**, *108*, 1515–1524. [CrossRef] [PubMed]

11. Winn, A.N.; Dusetzina, S.B. The association between trajectories of endocrine therapy adherence and mortality among women with breast cancer. *Pharmacoepidemiol. Drug Saf.* **2016**, *25*, 953–959. [CrossRef] [PubMed]

12. Yu, K.D.; Zhou, Y.; Liu, G.Y.; Li, B.; He, P.Q.; Zhang, H.W.; Lou, L.H.; Wang, X.J.; Wang, S.; Tang, J.H.; et al. A prospective, multicenter, controlled, observational study to evaluate the efficacy of a patient support program in improving patients' persistence to adjuvant aromatase inhibitor medication for postmenopausal, early stage breast cancer. *Breast Cancer Res. Treat.* **2012**, *134*, 307–313. [CrossRef] [PubMed]

13. Ziller, V.; Kyvernitakis, I.; Knoll, D.; Storch, A.; Hars, O.; Hadji, P. Influence of a patient information program on adherence and persistence with an aromatase inhibitor in breast cancer treatment—the compas study. *BMC Cancer* **2013**, *13*, 407. [CrossRef] [PubMed]

14. Neven, P.; Markopoulos, C.; Tanner, M.; Marty, M.; Kreienberg, R.; Atkins, L.; Franquet, A.; Gnant, M.; Neciosup, S.; Tesarova, P.; et al. The impact of educational materials on compliance and persistence rates with adjuvant aromatase inhibitor treatment: First-year results from the compliance of aromatase inhibitors assessment in daily practice through educational approach (cariatide) study. *Breast* **2014**, *23*, 393–399. [CrossRef] [PubMed]

15. Hadji, P.; Blettner, M.; Harbeck, N.; Jackisch, C.; Luck, H.J.; Windemuth-Kieselbach, C.; Zaun, S.; Kreienberg, R. The patient's anastrozole compliance to therapy (pact) program: A randomized, in-practice study on the impact of a standardized information program on persistence and compliance to adjuvant endocrine therapy in postmenopausal women with early breast cancer. *Ann. Oncol.* **2013**, *24*, 1505–1512. [CrossRef] [PubMed]

16. Markopoulos, C.; Neven, P.; Tanner, M.; Marty, M.; Kreienberg, R.; Atkins, L.; Franquet, A.; Gnant, M.; Neciosup, S.; Tesarova, P.; et al. Does patient education work in breast cancer? Final results from the global cariatide study. *Future Oncol.* **2015**, *11*, 205–217. [CrossRef] [PubMed]

17. Wagner, V.L.; Jing, W.; Boscoe, F.P.; Schymura, M.J.; Roohan, P.J.; Gesten, F.C. Improving adjuvant hormone therapy use in medicaid managed care-insured women, new york state, 2012–2014. *Prev. Chronic Dis.* **2016**, *13*, E120. [CrossRef] [PubMed]

18. Michie, S.; Abraham, C. Interventions to change health behaviours: Evidence-based or evidence-inspired? *Psychol. Health* **2004**, *19*, 29–49. [CrossRef]

19. Ekinci, E.; Nathoo, S.; Korattyil, T.; Vadhariya, A.; Zaghloul, H.A.; Niravath, P.A.; Abughosh, S.M.; Trivedi, M.V. Interventions to improve endocrine therapy adherence in breast cancer survivors: What is the evidence? *J. Cancer Surviv.* **2018**, *12*, 348–356. [CrossRef] [PubMed]

20. Pellegrini, I.; Sarradon-Eck, A.; Soussan, P.B.; Lacour, A.C.; Largillier, R.; Tallet, A.; Tarpin, C.; Julian-Reynier, C. Women's perceptions and experience of adjuvant tamoxifen therapy account for their adherence: Breast cancer patients' point of view. *Psycho Oncol.* **2010**, *19*, 472–479. [CrossRef] [PubMed]

21. Harrow, A.; Dryden, R.; McCowan, C.; Radley, A.; Parsons, M.; Thompson, A.M.; Wells, M. A hard pill to swallow: A qualitative study of women's experiences of adjuvant endocrine therapy for breast cancer. *BMJ Open* **2014**, *4*. [CrossRef] [PubMed]

22. Verbrugghe, M.; Verhaeghe, S.; Decoene, E.; De Baere, S.; Vandendorpe, B.; Van Hecke, A. Factors influencing the process of medication (non-)adherence and (non-)persistence in breast cancer patients with adjuvant antihormonal therapy: A qualitative study. *Eur. J. Cancer Care* **2017**, *26*, e12339. [CrossRef] [PubMed]

23. Wells, K.J.; Pan, T.M.; Vazquez-Otero, C.; Ung, D.; Ustjanauskas, A.E.; Munoz, D.; Laronga, C.; Roetzheim, R.G.; Goldenstein, M.; Carrizosa, C.; et al. Barriers and facilitators to endocrine therapy adherence among underserved hormone-receptor-positive breast cancer survivors: A qualitative study. *Support. Care Cancer* **2016**, *24*, 4123–4130. [CrossRef] [PubMed]

24. Van Londen, G.J.; Donovan, H.S.; Beckjord, E.B.; Cardy, A.L.; Bovbjerg, D.H.; Davidson, N.E.; Morse, J.Q.; Switzer, G.E.; Verdonck-de Leeuw, I.M.; Dew, M.A. Perspectives of postmenopausal breast cancer survivors on adjuvant endocrine therapy-related symptoms. *Oncol. Nurs. Forum* **2014**, *41*, 660–668. [CrossRef] [PubMed]

25. Iacorossi, L.; Gambalunga, F.; Fabi, A.; Giannarelli, D.; Marchetti, A.; Piredda, M.; De Marinis, M.G. Adherence to oral administration of endocrine treatment in patients with breast cancer: A qualitative study. *Cancer Nurs.* **2018**, *41*, E57–E63. [CrossRef] [PubMed]

26. Wickersham, K.; Happ, M.B.; Bender, C.M. Keeping the boogie man away: Medication self-management among women receiving anastrozole therapy. *Nurs. Res. Pract.* **2012**, *2012*, 9. [CrossRef] [PubMed]

27. Wouters, H.; van Geffen, E.C.G.; Baas-Thijssen, M.C.; Krol-Warmerdam, E.M.; Stiggelbout, A.M.; Belitser, S.; Bouvy, M.L.; van Dijk, L. Disentangling breast cancer patients' perceptions and experiences with regard to endocrine therapy: Nature and relevance for non-adherence. *Breast* **2013**, *22*, 661–666. [CrossRef] [PubMed]

28. Cahir, C.; Dombrowski, S.U.; Kelly, C.M.; Kennedy, M.J.; Bennett, K.; Sharp, L. Women's experiences of hormonal therapy for breast cancer: Exploring influences on medication-taking behaviour. *Support. Care Cancer* **2015**, *23*, 3115–3130. [CrossRef] [PubMed]

29. Brauer, E.R.; Ganz, P.A.; Pieters, H.C. "Winging it": How older breast cancer survivors persist with aromatase inhibitor treatment. *J. Oncol. Pract.* **2016**, *12*, e991–e1000. [CrossRef] [PubMed]

30. Lambert, L.K.; Balneaves, L.G.; Howard, A.F.; Gotay, C.C. Patient-reported factors associated with adherence to adjuvant endocrine therapy after breast cancer: An integrative review. *Breast Cancer Res. Treat.* **2018**, *167*, 615–633. [CrossRef] [PubMed]

31. Van der Laan, D.M.; Elders, P.J.M.; Boons, C.; Beckeringh, J.J.; Nijpels, G.; Hugtenburg, J.G. Factors associated with antihypertensive medication non-adherence: A systematic review. *J. Hum. Hypertens.* **2017**, *31*, 687–694. [CrossRef] [PubMed]

32. Capoccia, K.; Odegard, P.S.; Letassy, N. Medication adherence with diabetes medication: A systematic review of the literature. *Diabetes Educ.* **2016**, *42*, 34–71. [CrossRef] [PubMed]

33. Cane, J.; O'Connor, D.; Michie, S. Validation of the theoretical domains framework for use in behaviour change and implementation research. *Implement. Sci.* **2012**, *7*. [CrossRef] [PubMed]

34. Eldredge, L.K.B.; Markham, C.M.; Ruiter, R.A.C.; Kok, G.; Parcel, G.S. *Planning Health Promotion Programs: An Intervention Mapping Approach*; Wiley: Hoboken, NJ, USA, 2016.

35. Michie, S.; Atkins, L.; West, R. *The Behaviour Change Wheel: A Guide to Designing Interventions*; Silverback: Stuttgart, Germany, 2014.

36. Godin, G.; Kok, G. The theory of planned behavior: A review of its applications to health-related behaviors. *AJHP* **1996**, *11*, 87–98. [CrossRef] [PubMed]

37. Armitage, C.J.; Conner, M. Efficacy of the theory of planned behaviour: A meta-analytic review. *Br. J. Soc. Psychol.* **2001**, *40*, 471–499. [CrossRef] [PubMed]

38. Rich, A.; Brandes, K.; Mullan, B.; Hagger, M.S. Theory of planned behavior and adherence in chronic illness: A meta-analysis. *J. Behav. Med.* **2015**, *38*, 673–688. [CrossRef] [PubMed]

39. Zoellner, J.; Krzeski, E.; Harden, S.; Cook, E.; Allen, K.; Estabrooks, P.A. Qualitative application of the theory of planned behavior to understand beverage behaviors among adults. *J. Acad. Nutr. Diet.* **2012**, *112*, 1774–1784. [CrossRef] [PubMed]

40. Ajzen, I. The theory of planned behavior. *Organ. Behav. Hum. Decis. Process.* **1991**, *50*, 179–211. [CrossRef]

41. Krueger, R.A.; Casey, M.A. *Focus Groups: A Practical Guide for Applied Research*; SAGE Publications: Thousand Oaks, CA, USA, 2014.

42. Green, J.; Thorogood, N. *Qualitative Methods for Health Research*; SAGE Publications: Thousand Oaks, CA, USA, 2013.

43. Miles, M.B.; Huberman, A.M.; Saldana, J. *Qualitative Data Analysis*; SAGE Publications: Thousand Oaks, CA, USA, 2013.

44. Saldana, J. *The Coding Manual for Qualitative Researchers*; SAGE Publications: Thousand Oaks, CA, USA, 2012.

45. Paillé, P.; Mucchielli, A. *L'analyse Qualitative en Sciences Humaines et Sociales*; Armand Colin: Paris, French, 2012; p. 424.

46. Rosenstock, I.M.; Strecher, V.J.; Becker, M.H. Social learning theory and the health belief model. *Health Educ. Quart.* **1988**, *15*, 175–183. [CrossRef]

47. Sheeran, P.; Orbell, S. Augmenting the theory of planned behavior: Roles for anticipated regret and descriptive norms. *J. Appl. Soc. Psychol.* **1999**, *29*, 2107–2142. [CrossRef]

48. Godin, G. *Les Comportements Dans le Domaine de la Santé*; Presses de l'Université de Montréal: Montréal, QC, Canada, 2013.

49. Conner, M.; Armitage, C.J. Extending the theory of planned behavior: A review and avenues for further research. *J. Appl. Soc. Psychol.* **1998**, *28*, 1429–1464. [CrossRef]

50. Chlebowski, R.T.; Kim, J.; Haque, R. Adherence to endocrine therapy in breast cancer adjuvant and prevention settings. *Cancer Prev. Res.* **2014**, *7*, 378–387. [CrossRef] [PubMed]

51. Van Liew, J.R.; Christensen, A.J.; de Moor, J.S. Psychosocial factors in adjuvant hormone therapy for breast cancer: An emerging context for adherence research. *J. Cancer Surviv.* **2014**, *8*, 521–531. [CrossRef] [PubMed]

52. Heisig, S.R.; Shedden-Mora, M.C.; von Blanckenburg, P.; Schuricht, F.; Rief, W.; Albert, U.S.; Nestoriuc, Y. Informing women with breast cancer about endocrine therapy: Effects on knowledge and adherence. *Psycho Oncol.* **2015**, *24*, 130–137. [CrossRef] [PubMed]

53. Horne rR Concordance, Adherence and Compliance in Medicine Taking. In National Co-Ordinating Centre for NHS Service Delivery and Organisation r, 2005. Available online: http://www.netscc.ac.uk/hsdr/files/project/SDO_FR_08-1412-076_V01.pdf (accessed on 6 June 2018).

54. Abbott, R.; Edwards, S.; Whelan, M.; Edwards, J.; Dranitsaris, G. Are community pharmacists equipped to ensure the safe use of oral anticancer therapy in the community setting? Results of a cross-country survey of community pharmacists in canada. *J. Oncol. Pharm. Pract.* **2014**, *20*, 29–39. [CrossRef] [PubMed]

55. Kennelty, K.A.; Chewning, B.; Wise, M.; Kind, A.; Roberts, T.; Kreling, D. Barriers and facilitators of medication reconciliation processes for recently discharged patients from community pharmacists' perspectives. *RSAP* **2015**, *11*, 517–530. [CrossRef] [PubMed]

56. Laliberte, M.C.; Perreault, S.; Damestoy, N.; Lalonde, L. Ideal and actual involvement of community pharmacists in health promotion and prevention: A cross-sectional study in Quebec, Canada. *BMC Public Health* **2012**, *12*, 192. [CrossRef] [PubMed]

57. Lea, V.M.; Corlett, S.A.; Rodgers, R.M. Workload and its impact on community pharmacists' job satisfaction and stress: A review of the literature. *Int. J. Pharm. Pract.* **2012**, *20*, 259–271. [CrossRef] [PubMed]

58. Bharadia, R.; Lorenz, K.; Cor, K.; Simpson, S.H. Financial remuneration is positively correlated with the number of clinical activities: An example from diabetes management in alberta community pharmacies. *Int. J. Pharm. Pract.* **2018**, *26*, 77–80. [CrossRef] [PubMed]

59. Guillaumie, L.; Moisan, J.; Grégoire, J.P.; Villeneuve, D.; Beaucage, C.; Bujold, M.; Lauzier, S. Perspective of community pharmacists on their practice with patients who have an antidepressant drug treatment: Findings from a focus group study. *Res. Social. Adm. Pharm.* **2015**, *11*, e43–e56. [CrossRef] [PubMed]

20

The Role of Pharmacists in General Practice in Asthma Management

Louise S. Deeks [1], Sam Kosari [1,*], Katja Boom [1], Gregory M. Peterson [1,2], Aaron Maina [1], Ravi Sharma [3] and Mark Naunton [1]

[1] Discipline of Pharmacy, Faculty of Health, University of Canberra, Bruce, Canberra, ACT 2601, Australia; louise.deeks@canberra.edu.au (L.S.D.); katjaboom@hotmail.com (K.B.); g.peterson@utas.edu.au (G.M.P.); aaron.maina@gmail.com (A.M.); mark.naunton@canberra.edu.au (M.N.)
[2] Faculty of Health, University of Tasmania, Hobart, TAS 7001, Australia
[3] UCL School of Pharmacy, London WC1N 1AX, UK; ravi.sharma4@nhs.net
*   Correspondence: sam.kosari@canberra.edu.au

Abstract: Background: Asthma is principally managed in general practice. Appropriate prescribing and medication use are essential, so general practice pharmacists appear suitable to conduct asthma management consultations. This pilot study aimed to evaluate the asthma management role of a pharmacist in general practice. **Methods**: Analysis of an activity diary and stakeholder interviews were conducted to identify interventions in asthma management; determine whether asthma control changed following pharmacist input; and determine acceptability of asthma management review by a pharmacist in one general practice in Canberra, Australia. **Results**: Over 13 months, the pharmacist saw 136 individual patients. The most common activities were asthma control assessment; recommendations to adjust medication or device; counselling on correct device use; asthma action plan development and trigger avoidance. For patients with multiple consultations, the mean Asthma Control Test score improved from the initial to last visit (14.4 ± 5.2 vs. 19.3 ± 4.7, $n = 23$, $p < 0.0001$). Eight of the 19 (42%) patients moved from having poor to well-controlled asthma. Case studies and qualitative data indicated probable hospital admission avoidance and stakeholder acceptability of asthma management by a practice pharmacist. **Conclusions**: This pilot study demonstrated it is feasible, acceptable and potentially beneficial to have a general practice pharmacist involved in asthma management. Fuller evaluation is warranted.

Keywords: primary health care; asthma; general practice; pharmacists; patient education

1. Introduction

Asthma is a common chronic condition that is principally managed in general practice. A 2014–2015 survey determined that of the 10.8% of Australians who had asthma, almost two-thirds (60.9%) had consulted a general practitioner (GP) in the previous 12 months for their condition and 6.0% had consulted a specialist [1]. However, one in four of the asthma patients surveyed reported poor symptom control over the previous 12 months [1], so there may be scope for improvement of asthma management in general practice. Reasons identified for possible suboptimal management included variable adherence to prescribing guidelines and poor utilisation of asthma action plans [2]. Improved asthma control is associated with better quality of life, increased productivity and savings to the health system [3].

Incorrect medication selection and use can lead to poor asthma management and adverse outcomes [4–6]. Pharmacists have demonstrated that they can improve asthma control through increasing the appropriate use of medication [7]. Given that most of the asthma care is delivered in general practice, pharmacists in this setting may provide an opportunity to work collaboratively with GPs, nurses and other healthcare professionals to improve asthma management. While not as developed as in the United Kingdom, the role of pharmacists in general practice is becoming more established in Australia. This was recognized by the Australian Government, who announced some funding via The Workforce Incentive Program in 2018 [8]. It was identified that one of the practice pharmacists' roles would be supporting patients with chronic health conditions [8]. This is consistent with other countries such as England [9]. The National Health Service (NHS) in England states that one of the aims of the clinical pharmacist in general practice is to manage patients with long-term conditions [9].

General practices in Australia are encouraged to engage with asthma patients via the Asthma Cycle of Care, a Medicare Benefits Schedule (MBS) claimable activity for GPs. This comprises two asthma-related consultations within a 12-month period for patients diagnosed with moderate to severe asthma. An Asthma Cycle of Care requires a documented diagnosis, assessment of asthma control and severity, a review of the patient's use and access to asthma medication and devices, development and subsequent review of a written asthma action plan, and asthma self-management education [10]. The severity of asthma at a point in time can be determined by administering the Asthma Control Test (ACT). The ACT is a patient questionnaire about symptoms, medication use, quality of life and perceived control over the previous 4 weeks. Each of the five questions is assigned a minimum score of 1 and a maximum score of 5, providing a total score between 5 and 25. An ACT score of 19 or below indicates that asthma management needs improvement, while 20 or more indicates good control [11,12].

Practice nurses usually conduct the Asthma Cycle of Care activities, but pharmacists also possess the necessary skills. The aim of this pilot study was to describe interventions in asthma management by one general practice pharmacist, subsequent changes in asthma control and the acceptability of this model of care. This study was nested within a trial conducted in the Australian Capital Territory, Australia [13,14], which was funded by the Capital Health Network, the local Primary Health Network.

2. Materials and Methods

Five part-time (15.2–16 h per week) non-dispensing pharmacists were employed by three general practices in the Australian Capital Territory from February 2016. The three practices recruited their own pharmacists without any involvement of the research team, and they had not previously had a pharmacist within the practice. The pharmacists were subsequently utilized according to their own individual skillset and local workplace needs, as independently determined by each practice. Each general practice pharmacist maintained a daily activity diary, the analysis of which has been described elsewhere [13]. Stakeholder experiences with the pharmacists in general practice have also been published [14].

A sub-analysis of the activity diary from one of the pharmacists, who had selected asthma management as an area of focus, and the stakeholder perspectives were conducted to identify which interventions were conducted; determine whether asthma control had improved following pharmacist input, by comparing ACT results at the initial consultation with those at following consultations; and to determine the acceptability of a general practice pharmacist in asthma management.

The initial sub-analysis of the activity diary was conducted by one researcher (AM) and checked by two other researchers (LD, SK). Changes in ACT scores (first to last consultation) were compared for each individual using a paired t-test, while the Fisher's exact test was used to examine changes in the distribution of patients across categories of asthma control.

Feedback about pharmacist-provided asthma care was obtained from the semi-structured interviews that were conducted by one researcher (LD) with patients, GPs and the practice pharmacist. These interviews were audio-recorded and transcribed verbatim by a professional transcribing agency, with LD checking the transcripts for accuracy. The transcripts were imported into NVivo (version 10.2.2, QSR, Melbourne, VIC, Australia). Two researchers (LD, SK) conducted the thematic analysis by reading the transcripts and adding codes to the data to identify emerging themes that described the data. Each researcher worked independently initially to reduce any bias, then agreed on emerging themes and resolved any discrepancies by discussion.

Case studies were identified in consultation with the practice pharmacist. The University of Canberra Human Ethics Research Committee approved the study (Project number 15-235).

3. Results

3.1. Activity Diary

Activity diary data was collected from 23 May until 25 November, 2016 and from 15 May until 15 December, 2017. Patients with asthma were either identified and invited to attend for review by the practice pharmacist or referred to the practice pharmacist by the GPs or other members of practice staff. GPs, nurses and receptionists suggested that patients consult with the practice pharmacist if they had concerns about asthma control, compliance with inhalation devices, device selection or requirements for training in device use. The patients' ages ranged from 17 months to 84 years.

3.1.1. Interventions by the Pharmacist

Overall, 87.5% (119/136) patients who consulted with the practice pharmacist had their asthma control recorded on their first visit and, in general, they had relatively poor asthma control (mean ACT score of 18 ± 5.3; Table 1). The pharmacist conducted activities such as issuing asthma action plans, educating patients, recommending to step up/down therapy, reviewing inhaler technique and making other relevant recommendations such as device changes (e.g., dry-powder to metered-dose inhaler). Step up of therapy comprised increasing or starting corticosteroid/long-acting beta agonist combination inhaler; corticosteroid inhaler; short-acting muscarinic antagonist inhaler; oral corticosteroid; oral montelukast; or long-acting muscarinic antagonist inhaler. Step down of therapy comprised reducing or stopping corticosteroid/long-acting beta agonist combination inhaler; corticosteroid inhaler; or long-acting muscarinic antagonist inhaler. Asthma plans were provided and discussed with all patients. The pharmacist made comprehensive entries into the patients' clinical notes and discussed prescribing recommendations, the ACT results and the asthma plans with each patient's GP during or as soon as possible after the consultation. Follow up consultations were arranged with the GP, pharmacist or nurse to monitor progress with alterations to management where necessary. Data from the practice pharmacist asthma consultations is shown in Table 1. Illustrative case studies are provided in Appendix A.

For patients below 6 years of age, the pharmacist mainly talked with the accompanying adult, but involved the children as much as possible. The pharmacist tried to make it fun and engaging for the child e.g. showed pictures or used drawings. The pharmacist also gave stickers that could be placed on inhalers if the child answered questions correctly. Educational games/videos/apps were used for different age groups. Teenagers were usually given an emergency spacer (flat paper spacer) for when they were going out.

Table 1. Summarised data from the practice pharmacist asthma consultations.

	Consultations	ACT Values (Mean ± SD)
Number of consultations	166	
Number of patients	136	
Age (years): mean ± SD	33 ± 25 *	
Gender of patients	87 females, 47 males *	
Number of consultations with asthma action plan issued or reviewed	144 (86.7%)	
Number of patients with ACT score recorded on first visit	119 (87.5%)	18 ± 5.3
Number of consultations where step down of therapy was recommended	25 (15.1%)	21 ± 4.0
Number of consultations where step up of therapy was recommended	37 (22.3%)	14 ± 5.2
Number of consultations where device change was recommended	22 (13.3%)	
Number of consultations where spacer was added	40 (24.1%)	
Number of consultations where advice about allergy management was given	14 (8.4%)	
Number of consultations where advice about managing adverse drug reactions was given	12 (7.2%)	
Number of consultations where smoking cessation advice was given	7 (4.2%; all the smokers in the cohort)	
Number of consultations where other interventions were made ($n=$ / < 5 for each)	exercise(5), thunderstorm asthma(3), referral for bone mineral density measurement(2), recommending influenza vaccination(2), influenza vaccine administration(1), peak flow monitoring(1), sleep hygiene advice(1), spirometry testing(1), prioritising treatment due to cost of medications(1)	

* 2 not specified.

3.1.2. Changes in ACT Scores Following the Pharmacist's Interventions

A subset of 26 patients (19.1%) were seen more than once by the pharmacist during the data collection periods. Following the pharmacist's interventions, ACT scores improved for 19 patients, worsened for three patients, were unchanged for one patient and data was incomplete for three patients. The mean ACT score for this subset of patients was 14.4 (SD = 5.2) at the first visit and 19.3 (SD = 4.7) at the most recent visit ($n = 23$, t = 5.43, $p < 0.0001$). Prior to the pharmacist review, 17% (4/23) patients had good asthma control (ACT > 19), increasing to 52% (12/23) afterwards (Fisher's exact test $p = 0.03$). In total, 42% (8/19) patients with poor control moved to well-controlled asthma following review by the practice pharmacist.

3.2. Perceptions of Asthma Care Provided by Practice Pharmacist

The themes and data demonstrated that asthma care by the practice pharmacist was acceptable to patients, GPs and the practice pharmacist (see Table 2). At least one avoided hospital admission was attributed to the practice pharmacist's interventions. The GPs also reported that the practice pharmacist had educated them about asthma.

Table 2. The perceptions of asthma care provided by practice pharmacist.

Themes	Illustrative Quotes
Satisfaction of patients, GPs and pharmacists	*"They actually made some adjustment—well the GP had made some adjustment to my medication and both of them want to review that together with me and see how that actually goes and whether that sort of caused much of a change in the way in which my breathing with my asthma has actually improved a lot".* (Patient, 2016) *"One of the most satisfying things is also the asthma cycle of care. Seeing them coming back you look at their asthma, you give their education, they're coming back and they're saying they're feeling so much better".* (Practice Pharmacist, 2016) *"I think some of the patients have really valued that and got better asthma control so that has been really good".* (GP2, 2018) *"Patients who have poor adherence that I wasn't aware of and their asthma is so much better now because they're actually taking their preventers, which is a revelation to them. I think patients have found the interactions with [the pharmacist] very helpful around asthma".* (GP1, 2016) *"One's [patients] that have come in for asthma reviews have been very pleased".* (GP1, 2018)
Improved care and avoided hospital admission	*"There is a one asthma patient that I have had who was really difficult and basically tolerated really poorly controlled asthma. She would only come in when she was very bad. Again, [the pharmacist] got her in and emphasised the preventative part of it, and I think that's prevented even hospital admissions as well as improved the lady's quality of life".* (GP1, 2018)
Pharmacist as an expert in asthma care	*"I think that whole process has really sharpened me up in terms of the kinds of ways that we do provide this asthma cycle of care. She's providing extra knowledge into that space and I guess it's helping the patients with their inhaler technique. She's taught me some things about inhaler techniques that I didn't know".* (GP1, 2016) *"If somebody comes in for asthma, everybody, even the reception, think about me".* (Practice Pharmacist, 2018)

4. Discussion

4.1. Summary

This pilot study demonstrated that it is feasible, acceptable and beneficial to have a pharmacist in general practice focusing on asthma management. Following practice pharmacist review, 42% (8/19) of patients moved from poor to well-controlled asthma, while case studies and qualitative data indicated probable hospital admission avoidance and acceptability to stakeholders. The GPs had not previously routinely issued asthma action plans or recorded asthma control scores for patients, so this was an added benefit of pharmacist involvement.

4.2. Strengths and Limitations

Data from one pharmacist was analyzed, so all patients received a comparable level of care and completion of the ACT was consistent. The practice pharmacist was a generalist and not an asthma specialist; this can be perceived as advantageous, being more representative of likely future care models. On the other hand, the pharmacist had additional medication review qualifications [15] and was experienced.

We were reliant on the pharmacist accurately self-reporting activities. The general practice population was from one city, so may not be representative of the wider Australian population. In some countries, pharmacists are permitted to prescribe medication but this is not the case in Australia, where this study was conducted; findings may have been different had there been pharmacist prescribing. We acknowledge that the improvements in asthma control in our pilot study may have been affected by other factors, such as seasonal variability of asthma triggers or interventions by other health care professionals. The nature of the study meant there was no control group, although previous studies with a control group have demonstrated pharmacist effectiveness in improving asthma symptoms [16,17].

4.3. Comparison with Existing Literature

Improvements in asthma clinical markers in this study are consistent with the improved clinical indicators following practice pharmacist intervention in other chronic conditions [18], and with that found in a systematic review of pharmacists' effect on asthma control in settings not including general practice [7]. An English study demonstrated that a specialist respiratory pharmacist visiting a general practice could reduce asthma exacerbations and associated costs [19]. In addition, Gums et al. reported that a physician–pharmacist collaborative asthma care model in USA primary care medical offices reduced asthma-related emergency department visits and hospitalizations, and improved both asthma control and quality of life [20].

All the patients who saw the pharmacist received asthma action plans, an intervention recommended by the Australian asthma guidelines [21]. The use of written action plans to enable patients to adjust their medication seems to be more effective in improving health outcomes than other self-management strategies [22]; however, quality evidence is lacking [23]. A project conducted in Minnesota urban community clinics resulted in more patients having optimal asthma control (ACT $\geq$ 20), by increasing completion of asthma action plans and educating patients about using the plan [24]. This contrasts to the findings of a review in 2017, which concluded that asthma action plans have no effect on hospital attendance due to asthma, asthma symptom scores or adverse events [23].

Good healthcare teamwork in non-acute settings has been linked with better patient impact [25]. The practice pharmacist in this pilot study managed asthma within a multidisciplinary team to achieve shared goals. This approach is recommended in the Australian Asthma Handbook, 'effective asthma management involves the whole primary care team, working with the person and also their family or carer where appropriate' [21]. Gums et al. determined that pharmacist and doctor collaboration can improve asthma outcomes [20] and this is consistent with our findings.

Lack of adherence to prescribing guidelines is also associated with poor asthma control [2]. The pharmacist in this study made recommendations using prescribing guidelines. Pharmacists have demonstrated that they can enhance adherence to guidelines in other conditions (e.g., type 2 diabetes and heart failure) [26,27], so it is reasonable to suggest that practice pharmacists may improve adherence to asthma prescribing guidelines.

4.4. Implications for Research

Future well-designed studies are required to confirm the promising results reported here and extend to outcome measures such as hospital admissions, quality of life and cost-effectiveness.

Author Contributions: The contributions of the authors were: conceptualization, L.S.D., M.N., S.K.; methodology, L.S.D., S.K., M.N., K.B.; formal analysis, A.M., S.K., L.S.D., G.M.P.; supervision, S.K.; writing—original draft preparation, L.S.D.; writing—review and editing, L.S.D., G.M.P., M.N., S.K., R.S.; project administration, S.K., K.B., M.N.; funding acquisition, M.N., S.K., L.S.D.

Funding: This research was funded by the Capital Health Network using money provided by the Australian Government under the Primary Health Network Program.

Acknowledgments: We would like to acknowledge the staff and patients at the participating general practice for their cooperation during this pilot.

Appendix A

Appendix A.1 Case Study One

The pharmacist saw a 4-year-old boy and his mother for a GP-initiated asthma review. His medical history included hayfever and eczema. His medication use included: fluticasone 50 mg metered dose inhaler two puffs twice a day via spacer, montelukast 4mg once a day, salbutamol 100 mg metered dose inhaler two puffs when needed for breathlessness via spacer. The patient's mother reported that her son had an asthma exacerbation the previous week, probably caused by a cold. She administered montelukast 4 mg daily for 3 days and then stopped because her son had become aggressive and had started having tantrums. The pharmacist explained that behavioral changes can be a rare side effect from the montelukast. Following discussion with the GP, another trial of montelukast was recommended when the child's asthma was well-controlled. Over the course of a week, the boy's asthma improved (ACT 11/25 to 19/25). The pharmacist counselled the patient and his mother about asthma medication, triggers and symptoms. One of the identified triggers was uncontrolled hayfever with nasal congestion being his main symptom. The pharmacist suggested a trial of a beclomethasone nasal spray and advised the boy and his mother about limiting time outdoors when the pollen count was high. Asthma inhaler technique was optimised, and written information about asthma and inhaler technique was provided. The mother was unaware of the need to shake the inhaler prior to use, this was reinforced by the pharmacist. The patient and his mother were counselled about the asthma action plan written by the pharmacist, including that if asthma worsens then to start fluticasone.

Appendix A.2 Case Study Two

A 46-year-old female had attended the hospital emergency department (ED) with an asthma exacerbation one week before her unscheduled initial pharmacist consultation. Her medications were salbutamol CFC-Free 100 mg/dose inhaler 2–6 puffs four times a day and when needed, ipratropium 21 mg/dose inhaler 4 puffs up to four times a day, fluticasone/eformoterol 250/10 inhaler 2 puffs twice a day. Her ACT score was 6/25 at review. The pharmacist provided education about asthma symptoms, discussed possible triggers and provided medication counselling using the lay terms 'reliever' and 'preventer'. The pharmacist optimised inhaler technique and provided a GP-approved asthma action plan. The patient was reviewed by the pharmacist one week later and her ACT score had improved by 7 points (13/25). The pharmacist recommended that salbutamol (100 microgram/dose) be reduced from 6 to 4 puffs four times a day and when needed, with the plan to reduce further as asthma control improved. The pharmacist reinforced the importance of continuing with twice daily use of the steroid inhaler. The asthma action plan was adjusted accordingly.

Three weeks later the patient presented to the pharmacist with worsening of asthma (ACT 7/25). Following refusal to attend ED, the pharmacist collaborated with the GP to initiate oral prednisolone.

Since the pharmacist involvement in her asthma care there have been no hospital attendances; whereas in the same timeframe during the previous year there were two asthma-related ED attendances.

Appendix A.3 Case Study Three

A 62-year-old male had a practice pharmacist appointment for a chronic obstructive pulmonary disease (COPD) review. He was an ex-smoker with no other chronic conditions. His current medications were tiotropium dry powder inhaler 18 mg daily, indacaterol dry powder inhaler 150 micrograms daily, and salbutamol 100 mg 2 puffs when needed for breathlessness. The pharmacist suspected that the patient may have undiagnosed asthma. The pharmacist administered the COPD assessment test (CAT) [28] with the patient. The COPD CAT assesses current health status relating to COPD and impact on quality of life. It is eight questions, each with scores of 0–5, and the maximum total score of 40 [29]. The COPD CAT score relates to impact of COPD and are considered as very high (> 30), high (> 20), medium (10–20) and low (< 10) [29]. The COPD CAT score for the patient was 21. He was experiencing shortness of breath (SOB) and had disrupted sleep. His triggers were listed as cold and flu but the SOB also worsened when he was exposed to dust at work. In consultation with the GP, the practice pharmacist advised the patient to trial an inhaled corticosteroid, ciclesonide 80 mg metered dose inhaler, 2 puffs daily using a spacer. The practice pharmacist counselled the patient on his new medication and inhaler technique. The pharmacist wrote an asthma action plan and explained to the patient how to use the plan. Using the nSpire™ PiKo-6 electronic FEV1/FEV6 meter, the pharmacist assessed respiratory function prior to commencement of the inhaled corticosteroid using the patient's height (170 cm) to determine predicted values (see Table A1).

Two weeks later, the pharmacist reviewed the patient's response to the inhaled corticosteroid trial (COPD CAT score = 0/40 and asthma ACT = 20/25). His respiratory function tests were repeated (see Table 1). The diagnosis was changed from COPD to asthma as a result of the pharmacist review. In consultation with the GP, the practice pharmacist advised the patient to stop tiotropium and later indacterol. The asthma action plan was adjusted by the pharmacist accordingly. The pharmacist and patient discussed asthma symptoms, triggers and inhalers.

Table A1. Respiratory function test results.

Test	Predicted	Pre Corticosteroid (% Predicted)	Post Corticosteroid (% Predicted)
FEV1	3.01	2.22 (73%)	3.29 (109%)
FEV6	3.75	3.05 (81%)	4.21 (112%)
FEV1/FEV6		0.73	0.78
PEFR		471	469

FEV1 is forced expiratory volume in 1 s; FEV6 is forced expiratory volume in 6 s (used as an alternative to forced vital capacity); PEFR is peak expiratory flow rate.

References

1. Australian Bureau of Statistics. Australian Health Survey: Health Service Usage and Health Related Actions, 2014–2015. Available online: http://www.abs.gov.au/ausstats/abs@.nsf/Lookup/by%20Subject/4364.0.55.002~2014-15~Main%20Features~Asthma~10003 (accessed on 28 June 2018).

2. Reddel, H.K.; Valenti, L.; Easton, K.L.; Gordon, J.; Bayram, C.; Miller, G.C. Assessment and management of asthma and chronic obstructive pulmonary disease in Australian general practice. *Aust. Fam. Phys.* **2017**, *46*, 413–419.

3. Pavord, I.D.; Mathieson, N.; Scowcroft, A.; Pedersini, R.; Isherwood, G.; Price, D. The impact of poor asthma control among asthma patients treated with inhaled corticosteroids plus long-acting β 2-agonists in the United Kingdom: A cross-sectional analysis. *NPJ Prim. Care Respir. Med.* **2017**, *27*. [CrossRef] [PubMed]

4. Haughney, J.; Price, D.; Kaplan, A.; Chrystyn, H.; Horne, R.; May, N.; Moffat, M.; Versnel, J.; Shanahan, E.R.; Hillyer, E.V.; et al. Achieving asthma control in practice: Understanding the reasons for poor control. *Respir. Med.* **2008**, *102*, 1681–1693. [CrossRef] [PubMed]

5. Anis, A.H.; Lynd, L.D.; Wang, X.H.; King, G.; Spinelli, J.J.; Fitzgerald, M.; Bai, T.; Paré, P. Double trouble: Impact of inappropriate use of asthma medication on the use of health care resources. *CMAJ* **2001**, *164*, 625–631. [PubMed]

6. Laforest, L.; Licaj, I.; Devouassoux, G.; Chatte, G.; Martin, J.; Van Ganse, E. Asthma drug ratios and exacerbations: Claims data from universal health coverage systems. *Eur. Respir. J.* **2014**, *43*, 1378–1386. [CrossRef] [PubMed]

7. Garcia-Cardenas, V.; Armour, C.; Benrimoj, S.I.; Martinez-Martinez, F.; Rotta, I.; Fernandez-Llimos, F. Pharmacists' interventions on clinical asthma outcomes: A systematic review. *Eur. Respir. J.* **2016**, *47*, 1134–1143. [CrossRef] [PubMed]

8. Australian Government Department of Health. Budget 2018–2019 Stronger Rural Health—Recruitment and Retention—Workforce Incentive Program. Available online: http://www.health.gov.au/internet/budget/publishing.nsf/Content/budget2018-factsheet28.htm (accessed on 9 May 2018).

9. NHS England. Clinical Pharmacists in General Practice. Available online: https://www.england.nhs.uk/gp/gpfv/workforce/building-the-general-practice-workforce/cp-gp/ (accessed on 18 May 2017).

10. Capital Health Network. Frequently Used Desktop Guide to Item Numbers for General Practice Services. Available online: https://www.chnact.org.au/medicare-benefits-schedule (accessed on 14 October 2016).

11. Nathan, R.A.; Sorkness, C.A.; Kosinski, M.; Schatz, M.; Li, J.T.; Marcus, P.; Murray, J.J.; Pendergraft, T.B. Development of the asthma control test: A survey for assessing asthma control. *J. Allergy Clin. Immunol.* **2004**, *113*, 59–65. [CrossRef] [PubMed]

12. Thomas, M.; Kay, S.; Pike, J.; Williams, A.; Rosenzweig, J.R.; Hillyer, E.V.; Price, D. The Asthma Control Test (ACT) as a predictor of GINA guideline-defined asthma control: Analysis of a multinational cross-sectional survey. *Prim. Care Respir. J.* **2009**, *18*, 41–49. [CrossRef] [PubMed]

13. Naunton, M.; Han, G.T.; Kyle, G.; Davey, R.; Dawda, P.; Goss, J.; Porritt, J.; Kosari, S. What can pharmacists do in general practice? A pilot trial. *Aust. J. Gen. Pract.* **2018**, *47*, 545–549.

14. Deeks, L.S.; Kosari, S.; Naunton, M.; Cooper, G.; Porritt, J.; Davey, R.; Dawda, P.; Goss, J.; Kyle, G. Stakeholder perspectives about general practice pharmacists in the Australian Capital Territory: A qualitative pilot study. *Aust. J. Prim. Health* **2018**. [CrossRef] [PubMed]

15. Australian Association of Consultant Pharmacy. How to Become Accredited. Available online: https://aacp.com.au/how-to-become-accredited/ (accessed on 1 August 2018).

16. Mehuys, E.; Van Bortel, L.; De Bolle, L.; Van Tongelen, I.; Annemans, L.; Remon, J.P.; Brusselle, G. Effectiveness of pharmacist intervention for asthma control improvement. *Eur. Respir. J.* **2008**, *31*, 790–799. [CrossRef] [PubMed]

17. Barbanel, D.; Eldridge, S.; Griffiths, C. Can a self-management programme delivered by a community pharmacist improve asthma control? A randomised trial. *Thorax* **2003**, *58*, 851–854. [CrossRef] [PubMed]

18. Tan, E.C.K.; Stewart, K.; Elliott, R.A.; George, J. Pharmacist services provided in general practice clinics: A systematic review and meta-analysis. *Res. Soc. Adm. Pharm.* **2014**, *10*, 608–622. [CrossRef] [PubMed]

19. Khachi, H. P56 Impact Of Pharmacist-led Asthma and Copd Reviews In General Practice. *Thorax* **2014**, *69*, A98–A99. [CrossRef]

20. Gums, T.H.; Carter, B.L.; Milavetz, G.; Buys, L.; Rosenkrans, K.; Uribe, L.; Coffey, C.; MacLaughlin, E.J.; Young, R.B.; Ables, A.Z.; et al. Physician-pharmacist collaborative management of asthma in primary care. *Pharmacotherapy* **2014**, *34*, 1033–1042. [CrossRef] [PubMed]

21. National Asthma Council Australia. Australian Asthma Handbook—Quick Reference Guide, Version 1.1. Melbourne. 2015. Available online: http://www.asthmahandbook.org.au (accessed on 28 June 2018).

22. Gibson, P.G.; Powell, H.; Wilson, A.; Abramson, M.J.; Haywood, P.; Bauman, A.; Hensley, M.J.; Walters, E.H.; Roberts, J.J. Self-management education and regular practitioner review for adults with asthma. *Cochrane Database Syst. Rev.* **2003**, CD001117. [CrossRef] [PubMed]

23. Gatheral, T.L.; Rushton, A.; Evans, D.J.; Mulvaney, C.A.; Halcovitch, N.R.; Whiteley, G.; Eccles, F.J.; Spencer, S. Personalised asthma action plans for adults with asthma. *Cochrane Database Syst. Rev.* **2017**, *4*, CD011859. [CrossRef] [PubMed]

24. Akhter, L.S.; Monkman, J.L.; Vang, G.; Pfeiffer, J. Improving Asthma Control through Asthma Action Plans: A Quality Improvement Project at a Midwest Community Clinic. *J. Community Health Nurs.* **2017**, *34*, 136–146. [CrossRef] [PubMed]

25. Miller, C.J.; Kim, B.; Silverman, A.; Bauer, M.S. A systematic review of team-building interventions in non-acute healthcare settings. *BMC Health Serv. Res.* **2018**, *8*, 146. [CrossRef] [PubMed]

26. Gilani, F.; Majumdar, S.R.; Johnson, J.A.; Tsuyuki, R.T.; Lewanczuk, R.Z.; Spooner, R.; Simpson, S.H. Adding pharmacists to primary care teams increases guideline-concordant antiplatelet use in patients with type 2 diabetes: Results from a randomized trial. *Ann. Pharmacother.* **2013**, *47*, 43–48. [CrossRef] [PubMed]

27. Ziman, M.E.; Bui, H.T.; Smith, C.S.; Tsukiji, L.A.; Asmatey, V.M.; Chu, S.B.; Miano, J.S. The pharmacists' role in improving guideline compliance for thyroid function testing in patients with heart failure. *J. Pharm. Pract.* **2012**, *25*, 195–200. [CrossRef] [PubMed]

28. Jones, P.W.; Harding, G.; Berry, P.; Wiklund, I.; Chen, W.-H.; Kline Leidy, N. Development and first validation of the COPD Assessment Test. *Eur. Respir. J.* **2009**, *34*, 648–654. [CrossRef] [PubMed]

29. CAT Development Steering Group. Health Professional User Guide. CAT COPD Assessment Test. Expert Guidance on Frequently Asked Questions Issue 3. February 2012. Available online: http://www.catestonline.org (accessed on 27 June 2018).

Permissions

List of Contributors

Sherine Ismail, Sara Al Khansa, Mohammed Aseeri and Hani Alhamdan
King Abdullah International Medical Research Center, King Saud bin Abdulaziz University for Health Sciences, Pharmaceutical Care Department, King Abdulaziz Medical City, Ministry of National Guard Health Affairs, Jeddah 21423, Saudi Arabia

K. H. Mujtaba Quadri
National University of Medical Sciences, The Mall, Rawalpindi 44000, Pakistan

Nurain Suleiman
Pharmaceutical Services Division, Johor State Health Department, 81200 Johor Bahru, Johor, Malaysia
Kulliyyah of Pharmacy, International Islamic University Malaysia, 25710 Kuantan, Pahang, Malaysia

Siti Hadijah Shamsudin
Kulliyyah of Pharmacy, International Islamic University Malaysia, 25710 Kuantan, Pahang, Malaysia

Razman Mohd Rus and Samsul Draman
Kulliyyah of Medicine, International Islamic University Malaysia, 25710 Kuantan, Pahang, Malaysia

Mai Nurul Ashikin Taib
Ara Damansara Medical Centre, 40150 Shah Alam, Selangor, Malaysia

Barbara Mc Kenzie and Alyson Brown
School of Pharmacy and Life Sciences, Robert Gordon University, Aberdeen AB10 7GJ, Scotland, UK

Alan Kearney, Ciaran Halleran, Derina Byrne and Jennifer Haugh
Pharmacy Department, Mercy University Hospital, Cork T12 WE28, Ireland

Elaine Walsh
Department of General Practice, School of Medicine, University College Cork, Cork T12 YN60, Ireland

Laura J. Sahm
Pharmacy Department, Mercy University Hospital, Cork T12 WE28, Ireland
The Pharmaceutical Care Research Group, School of Pharmacy, University College Cork, Cork T12 YN60, Ireland

Hayley Croft and Jennifer Schneider
School of Biomedical Sciences and Pharmacy, Faculty of Health and Medicine, The University of Newcastle, Callaghan, NSW 2308, Australia

Conor Gilligan
School of Medicine and Public Health, The University of Newcastle, Callaghan, NSW 2308, Australia

Rohan Rasiah
Western Australian Centre Rural Health, Geraldton, WA 6530, Australia

Tracy Levett-Jones
Faculty of Health, University of Technology Sydney, Ultimo, NSW 2007, Australia

Conxita Mestres
School of Health Sciences Blanquerna, University Ramon Llull, Padilla 326, 08025 Barcelona, Spain

Anna Agustí
Pharmacy Service, HSS Mutuam Girona, Avinguda de França 64, 17007 Girona, Spain

Marta Hernandez and Blanca Llagostera
Pharmacy Service, EAR Grup Mutuam, Ausias March 39, 08010 Barcelona, Spain

Laura Puerta
Pharmacy Service, HSS Mutuam Güell, Mare de Deu de la Salut 49, 08024 Barcelona, Spain

Conxita Mestres
School of Health Sciences Blanquerna, University Ramon Llull, Padilla 326, 08025 Barcelona, Spain

Anna Agustí
Pharmacy Service, HSS Mutuam Girona, Avinguda de França 64, 17007 Girona, Spain

Marta Hernandez and Blanca Llagostera
Pharmacy Service, EAR Grup Mutuam, Ausias March 39, 08010 Barcelona, Spain

Laura Puerta
Pharmacy Service, HSS Mutuam Güell, Mare de Deu de la Salut 49, 08024 Barcelona, Spain

Magdalena Iorga
Department of Behavioral Sciences, University of Medicine and Pharmacy "Grigore T. Popa", Iasi 700115, Romania

Corina Dondas
Department of Career Counseling, University of Medicine and Pharmacy "Grigore T. Popa", Iasi 700115, Romania

Camelia Soponaru
Department of Psychology, University "Alexandru Ioan Cuza", Iasi 700506, Romania

Ioan Antofie
Department of Hospital Pharmacy, C.F. Hospital, Cluj-Napoca 599597, Romania

Michael C. Thomas and Peter J. Hughes
McWhorter School of Pharmacy, Samford University, Birmingham, AL 35229, USA

Petr Nachtigal and Tomáš Šimůnek
Faculty of Pharmacy, Charles University, Akademika Heyrovského 1203, Hradec Králové 500 05, Czech Republic

Jeffrey Atkinson
Pharmacolor Consultants Nancy, 12 rue de Versigny, 54600 Villers, France

Christopher Harlow
St. Matthews Community Pharmacy, Louisville, KY 40207, USA

Catherine Hanna
American Pharmacy Services Corporation, Frankfort, KY 40601, USA

Lynne Eckmann
Wheeler Pharmacy, Home Connection, Lexington, KY 40507, USA

Yevgeniya Gokun
General Dynamics Information Technology, Little Rock, AR 72205, USA

Faika Zanjani
Department of Behavioral and Community Health, University of Maryland School of Public Health, College Park, MD 20742, USA

Karen Blumenschein and Holly Divine
Department of Pharmacy Practice and Science, University of Kentucky College of Pharmacy Lexington, KY 40536, USA

Rie Kubota, Kiyoshi Shibuya, Yoichi Tanaka, Manahito Aoki, Megumi Shiomi, Wataru Ando, Katsuya Otori and Takako Komiyama
Research and Education Center for Clinical Pharmacy, School of Pharmacy, Kitasato University 5-9-1 Shirokane, Minato-ku, Tokyo 108-8641, Japan

Brian Isetts
Department of Pharmaceutical Care and Health Systems, University of Minnesota College of Pharmacy, 308 Harvard St., SE Minneapolis, MN 55455, USA

Nina Katajavuori, Outi Salminen, Katariina Vuorensola, Helena Huhtala, Pia Vuorela and Jouni Hirvonen
Faculty of Pharmacy, University of Helsinki, 00014 Helsinki, Finland

Md. Omar Reza Seam, Rita Bhatta, Bijoy Laxmi Saha, Abhijit Das, Md. Monir Hossain and Palash Karmakar
Department of Pharmacy, Noakhali Science and Technology University, Sonapur, Noakhali 3814, Bangladesh

S. M. Naim Uddin
Department of Pharmacy, University of Chittagong, Chittagong 4331, Bangladesh

M. Shahabuddin Kabir Choudhuri and Mohammad Mafruhi Sattar
Department of Pharmacy, Jahangirnagar University, Savar, Dhaka 1342, Bangladesh

Marketa Marvanova
Department of Pharmacy Practice, School of Pharmacy/College of Health Professions, North Dakota State University, Department 2650, Fargo, ND 58108-6050, USA

Paul Jacob Henkel
Department of Geographical and Historical Studies, University of Eastern Finland, FI-80101 Joensuu, Finland

Mitch Blair
Department of Paediatrics, Imperial College London, London SW7 2AZ, UK

Arjun Menon
Imperial College School of Medicine, Imperial College London, London SW7 2AZ, UK

Damilola T. Olufemi-Yusuf and Sophie Beaudoin Gabriel
Faculty of Pharmacy and Pharmaceutical Sciences, University of Alberta, Edmonton, AB T6G 1C9, Canada

Tatiana Makhinova and Lisa M. Guirguis
Faculty of Pharmacy and Pharmaceutical Sciences, University of Alberta, Edmonton, AB T6G 1C9, Canada
Asthma Working Group of the Respiratory Health Strategic Clinical Network, Alberta Health Services, Calgary, AB T2W 1S7, Canada

Brittany Humphries
Population Health and Optimal Health Practices, CHU de Quebec–Université Laval Research Centre, Hôpital du Saint-Sacrement, 1050 chemin Ste-Foy, Quebec, QC G1S 4L8, Canada

Faculty of Pharmacy, Université Laval, 1050 avenue de la Médecine, Quebec, QC G1V 0A6, Canada
Department of Health Research Methods, Evidence and Impact, McMaster University, 1280 Main StreetWest, Hamilton, ON L8S 4K1, Canada

Stéphanie Collins
Population Health and Optimal Health Practices, CHU de Quebec–Université Laval Research Centre, Hôpital du Saint-Sacrement, 1050 chemin Ste-Foy, Quebec, QC G1S 4L8, Canada
Faculty of Pharmacy, Université de Montréal, 2940 Chemin de Polytechnique, Montréal, QC H3T 1J4, Canada

Laurence Guillaumie
Population Health and Optimal Health Practices, CHU de Quebec–Université Laval Research Centre, Hôpital du Saint-Sacrement, 1050 chemin Ste-Foy, Quebec, QC G1S 4L8, Canada
Faculty of Nursing, Université Laval, Quebec, 1050 avenue de la Médecine, Quebec, QC G1V 0A6, Canada

Julie Lemieux and Louise Provencher
Oncology Research Unit, CHU de Quebec–Université Laval Research Centre, Hôpital du Saint-Sacrement, 1050 chemin Ste-Foy, Quebec, QC G1S 4L8, Canada
Centre des maladies du sein Deschênes-Fabia, CHU de Quebec–Université Laval, Hôpital du Saint-Sacrement, 1050 chemin Ste-Foy, Quebec, QC, G1S 4L8, Canada

Anne Dionne
Faculty of Pharmacy, Université Laval, 1050 avenue de la Médecine, Quebec, QC G1V 0A6, Canada
Oncology Research Unit, CHU de Quebec–Université Laval Research Centre, Hôpital du Saint-Sacrement, 1050 chemin Ste-Foy, Quebec, QC G1S 4L8, Canada

Centre des maladies du sein Deschênes-Fabia, CHU de Quebec–Université Laval, Hôpital du Saint-Sacrement, 1050 chemin Ste-Foy, Quebec, QC, G1S 4L8, Canada

Jocelyne Moisan
Population Health and Optimal Health Practices, CHU de Quebec–Université Laval Research Centre, Hôpital du Saint-Sacrement, 1050 chemin Ste-Foy, Quebec, QC G1S 4L8, Canada
Faculty of Pharmacy, Université Laval, 1050 avenue de la Médecine, Quebec, QC G1V 0A6, Canada

Sophie Lauzier
Population Health and Optimal Health Practices, CHU de Quebec–Université Laval Research Centre, Hôpital du Saint-Sacrement, 1050 chemin Ste-Foy, Quebec, QC G1S 4L8, Canada
Faculty of Pharmacy, Université Laval, 1050 avenue de la Médecine, Quebec, QC G1V 0A6, Canada
Centre des maladies du sein Deschênes-Fabia, CHU de Quebec–Université Laval, Hôpital du Saint-Sacrement, 1050 chemin Ste-Foy, Quebec, QC, G1S 4L8, Canada

Louise S. Deeks, Sam Kosari, Katja Boom, Aaron Maina and Mark Naunton
Discipline of Pharmacy, Faculty of Health, University of Canberra, Bruce, Canberra, ACT 2601, Australia

Gregory M. Peterson
Discipline of Pharmacy, Faculty of Health, University of Canberra, Bruce, Canberra, ACT 2601, Australia
Faculty of Health, University of Tasmania, Hobart, TAS 7001, Australia

Ravi Sharma
UCL School of Pharmacy, London WC1N 1AX, UK

Index

CPSIA information can be obtained
at www.ICGtesting.com
Printed in the USA
BVHW011940280619
552133BV00014B/35/P